Dermatology Atlas for Skin of Color

Diane Jackson-Richards • Amit G. Pandya
Editors

Dermatology Atlas for Skin of Color

Springer

Editors
Diane Jackson-Richards, MD
Department of Dermatology
Multicultural Dermatology Center
Henry Ford Hospital
Detroit, MI
USA

Amit G. Pandya, MD
Department of Dermatology
University of Texas Southwestern
Medical Center
Dallas, TX
USA

ISBN 978-3-642-54445-3 ISBN 978-3-642-54446-0 (eBook)
DOI 10.1007/978-3-642-54446-0
Springer Heidelberg New York Dordrecht London

Library of Congress Control Number: 2014943110

Printed on acid-free paper

Springer is part of Springer Science+Business Media (www.springer.com)

In loving memory of my son, Paul Brandon Martin

–Diane Jackson-Richards

To my wife Alma, my sons Anil and Alberto and my parents Girish and Tanman for their love, support, and encouragement throughout my life

–Amit G. Pandya

Foreword

> America is not like a blanket – one piece of unbroken cloth. America is more like a quilt – many patches, many pieces, many colors, many sizes, all woven together by a common thread.
>
> – Jesse Jackson

Our common thread in dermatology is the diversity of skin diseases. This diversity is influenced by the color of one's skin. Darker skin types constitute the majority of the global population. They are an integral part of the many pieces, sizes and colors of the global fabric of society. They include Hispanics, Latinos, Africans, African Americans, Caribbean, Native Americans, East Indians, Malaysians, Vietnamese, Indonesians, Koreans and Chinese. In America, mass migration and miscegenation has changed the face of the American canvas. By the year 2050, 50 % of Americans will be considered "people of color".

Multiple studies have documented morphologic and physiologic differences in darker skinned individuals as compared to Caucasians. Moreover, these differences can significantly influence the frequency and clinical manifestations of skin diseases. From a historical perspective, until recently, textbooks of dermatology did not focus on the often unique presentation of skin diseases in people of color. However, there has been a recent paradigm shift with new textbooks devoted exclusively to skin diseases in darker racial ethnic groups.

Accolades and congratulations to Drs. Diane Jackson-Richards and Amit G. Pandya for they have edited a very special and unique *Atlas for Skin of Color*. Their work is a magnificent display of clinical images and succinct discussions of skin diseases in this group of patients.

Atlas for Skin of Color will be an invaluable resource for Dermatologists, Internists, Family Physicians and any clinician interested in the unique clinical presentations and manifestations and treatment of skin diseases in darker racial ethnic groups.

Los Angeles, CA, USA Pearl E. Grimes, MD

Preface

What is skin of color? The tent is large, encompassing many ethnic and racial groups, including Asians, Hispanics, Middle Easterners, Native Americans, Pacific Islanders, and those of African descent. Although these individuals characteristically have Fitzpatrick phototypes IV, V, and VI, the range of skin tones is infinite, producing a spectrum of colors throughout the world. In addition to skin tones, there is a wide range of hair textures, from thin, oily, and straight to extremely curly, dry, and thick. Populations with brown and black skin are increasing rapidly throughout the world. In the USA, this increase is occurring so rapidly that persons with skin of color will comprise the majority of the population by 2050. As this change occurs, there will be a need for more physicians and other healthcare providers to recognize the myriad presentations of skin diseases in patients with skin of color. It is for this purpose that we have produced this Atlas.

Many dermatologic conditions are seen more commonly in those with skin of color. In addition, skin disorders are often clinically different in this population. Furthermore, these patients have unique responses to treatment which must be understood before embarking on a therapeutic plan. The presence of melanin and the unique reactivity of melanocytes are central to these unique presentations and reactions. For example, dermatomyositis is usually apparent in affected patients, due to the characteristic violaceous erythema on the face and hands. However, this finding may be obscured by melanin in patients with skin of color, requiring clinicians to use other clues to make the diagnosis. Similarly, lasers are quite useful for the treatment of pigmentary disorders in light-skinned patients but can cause unacceptable hyperpigmentation, hypopigmentation, or scarring in patients with skin of color. Certain disorders, such as skin cancers, are less common in patients with skin of color but may have serious consequences. These lesions can also be difficult to diagnose correctly or overlooked in pigmented skin due to their unusual appearance or unusual location.

Atlas for Skin of Color addresses these issues by providing over 400 images to help the reader understand the presentation of common skin disorders in pigmented patients. Each chapter includes a succinct discussion of the etiology, epidemiology, clinical presentation, and recommended treatment options for each disorder. It is our hope that this book will help physicians and other healthcare providers to improve their ability to recognize and treat skin diseases in patients with skin of color.

Detroit, MI, USA Diane Jackson-Richards, MD
Dallas, TX, USA Amit G. Pandya, MD

Contents

Contributors

Nnenna G. Agim, MD Department of Pediatric Dermatology, Children's Medical Center Dallas, Dallas, TX, USA

Lauren A. Baker, BS Department of Dermatology, University of Texas Southwestern Medical Center, Dallas, TX, USA

Gabriela Blanco, MD Department of Dermatology, University of Texas Southwestern Medical Center, Dallas, TX, USA

Kathryn A. Bowman, BS Department of Dermatology, University of Texas Southwestern Medical Center, Dallas, TX, USA

Benjamin F. Chong, MD Department of Dermatology, University of Texas Southwestern Medical Center, Dallas, TX, USA

Jack B. Cohen, DO, MD Department of Dermatology, Dallas County Health & Human Services, Dallas, TX, USA

Department of Dermatology, University of Texas Southwestern Medical Center, Dallas, TX, USA

Daniel Condie, BS Department of Dermatology, University of Texas Southwestern Medical Center, Dallas, TX, USA

Sharif Currimbhoy, BS Department of Dermatology, University of Texas Southwestern Medical Center, Dallas, TX, USA

Arturo Ricardo Dominguez, MD Department of Dermatology, University of Texas Southwestern Medical Center, Dallas, TX, USA

Thao Duong, MD Department of Internal Medicine, University of Texas Southwestern Medical Center, Dallas, TX, USA

Raechele Cochran Gathers, MD Department of Dermatology, Multicultural Dermatology Center, Henry Ford Hospital, Detroit, MI, USA

Donald Glass II, MD, PhD Department of Dermatology, University of Texas Southwestern Medical Center, Dallas, TX, USA

Shauna Goldman, BS Department of Dermatology, University of Texas Southwestern Medical Center, Dallas, TX, USA

Daniel Grabell, MBA Department of Dermatology, University of Texas Southwestern Medical Center, Dallas, TX, USA

Nan Guo, BS Department of Dermatology, University of Texas Southwestern Medical Center, Dallas, TX, USA

Richard H. Huggins, MD Department of Dermatology, Henry Ford Hospital, Detroit, MI, USA

Prescilia Isedeh, MD Department of Dermatology, Henry Ford Medical Center, Detroit, MI, USA

Diane Jackson-Richards, MD Department of Dermatology, Multicultural Dermatology Center, Henry Ford Hospital, Detroit, MI, USA

Heidi T. Jacobe, MD, MSCS Department of Dermatology, University of Texas Southwestern Medical Center, Dallas, TX, USA

Kathryn Kinser, BS Department of Dermatology, University of Texas Southwestern Medical Center, Dallas, TX, USA

Nita Kohli, MD, MPH Department of Dermatology, University Hospitals Case Medical Center-Case Western Reserve University, Cleveland, OH, USA

Tiffany J. Lieu, MD Department of Dermatology, University of Texas Southwestern Medical Center, Dallas, TX, USA

Henry W. Lim, MD Department of Dermatology, Henry Ford Medical Center, Henry Ford Hospital, Detroit, MI, USA

Bassel Mahmoud, MD Department of Dermatology, Multicultural Dermatology Center, Henry Ford Hospital, Detroit, MI, USA

Thomas Lee Department of Dermatology, University of Texas Southwestern Medical Center, Dallas, TX, USA

Tiffany T. Mayo, BS, MS, MD Department of Dermatology, University of Alabama, Birmingham, AL, USA

Mio Nakamura, BS Wayne State University, School of Medicine, Detroit, MI, USA

Department of Dermatology, Multicultural Dermatology Center, Henry Ford Hospital, Detroit, MI, USA

Padma Nallamothu, MD Department of Dermatology, Henry Ford Hospital/ Wayne State University Program, Detroit, MI, USA

Katherine Omueti Ayoade, MD, PhD Department of Dermatology, University of Texas Southwestern Medical Center, Dallas, TX, USA

Meredith Orseth, BS Department of Medicine, University of Virginia School of Medicine, University of Virginia Health System, Charlottesville, VA, USA

Amit G. Pandya, MD Department of Dermatology, University of Texas Southwestern Medical Center, Dallas, TX, USA

Pranita V. Rambhatla, MD Department of Dermatology, Henry Ford Hospital, Detroit, MI, USA

Tara Rao, MD Department of Dermatology, General Dermatology Clinic, University of Texas Southwestern Medical Center, Dallas, TX, USA

Stephanie Alexandra Savory, MD Department of Dermatology, University of Texas Southwestern Medical Center, Dallas, TX, USA

Divya Srivastava, MD Department of Dermatology, University of Texas Southwestern Medical Center, Dallas, TX, USA

Amanda Strickland, BS Department of Dermatology, University of Texas Southwestern Medical Center, Dallas, TX, USA

Amy Thorne, MFA, DO Department of Dermatology, University of New Mexico, Albuquerque, NM, USA

Ryan Thorpe, BS Department of Dermatology, University of Texas Southwestern Medical Center, Dallas, TX, USA

Alfred Wang, BS Department of Dermatology, University of Texas Southwestern Medical Center, Dallas, TX, USA

Part I

Pigmentary Disorders

Vitiligo

1

Sharif Currimbhoy and Amit G. Pandya

Contents

1.1 Introduction

Vitiligo is a chronic depigmenting skin disease that is caused by progressive autoimmune-mediated melanocyte destruction [1]. Although there is no predilection for skin type or race, lesions in patients with skin of color are more visible and thus cause a higher impact on quality of life [1–3]. The prevalence of vitiligo is estimated at 0.5–1 %, with half of patients presenting before the age of 20 and 95 % before the age of 40 [2]. The majority of cases of vitiligo are sporadic in nature with a positive family history of vitiligo found in 20–30 % of the patients [2]. Although men and women are affected by vitiligo at equal rates, there is a higher proportion of women who seek treatment [2]. The psychological impact of vitiligo can be severe, especially in patients with skin of color, and includes depression, low self-esteem, fear of rejection, and a decreased quality of life [2, 4]. Although no inciting factors for vitiligo have been confirmed, stress, skin trauma, severe sunburn, pregnancy, and emotional stress have been reported by patients as events which preceded the onset of vitiligo [2, 5]. Early diagnosis and treatment should be sought by patients and physicians to help maximize repigmentation [2].

S. Currimbhoy, BS
Department of Dermatology, University of Texas Southwestern Medical Center, 5939 Harry Hines Blvd, Dallas, TX 75235, USA
e-mail: sharif.currimbhoy@utsouthwestern.edu

A.G. Pandya, MD (✉)
Department of Dermatology,
University of Texas Southwestern Medical Center,
5323 Harry Hines Boulevard, Dallas, TX 75390, USA
e-mail: amit.pandya@utsouthwestern.edu

D. Jackson-Richards, A.G. Pandya (eds.), *Dermatology Atlas for Skin of Color*,
DOI 10.1007/978-3-642-54446-0_1, © Springer-Verlag Berlin Heidelberg 2014

1.2 Clinical Features

Vitiligo is separated into two main variants, each with a different presentation and clinical course. Non-segmental vitiligo (NSV), also called generalized vitiligo, is the most common form, seen in approximately 90 % of cases, and is generally more rapidly progressive in its course than segmental vitiligo [1]. Non-segmental vitiligo presents with depigmented macules and patches that occur in a bilateral distribution anywhere on the body but typically involves the face, axillary regions, dorsal hands, fingers, and feet (Fig. 1.1) [1–3]. Early lesions of vitiligo often have small depigmented lesions around larger lesions (Fig. 1.2). New areas of vitiligo commonly occur over joints particularly of the hands, elbows, and knees. When depigmentation occurs secondary to trauma or chronic pressure, it is known as the Koebner phenomenon (Fig. 1.3) [3]. Occasionally, the depigmentation can have a transitional stage, known as trichrome vitiligo, in which normal, hypopigmented, and depigmented skin is present in the same location (Fig. 1.4).

Segmental vitiligo (SV) is less common than NSV and typically begins at a younger age, with roughly 30 % of cases presenting during childhood [1]. Segmental vitiligo is characterized by unilateral or localized depigmentation that can spread along the distribution of a dermatome or along Blaschko's lines (Figs. 1.5 and 1.6) [1–3]. Spread of SV to the contralateral side of the body is rare, and lesions tend to be more stable than those of generalized vitiligo [3].

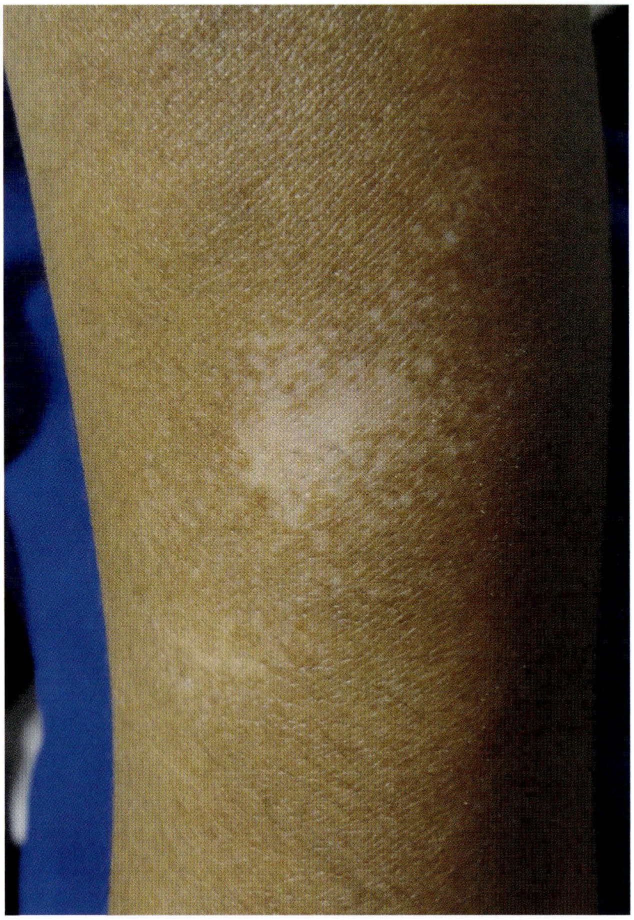

Fig. 1.2 Vitiligo of the forearm in a Hispanic female

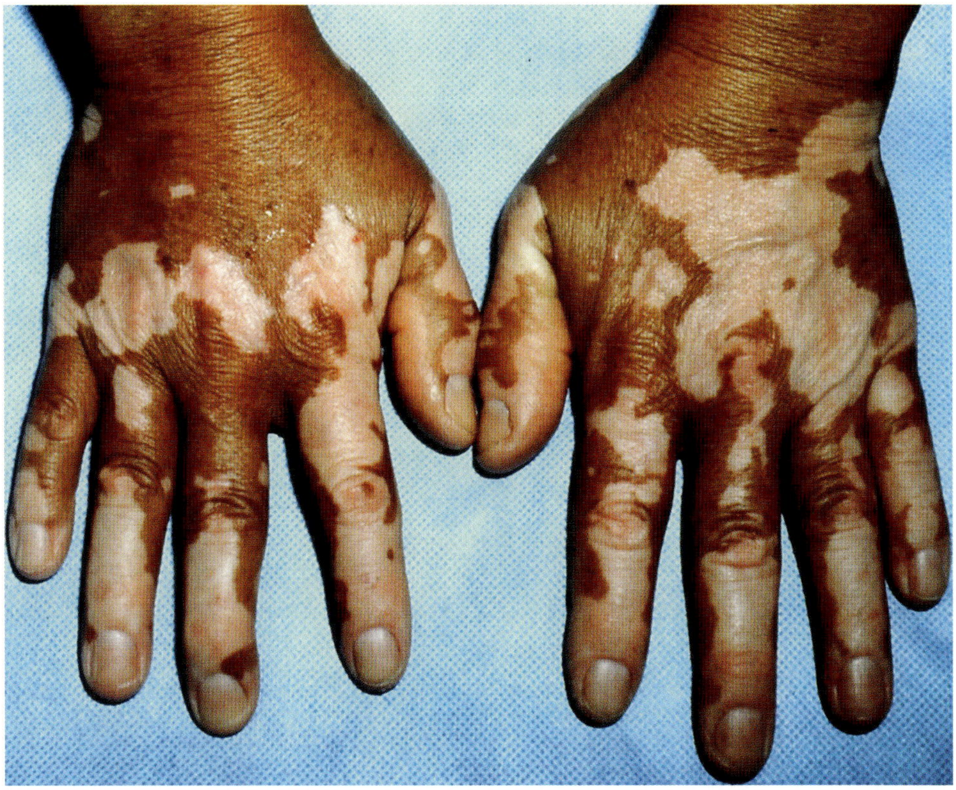

Fig. 1.1 Bilateral vitiligo in a Hispanic male

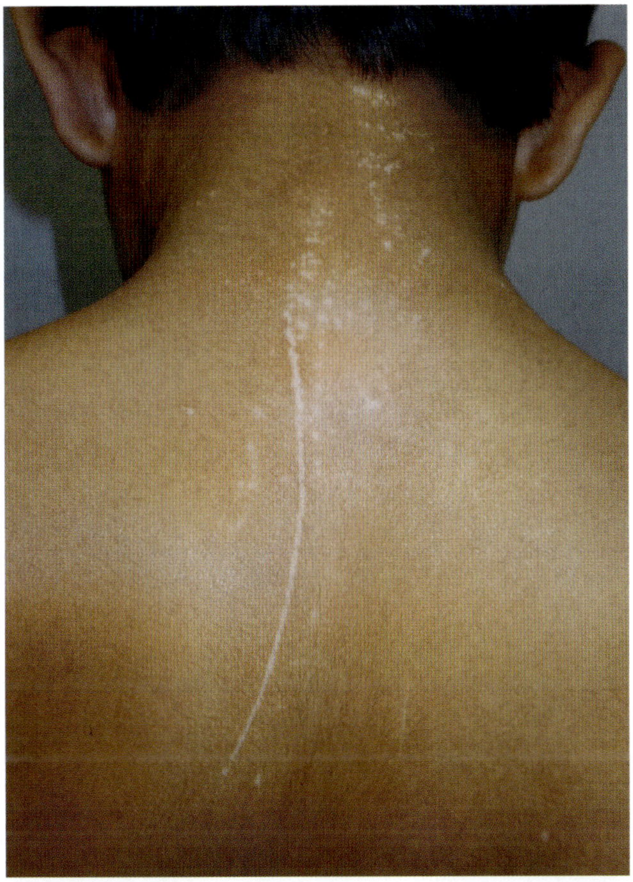

Fig. 1.3 Vitiligo of the back in a South Asian boy demonstrating the Koebner phenomenon after a scratch

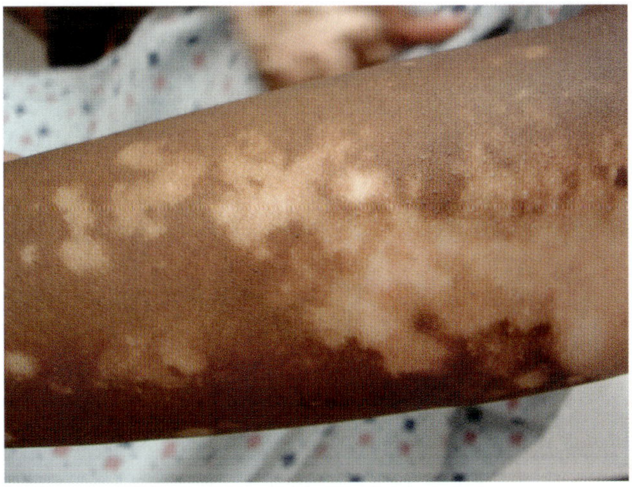

Fig. 1.4 Trichrome vitiligo on the arm of an African American female

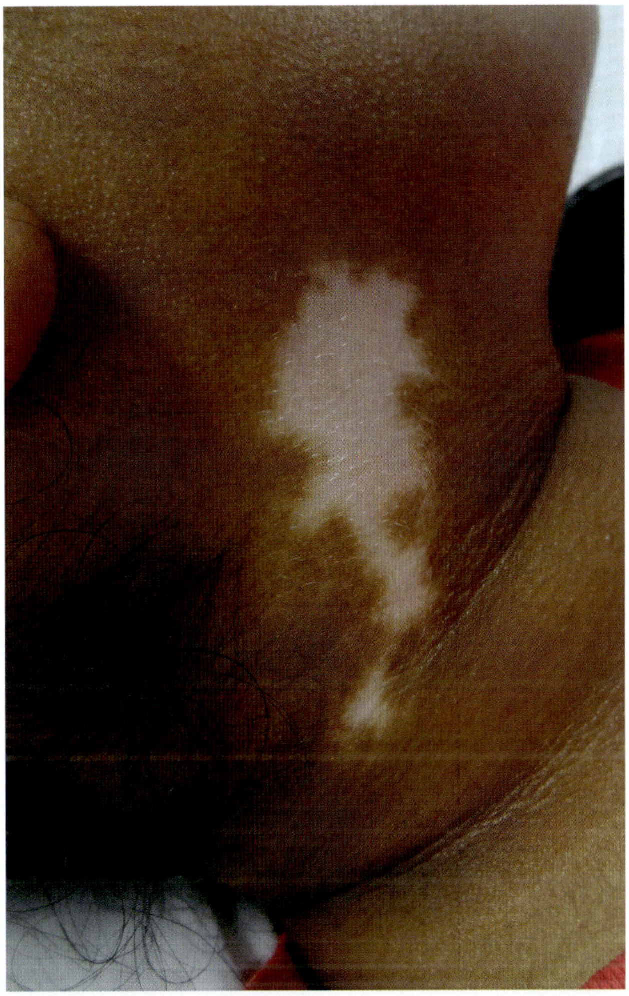

Fig. 1.5 Segmental vitiligo of the neck in a South Asian female

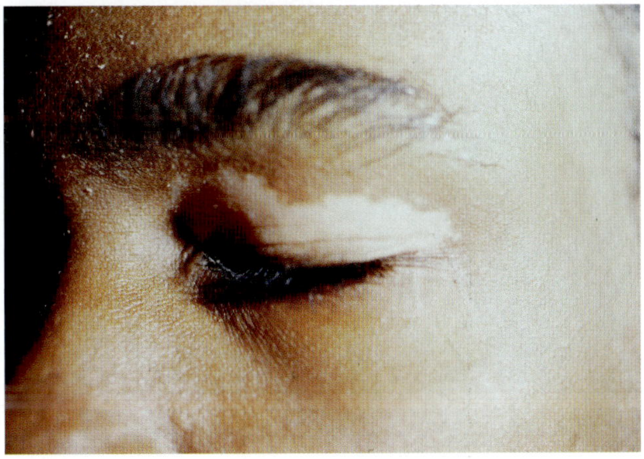

Fig. 1.6 Segmental vitiligo of the left upper eyelid in an African American male

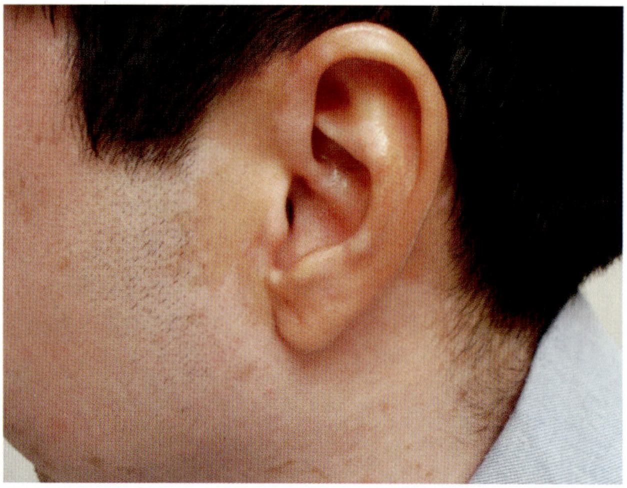

Fig. 1.7 Extensive vitiligo in a Filipino male with retention of hair pigment

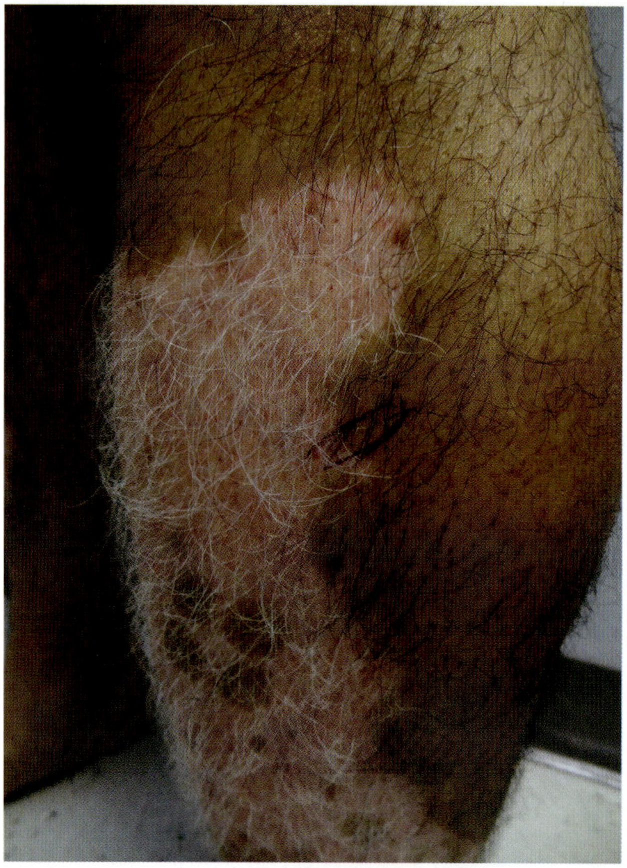

Fig. 1.8 Leukotrichia in a patch of vitiligo in a Hispanic male

In both segmental and non-segmental vitiligo, retention of hair pigment is a good prognostic sign (Fig. 1.7), whereas leukotrichia can be seen in areas of depigmentation and signifies a poorer prognosis regarding the prospects of repigmentation of that area (Fig. 1.8) [2]. In aggressive forms of vitiligo, patients may develop extensive depigmentation, covering the majority of their body surface area (Fig. 1.9).

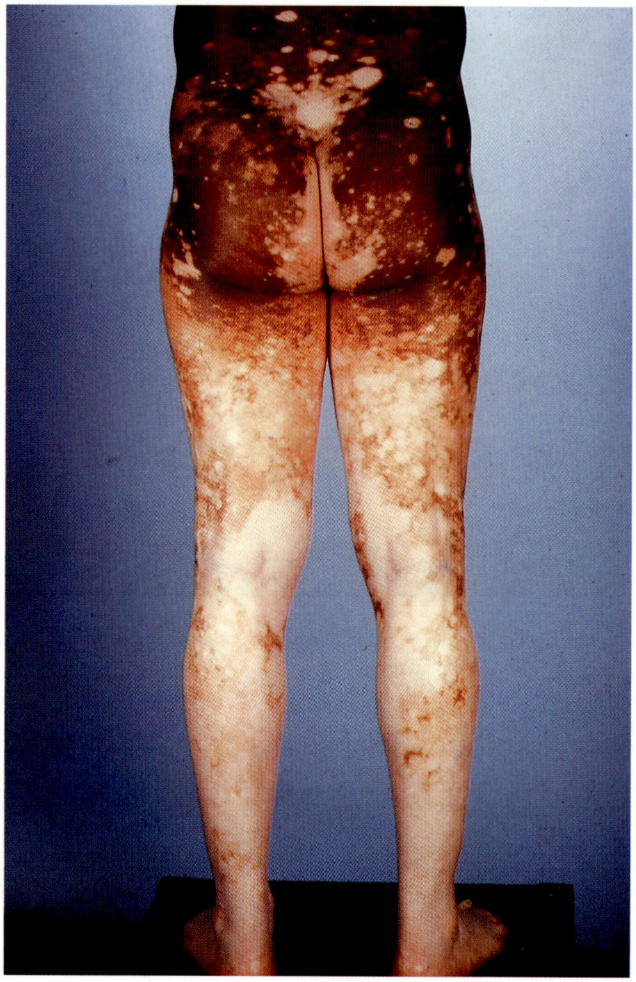

Fig. 1.9 Severe bilateral vitiligo in an African American male

1.3 Diagnosis and Differential Diagnosis

A diagnosis of vitiligo can usually be made simply by clinical examination, although the use of Wood's lamp may be used in patients with Fitzpatrick skin types I–III to highlight areas of depigmentation. The differential diagnosis for vitiligo includes tinea versicolor, pityriasis alba, post-inflammatory hypopigmentation, idiopathic guttate hypomelanosis, nevus depigmentosus, halo nevus, and piebaldism [1, 2].

1.4 Histopathological Features

Histologic examination of the skin from a lesion of vitiligo reveals lack of melanocytes, often with a sparse infiltrate of lymphocytes [2]. Immunohistochemical stains can be done, which reveal the absence of melanocytes in the depigmented lesion with large, sometimes vacuolated, melanocytes at the edges of the lesion, often with melanin granules still present within keratinocytes [2].

1.5 Natural History and Prognosis

The disease course of NSV is typically progressive, although the time frame and areas of spread are difficult to predict. As mentioned previously, areas with frequent trauma or pressure, such as the dorsal hands, waist, elbows, knees, and dorsal feet, have a higher chance of depigmentation and are common areas of involvement.

Segmental vitiligo tends to be more stable in its disease course, with rare spread to other distal body regions outside of the affected dermatome or Blaschko's lines [1, 2].

Thyroid dysfunction, hypothyroidism or hyperthyroidism, may be found in up to 18 % of patients, and screening is recommended for new patients [2]. Other less commonly associated autoimmune conditions seen in patients with non-segmental vitiligo include alopecia areata, psoriasis, pernicious anemia, diabetes mellitus type 1, and rheumatoid arthritis [2].

1.6 Treatment

Treatment options for vitiligo include both topical corticosteroids and immunomodulators, phototherapy with psoralen and ultraviolet A radiation (PUVA), narrowband ultraviolet B (NBUVB), and surgical modalities. The expectations for repigmentation should be discussed with patients, as all therapies require a long-term commitment and strict adherence to the treatment protocol. Potent topical corticosteroids are an effective therapy and have been shown to achieve greater than 75 % repigmentation in 56 % of patients with long-term use [1, 2]. Phototherapy with NBUVB, administered two to three times a week on alternating days, has been shown to achieve more than 75 % repigmentation in 63 % of patients after 1 year of treatment (Fig. 1.10). NBUVB has been shown to be superior to PUVA therapy with less side effects and is thus the treatment of choice for most patients [1]. Patients with skin of color, recent onset of

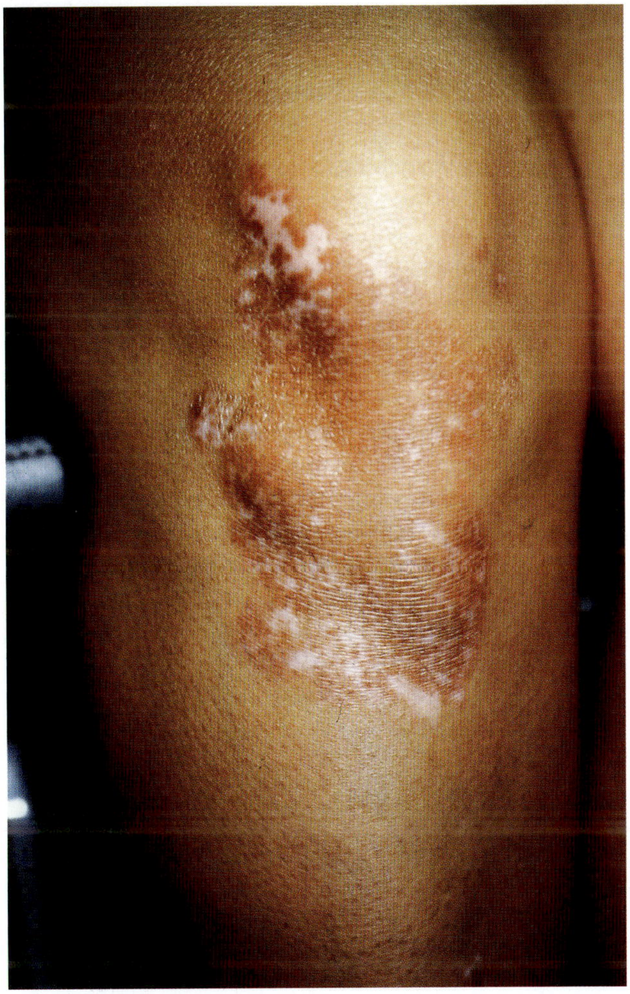

Fig. 1.10 Vitiligo of the right knee in a Hispanic female with repigmentation from phototherapy

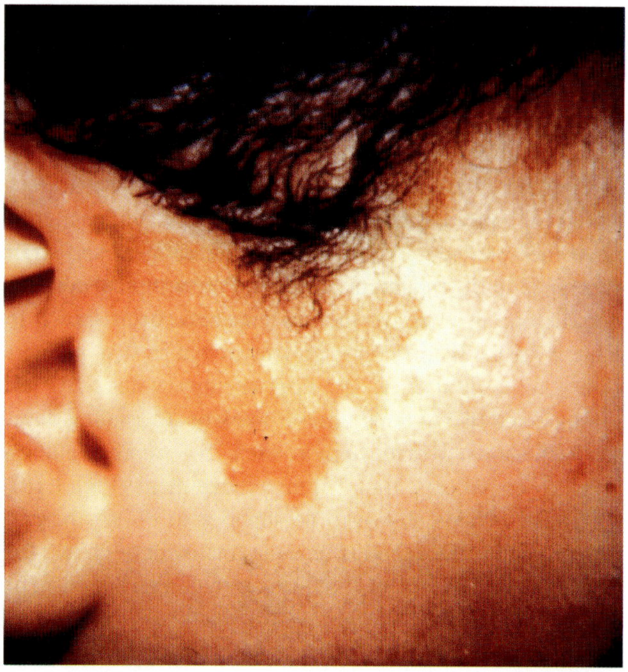

Fig. 1.11 Vitiligo of the right cheek in an African American female before depigmentation therapy

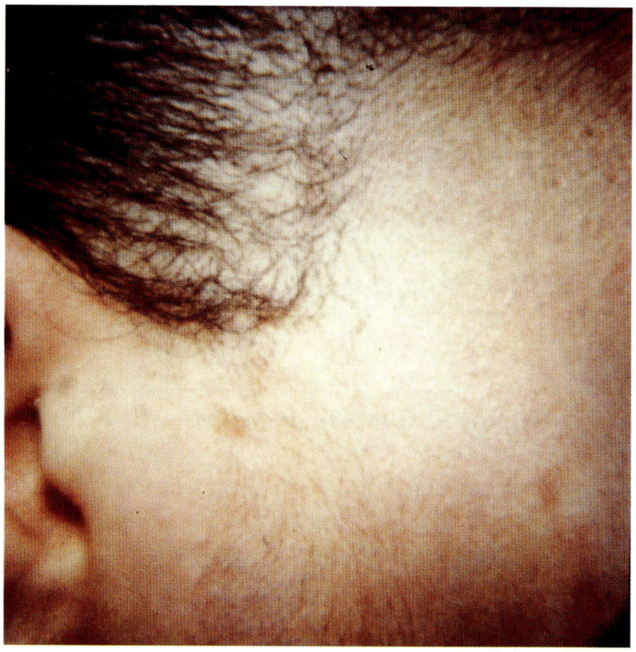

Fig. 1.12 Vitiligo of the right cheek in an African American female after depigmentation therapy

disease, and lesions on the face and trunk tend to respond best to phototherapy [2, 6]. Topical immunomodulators such as tacrolimus and pimecrolimus have a lower side effect profile than topical corticosteroid, although repigmentation with these therapies is mainly seen on the head and neck with repigmentation rates ranging from 26 to 72.5 % [2]. Surgical modalities with transplantation of unaffected skin to vitiliginous areas with punch grafting, epidermal blister grafting, split-thickness grafting, or autologous melanocyte suspension transplanting can be used for patients with stable vitiligo that is unresponsive to other therapies [2, 6]. Local treatment with topical monobenzyl ether of hydroquinone can be used in patients with severe depigmentation (>50 %) in order to achieve a more even appearance of the skin (Figs. 1.11 and 1.12) [2, 7]. Depigmentation treatment is more commonly used in patients with skin of color over areas that are visible to the public, such as the face and distal extremities [7].

References

1. Taïeb A, Picardo M. Clinical practice. Vitiligo. N Engl J Med. 2009;360(2):160–9.
2. Alikhan A, Felsten LM, Daly M, Petronic-rosic V. Vitiligo: a comprehensive overview Part I. Introduction, epidemiology, quality of life, diagnosis, differential diagnosis, associations, histopathology, etiology, and work-up. J Am Acad Dermatol. 2011;65(3):473–91.
3. Speeckaert R, Van Geel N. Distribution patterns in generalized vitiligo. J Eur Acad Dermatol Venereol. 2013. doi: 10.1111/jdv.12171. [Epub ahead of print].
4. Ongenae K, Van Geel N, De Schepper S, Naeyaert JM. Effect of vitiligo on self-reported health-related quality of life. Br J Dermatol. 2005;152(6):1165–72.
5. Alghamdi KM, Kumar A, Taïeb A, Ezzedine K. Assessment methods for the evaluation of vitiligo. J Eur Acad Dermatol Venereol. 2012;26(12):1463–71.
6. Syed ZU, Hamzavi IH. Role of phototherapy in patients with skin of color. Semin Cutan Med Surg. 2011;30(4):184–9.
7. Black W, Russell N, Cohen G. Depigmentation therapy for vitiligo in patients with Fitzpatrick skin type VI. Cutis. 2012;89(2):57–60.

Post-inflammatory Hypopigmentation

2

Shauna Goldman and Amit G. Pandya

Contents

2.1 Introduction

Post-inflammatory hypopigmentation is the partial to total loss of melanin following cutaneous inflammation or trauma. This very common acquired pigmentary disorder can be a sequela of numerous conditions, including inflammatory skin diseases, infections with cutaneous involvement, and therapeutic interventions [1]. Post-inflammatory hypopigmentation affects all types of skin without gender predilection [2]. In patients with skin of color, the contrast between the normal and hypopigmented skin may be especially prominent, often causing significant concern and distress, potentially more so than the condition which preceded it [3, 4].

Normal skin pigmentation relies on the production of melanin by melanocytes at the epidermal-dermal junction and the transfer of that melanin to surrounding keratinocytes. Post-inflammatory hypopigmentation likely reflects alterations to the constitutive melanocyte function by inflammatory mediators, cytokines, and growth factors at the epidermal-dermal junction [4, 5]. For example, interleukin 1 (IL-1), IL-6, and tumor necrosis factor-alpha (TNF-α) are molecules produced during common inflammatory dermatoses which have been demonstrated to inhibit proliferation and melanogenesis by human melanocytes in vitro [4, 5]. The response of an individual's melanocytes to the chemical milieu at the epidermal-dermal junction may be genetically determined [1].

S. Goldman, BS • A.G. Pandya, MD (✉)
Department of Dermatology,
University of Texas Southwestern Medical Center,
5323 Harry Hines Blvd., Dallas, TX 75390, USA
e-mail: shaunaeg@gmail.com; amit.pandya@utsouthwestern.edu

D. Jackson-Richards, A.G. Pandya (eds.), *Dermatology Atlas for Skin of Color*,
DOI 10.1007/978-3-642-54446-0_2, © Springer-Verlag Berlin Heidelberg 2014

2.2 Clinical Features

In general, the lesions of post-inflammatory hypopigmentation are circumscribed macules or patches with sharp to feathered margins (Figs. 2.1, 2.2, 2.3 and 2.4) [1, 2, 6]. Additional clinical features such as the color, distribution, and arrangement of lesions correspond to the type and severity of the inciting cutaneous disorder. For example, mild atopic dermatitis may be followed by slightly hypopigmented lesions [1], whereas complete loss of pigmentation often occurs in patients with discoid lupus erythematosus (Fig. 2.5) [2]. Likewise, the distribution and arrangement of these lesions depend on the configuration of the original inflammation or trauma. The post-inflammatory hypopigmentation of psoriasis, for example, takes the shape, distribution, and arrangement of the psoriasis lesions [2]. Similarly, post-inflammatory hypopigmentation secondary to lichen striatus appears in the same linear distribution as the primary inflammatory disorder (Fig. 2.6) [1, 2]. Depending on the original condition, the loss of pigmentation may become evident

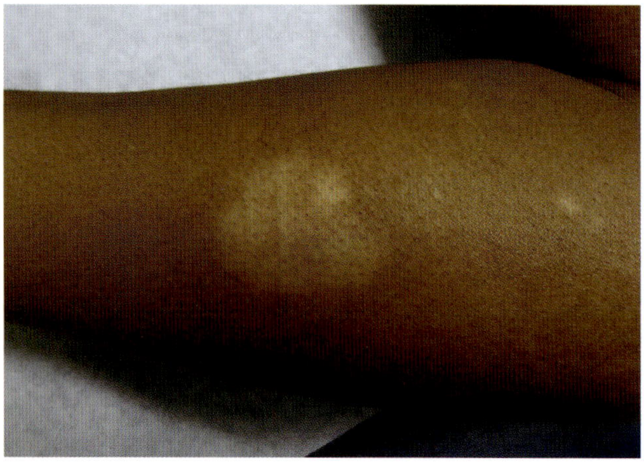

Fig. 2.1 Hypopigmented mycosis fungoides of the calf in an African American female

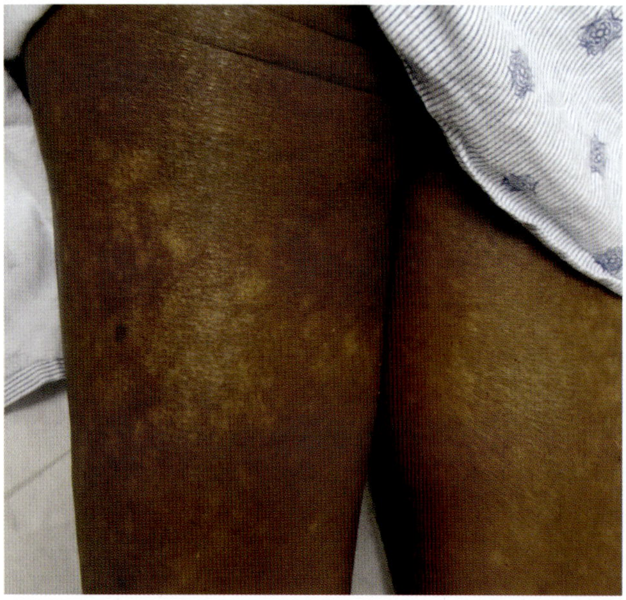

Fig. 2.2 Hypopigmented mycosis fungoides of the thighs in an African American female

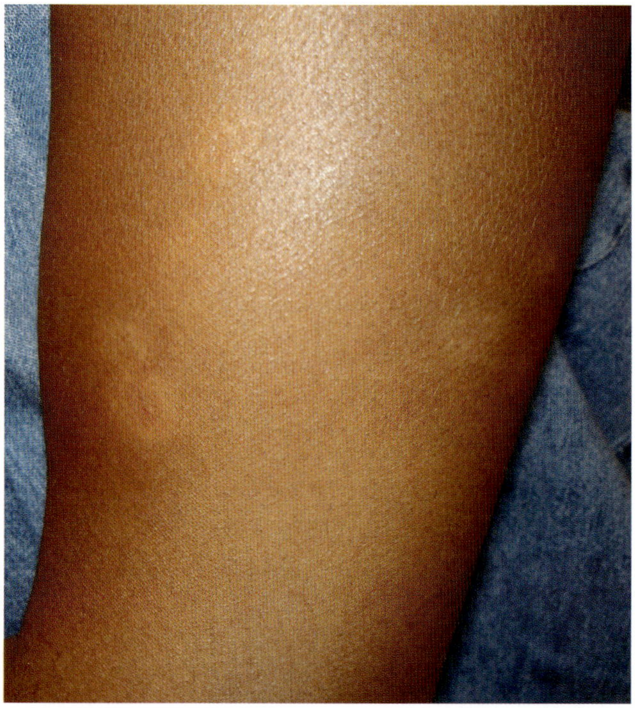

Fig. 2.3 Sarcoidosis on the arm of an African American female

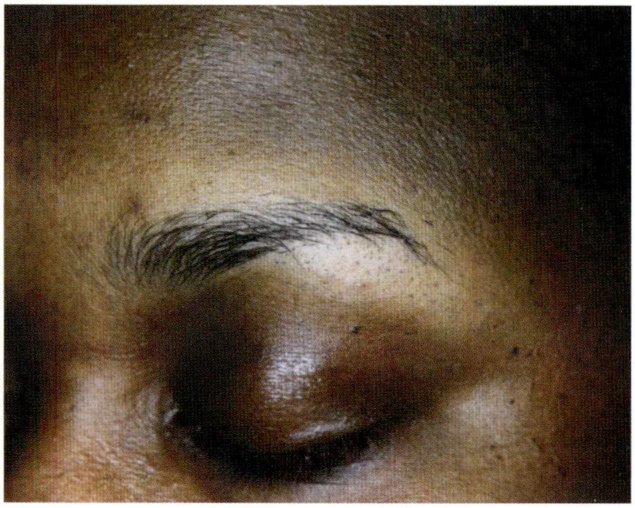

Fig. 2.4 Hypopigmentation from seborrheic dermatitis in an African American female

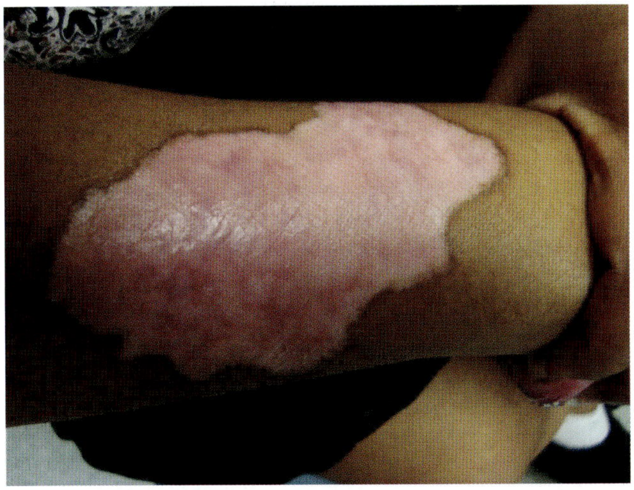

Fig. 2.5 Depigmentation from discoid lupus erythematosus in an African American female

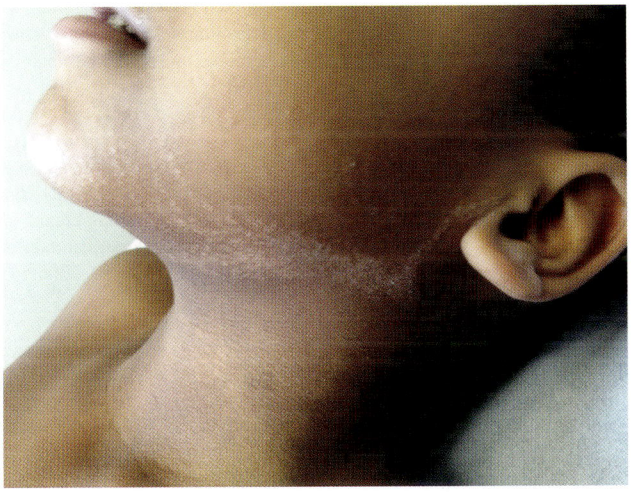

Fig. 2.6 Hypopigmentation from lichen striatus in an African American boy

during the active inflammation or over weeks to months following its resolution [6]. Despite the significant cosmetic and psychological concerns associated with post-inflammatory hypopigmentation, the lesions themselves are typically asymptomatic [1, 3].

2.3 Natural History and Prognosis

The clinical course of post-inflammatory hypopigmentation is largely dependent upon the inflammatory or traumatic process which preceded it. In most cases, the natural history of the lesions is characterized by improvement with time, especially when the primary process is promptly identified and treated. For example, post-inflammatory hypopigmentation due to mild atopic dermatitis may resolve within weeks to months, whereas cutaneous inflammation caused by discoid lupus erythematosus may leave severe hypopigmentation which may take years to resolve [1, 2]. Exposure to ultraviolet radiation, natural or artificial, can hasten repigmentation of lesions. When the inciting cutaneous inflammation results in irreversible loss of melanocytes, the post-inflammatory hypopigmentation can be permanent. Post-inflammatory hypopigmentation can also be a complication of dermatologic procedures, including cryotherapy, laser resurfacing, chemical peels, and dermabrasion [1, 2].

2.4 Histopathological Features

Biopsy of lesions may be helpful in the diagnosis of post-inflammatory hypopigmentation. Histopathological specimens of the hypopigmented lesions typically demonstrate decreased melanin in the epidermis [2]. Other nonspecific findings may include the presence of melanophages in the upper dermis and inflammatory infiltrate at the epidermal-dermal junction [1, 2]. Additional histopathological evidence, when present, may be useful for determining the preceding clinical condition [1, 2].

2.5 Diagnosis and Differential Diagnosis

The diagnosis of post-inflammatory hypopigmentation relies on a detailed history, as knowledge of any primary cutaneous disorders, previous therapeutic interventions, and other chemical exposures is crucial for a determination of the cause [1, 6]. While examination under Wood's lamp can be a useful diagnostic tool for evaluation of hypopigmented lesions, this may not yield as much diagnostic information in patients with darker skin due to lack of contrast between affected and normal skin [3]. Confocal laser scanning microscopy can provide additional information about the content and distribution of melanin at the epidermal-dermal junction to determine the cause of the hypopigmented macules [7]. Biopsy with subsequent histopathological analysis of the hypopigmented lesions and surrounding normal skin is also a valuable aid in diagnosis, especially for excluding sarcoidosis, mycosis fungoides, and leprosy, which may present with hypopigmented macules (Figs. 2.1–2.3) [1, 2].

The differential diagnosis of post-inflammatory hypopigmentation includes pityriasis alba, ash leaf macules of tuberous sclerosis, chemical leukoderma from job-related exposures, pityriasis versicolor, vitiligo, previous use of intralesional or potent topical corticosteroids, progressive macular hypomelanosis, leprosy, nevus depigmentosus, extramammary Paget's disease, mycosis fungoides, and sarcoidosis [2, 6, 7].

2.6 Treatment

The identification and treatment of the inciting inflammatory condition are the primary goals in the treatment of post-inflammatory hypopigmentation. These lesions typically demonstrate improvement with time; however, hypopigmentation may persist long after the underlying condition has been treated, especially in patients with skin of color [8, 9]. Topical administration of medium-potency corticosteroids and tars is the appropriate first-line therapy to stimulate melanogenesis [8]. Additional treatment strategies include cosmetic camouflage application, topical or oral psoralen plus UVA light (PUVA) therapy, narrowband UVB phototherapy (NBUVB), and excimer laser therapy [2–4, 8, 9]. Pimecrolimus 1 % cream has been shown to be efficacious in restoring skin pigmentation in a pilot trial of African American patients with post-inflammatory hypopigmentation secondary to seborrheic dermatitis [10]. Skin grafting can be considered in the treatment of severe cases of post-inflammatory hypopigmentation when there has been complete destruction of melanocytes [1–3].

References

1. Ruiz-Maldonado R, Orozco-Covarrubias ML. Post-inflammatory hypopigmentation and hyperpigmentation. Semin Cutan Med Surg. 1997;16:36–43.
2. Vachiramon V, Thadanipon K. Postinflammatory hypopigmentation. Clin Exp Dermatol. 2011;36:708–14.
3. Halder RM, Nandedkar MA, Neal KW. Pigmentary disorders in ethnic skin. Dermatol Clin. 2003;21:617–28.
4. Halder RM, Nootheti PK. Ethnic skin disorders overview. J Am Acad Dermatol. 2003;48(6 Suppl):S143–8.
5. Morelli JG, Norris DA. Influence of inflammatory mediators and cytokines on human melanocyte function. J Invest Dermatol. 1993;100:191S–5.
6. Kim NY, Pandya AG. Pigmentary diseases. Med Clin North Am. 1998;82:1185–207.
7. Xiang W, Xu A, Xu J, et al. In vivo confocal laser scanning microscopy of hypopigmented macules: a preliminary comparison of confocal images in vitiligo, nevus depigmentosus and postinflammatory hypopigmentation. Lasers Med Sci. 2010;25:551–8.
8. Halder RM, Richards GM. Management of dyschromias in ethnic skin. Dermatol Ther. 2004;17:151–7.
9. Lopez I, Ahmed A, Pandya AG. Topical PUVA for post-inflammatory hypopigmentation. J Eur Acad Dermatol Venereol. 2011;25:734–46.
10. High WA, Pandya AG. Pilot trial of 1 % pimecrolimus cream in the treatment of seborrheic dermatitis in African American adults with associated hypopigmentation. J Am Acad Dermatol. 2006;54:1083–8.

3 Pityriasis Alba

Meredith Orseth and Nnenna G. Agim

Contents

M. Orseth, BS
Department of Medicine, University of Virginia School of Medicine, University of Virginia Health System, 800739, Charlottesville, VA 22908, USA
e-mail: mlo3ef@virginia.edu

N.G. Agim, MD (✉)
Department of Pediatric Dermatology, Childrens's Medical Center Dallas, 2350 N Stemmons FWY, Dallas, TX 75207, USA
e-mail: nnenna.agim@childrens.com

3.1 Introduction

Pityriasis alba is a disorder of mild cutaneous inflammation resulting in disordered pigmentation characterized by hypopigmented macules, patches, and thin plaques with fine scale [1, 2]. Rare in adults, it affects an estimated 5 % of the pediatric population and is among the most common disorders of hypopigmentation seen in children. While people of all skin types are affected, it is more noticeable in those with more darkly pigmented skin [2–4]. Given its asymptomatic and generally limited nature, only a portion of individuals with pityriasis alba seek treatment. In many cases, however, areas of hypopigmentation are readily obvious and cause considerable distress for patients and their parents [2].

Strongly associated with atopy [1, 5], pityriasis alba is considered a minor criterion for diagnosing atopic dermatitis [6]. While little is known regarding the underlying pathogenesis, the decreased pigment of pityriasis alba is considered a post-inflammatory phenomenon following a low-grade eczematous reaction [1, 4]. Examination of the affected skin shows a decrease in the number of melanosomes, a characteristic finding in atopic dermatitis [7, 8]. Additionally, like atopic dermatitis, pityriasis alba has been linked with a loss-of-function filaggrin mutation. Given the integral role of filaggrin in the water-holding capacity of the stratum corneum, this explains xerosis as a frequently associated feature of both conditions [9].

Other associations of pityriasis alba have been investigated, with some sources suggesting that sun exposure habits, personal hygiene, and/or nutritional deficiencies are connected to the disease [1, 3, 5, 7]. While possible infectious etiologies have also been implicated, none are as of yet confirmed [1, 5].

D. Jackson-Richards, A.G. Pandya (eds.), *Dermatology Atlas for Skin of Color*,
DOI 10.1007/978-3-642-54446-0_3, © Springer-Verlag Berlin Heidelberg 2014

3.2 Clinical Features

The early lesions of pityriasis alba—mildly erythematous slightly scaly thin plaques with ill-defined margins—are seldom noticed. Instead, it is the resulting hypopigmented round to oval areas that are generally of concern to patients [5]. Slightly elevated with fine scale, plaques may be from 0.5 to 4 cm in diameter and number from one to several lesions [1–3]. The face, particularly the cheeks, is the most commonly involved site in children [1], although the lateral arms, shoulders, neck, and anterior thighs may also be affected (Figs. 3.1 and 3.2) [1–5]. While uncommon, widespread involvement may occur [5]. The lesions of pityriasis alba are typically asymptomatic, only occasionally associated with mild pruritus [2–4].

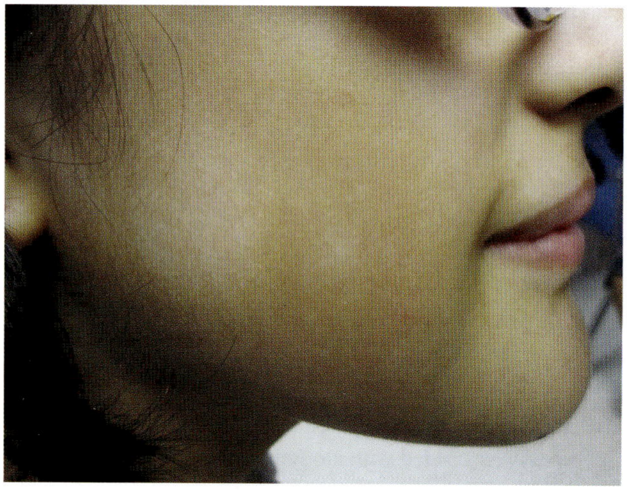

Fig. 3.1 Pityriasis alba on the face of a Hispanic girl

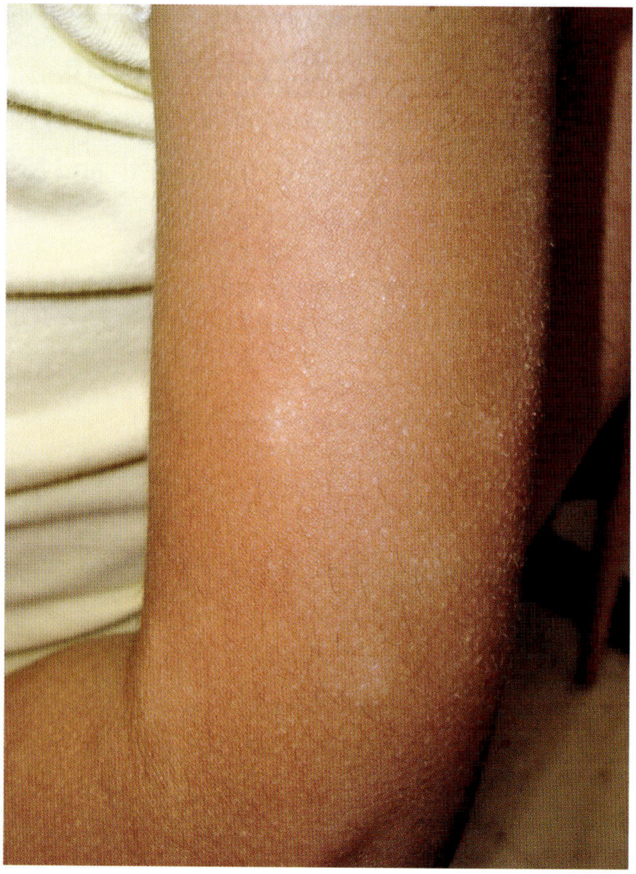

Fig. 3.2 Pityriasis alba on the arm of a Hispanic girl

3.3 Natural History and Prognosis

If untreated, pityriasis alba tends to be a relatively chronic condition with frequent relapses and a variable course. Although the disease most often resolves spontaneously prior to adulthood, repigmentation is a slow process that may take months to years to resolve in entirety [2–5]. Seasonal variation does occur, with plaques becoming more conspicuous in summer months when the affected areas do not tan like surrounding skin [1, 2]. In the dry winter months, plaques may become scaly and inflamed [5]. Although chronic and often a cosmetic burden, pityriasis alba is not associated with any complications or permanent disfigurement [2–5].

3.4 Histopathological Features

While rarely obtained, biopsy of skin affected by pityriasis alba shows a nonspecific picture consisting of spongiosis with exocytosis, hyperkeratosis, and dermal perivascular lymphocytic infiltration [5, 7, 8]. In early stages, follicular plugging, follicular spongiosis, and atrophic sebaceous glands may also be seen [8]. The quantity of melanocytes observed varies by report, with some sources suggesting fewer in number than normal skin, similar to atopic dermatitis [8]. Other studies indicate affected skin having a comparatively larger number of melanocytes that also appear damaged by electron microscopy [7]. Consistently, a reduced number of melanosomes are observed in lesions of pityriasis alba [7, 8].

3.5 Diagnosis and Differential Diagnosis

The diagnosis of pityriasis alba is made clinically, although certain laboratory tests (e.g., potassium hydroxide preparation) may be used to help differentiate it from other conditions. Biopsy is seldom indicated, only in specific cases when disorders such as sarcoidosis or mycosis fungoides must be excluded. Pityriasis alba is commonly mistaken for tinea versicolor and vitiligo [3, 7, 8]. In general, tinea versicolor differs from pityriasis alba in that facial involvement is less common; the hypopigmented lesions are smaller, more numerous, and often coalescing; and potassium hydroxide preparation is positive for yeast elements. Patches of vitiligo are more sharply demarcated than the lesions of pityriasis alba and completely lack scale and pigment [3]. Other disorders of hypopigmentation that should be considered in the differential diagnosis include follicular mucinosis, psoriatic leukoderma, mycosis fungoides, nevus depigmentosus, and nevus anemicus [3, 7, 8].

3.6 Treatment

Patients with pityriasis alba should be counseled that lesions will slowly improve on their own with time. If mild inflammation is present, topical corticosteroids or calcineurin inhibitors (i.e., 1 % pimecrolimus cream, 0.03 % or 0.1 % tacrolimus ointment) may be used [2, 3]. Other sources suggest using 0.1 % tacrolimus and 0.0003 % calcitriol ointments in conjunction [4]. Unfortunately, treatment of the hypopigmentation of pityriasis alba is difficult, and it has been shown that topical steroids and emollients are of similar efficacy [2, 3]. With the risk for side effects from chronic corticosteroid use, it is reasonable to treat only with lubrication and sun avoidance to prevent darkening of the skin surrounding the affected areas.

References

1. Weber BM, Sponchiado de Avila LG, Albaneze R, et al. Pityriasis alba: a study of pathogenic factors. J Eur Acad Dermatol Venereol. 2002;16(5):463–8.
2. Fujita WH, McCormick CL, Parneix-Spake A. An exploratory study to evaluate the efficacy of pimecrolimus cream 1 % for the treatment of pityriasis alba. Int J Dermatol. 2007;46(7):700–5.
3. Lin RL, Janniger CK. Pityriasis alba. Cutis. 2005;76(1):21–4.
4. Moreno-Cruz B, Torres-Álvarez B, Hernández-Blanco D, et al. Double-blind, placebo-controlled, randomized study comparing 0.0003 % calcitriol with 0.1 % tacrolimus ointments for the treatment of endemic pityriasis alba. Dermatol Res Pract. 2012;2012:303275. doi:10.1155/2012/303275. Epub 2012 Apr 22.
5. Vinod S, Singh G, Dash K, Grover S. Clinico epidemiological study of pityriasis alba. Indian J Dermatol Venereol Leprol [serial online] 2002 [cited 2013 Aug 10]; 68:338–40. Available from: http://www.ijdvl.com/text.asp?2002/68/6/338/11182
6. Hanifin JM, Rajka G. Diagnostic features of atopic dermatitis. Acta Derm Venereol Suppl (Stockh). 1980;92:44–7.
7. In SI, Yi SW, Kang HY, Lee ES, Sohn S, Kim YC. Clinical and histopathological characteristics of pityriasis alba. Clin Exp Dermatol. 2009;34(5):591–7. doi:10.1111/j.1365-2230.2008.03038.x. Epub 2008 Dec 15.
8. Vargas-Ocampo F. Pityriasis alba: a histologic study. Int J Dermatol. 1993;32:870–3.
9. Landeck L, Visser M, Kezic S, John SM. Genotype-phenotype associations in filaggrin loss-of-function mutation carriers. Contact Dermatitis. 2013;68(3):149–55.

Idiopathic Guttate Hypomelanosis

4

Katherine Omueti Ayoade and Amit G. Pandya

Contents

K.O. Ayoade, MD, PhD • A.G. Pandya, MD (✉)
Department of Dermatology, University of Texas Southwestern Medical Center, 5323 Harry Hines Boulevard, Dallas, TX 75390, USA
e-mail: katherine.ayoade@me.com; amit.pandya@utsouthwestern.edu

4.1 Introduction

Idiopathic guttate hypomelanosis (IGH) was first described by Costa in 1951 and was subsequently confirmed in a larger number of patients reported by Cummings and Cottel as well as Whitehead et al. in 1966 [1]. It is a common acquired leukoderma that is characterized by discrete porcelain white macules, measuring 2–5 mm in diameter; however, smaller macules or larger patches, 10–25 mm, have been observed [2–5]. Although benign and asymptomatic, affected individuals may seek medical attention for aesthetic reasons [3].

4.1.1 Epidemiology

The incidence of IGH in the population is about 80 % in persons over 70 [5]. Although IGH is more common in patients with advanced age, it has also been observed in young adults [1]. IGH is observed in all races, though it is more striking in individuals with darker skin [5, 6]. Female incidence appears to be higher, but this could be due to the fact that women are more likely to seek medical attention for aesthetic reasons [5].

4.1.2 Etiology

The etiology and pathogenesis of IGH are unknown. IGH has been hypothesized to be UV-induced, as it most commonly affects sun-exposed sites, such as the extremities, neck, and face [2]. Yet another hypothesis for the etiology of IGH is normal aging or photoaging. Other suggested contributing factors include genetics, trauma, and autoimmunity [3].

D. Jackson-Richards, A.G. Pandya (eds.), *Dermatology Atlas for Skin of Color*,
DOI 10.1007/978-3-642-54446-0_4, © Springer-Verlag Berlin Heidelberg 2014

4.2 Clinical Features

4.2.1 Distribution and Arrangement

Clinically, IGH consists of small hypopigmented and depigmented macules which are sometimes porcelain white, with discrete circumscribed borders (Figs. 4.1, 4.2, 4.3. 4.4, 4.5, 4.6, and 4.7). They are often scattered and usually observed on the exposed areas of the upper and lower extremities; however, they may appear on the face and neck. The macules of IGH measure about 2–5 mm in size but can be larger [5].

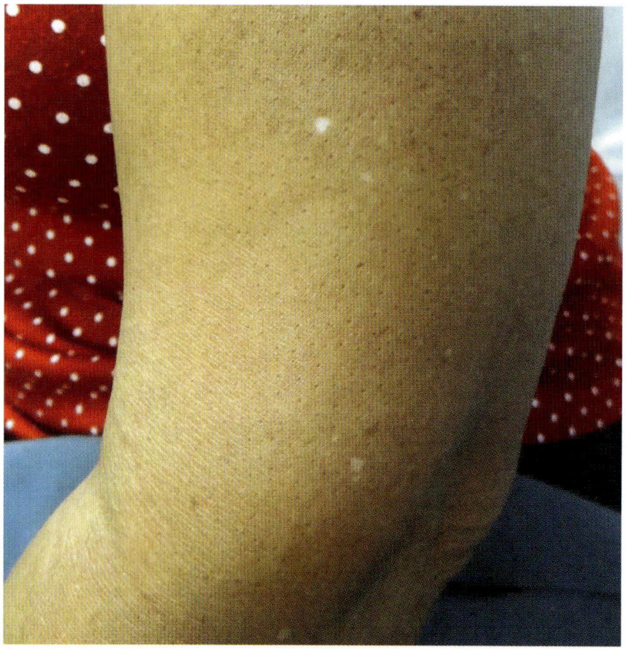

Fig. 4.1 IGH lesions on the upper arm of African-American female

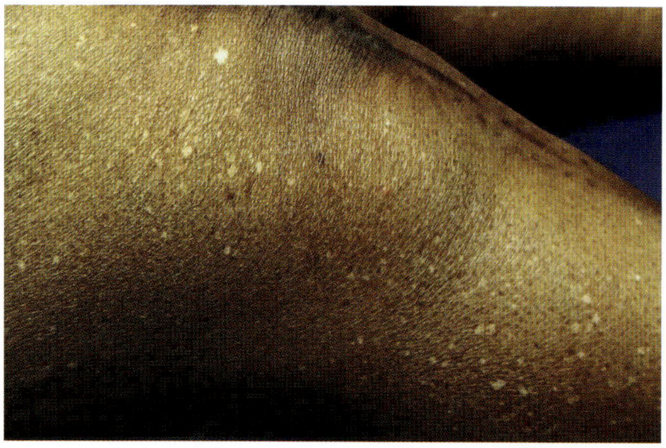

Fig. 4.2 Multiple lesions of IGH on the lower extremities of an African-American female

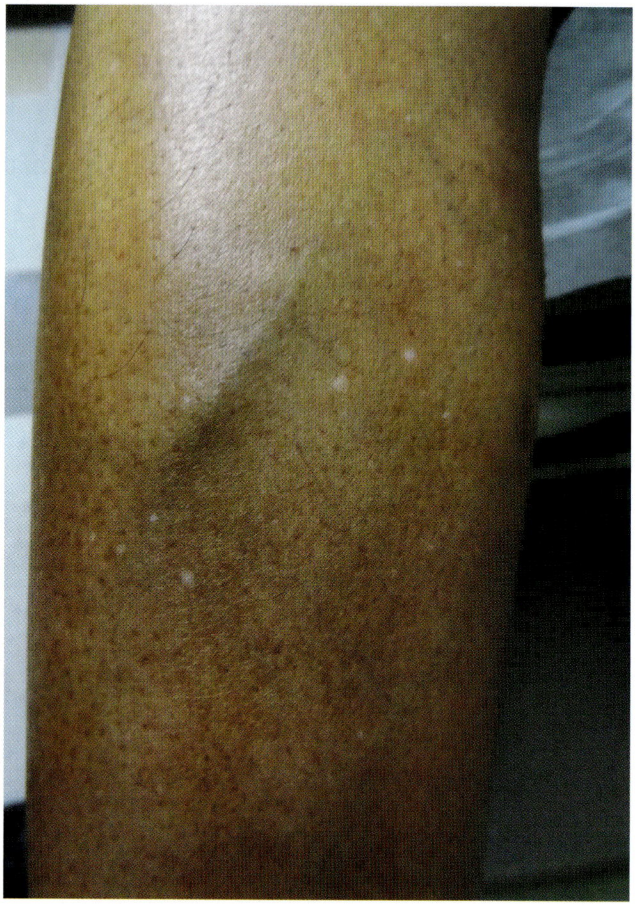

Fig. 4.3 IGH lesions on the shin of an African-American female

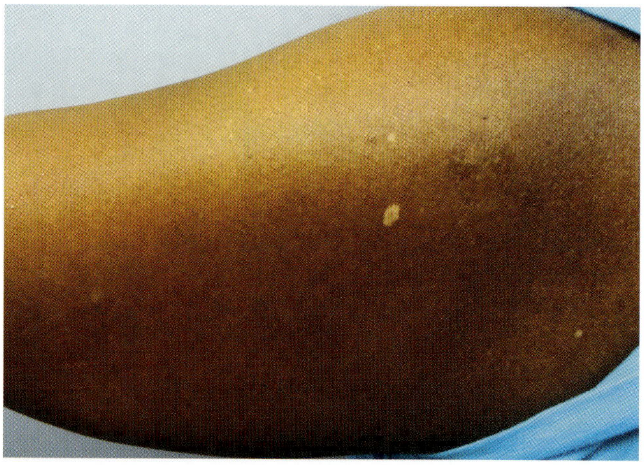

Fig. 4.4 IGH lesions on the posterior upper arm of an African-American female

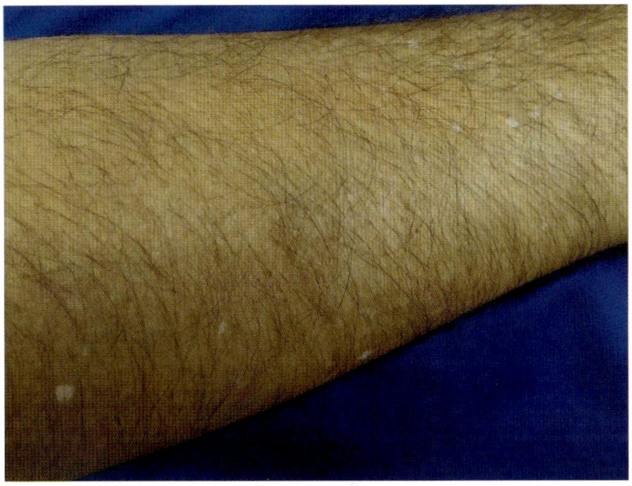

Fig. 4.5 IGH lesions on the dorsal forearm of a Latin American male

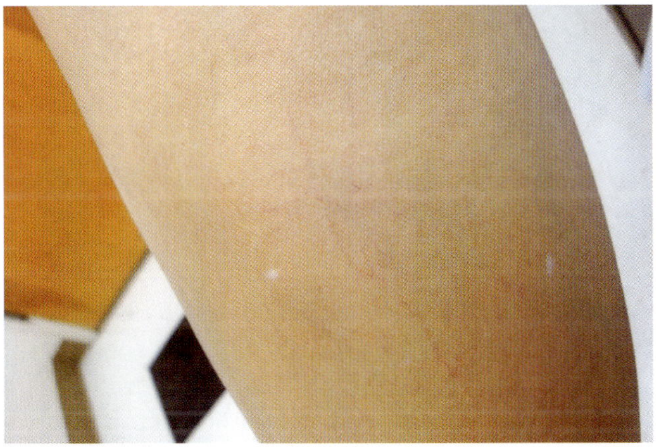

Fig. 4.6 Two lesions of IGH on the calf of a Filipino female

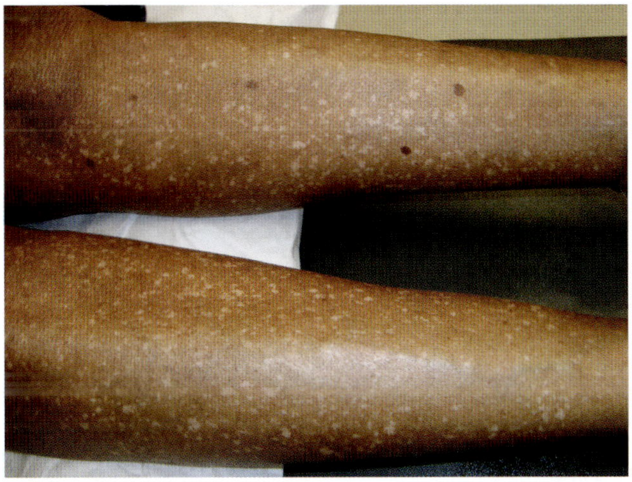

Fig. 4.7 Multiple lesions of IGH on the legs of an African-American female

4.3 Natural History and Prognosis

Once present, the macules of IGH may grow slightly but do not usually change much in size. The lesions do not coalesce and their surface is smooth but not atrophic. No spontaneous re-pigmentation has been observed [4, 5].

4.4 Histopathological Features

The main histological feature is variable loss of melanin granules in epidermal keratinocytes. A decrease in the absolute number of melanocytes is also observed [4, 7]. Other histopathological findings include hyperkeratosis and epidermal atrophy, including flattening of the rete pegs [4].

4.5 Diagnosis and Differential Diagnosis

IGH can mimic several skin disorders of pigmentation. The differential diagnosis includes post-inflammatory hypopigmentation, vitiligo, lichen sclerosis, pityriasis lichenoides chronica, pityriasis alba, atrophie blanche, leprosy, leukoderma following PUVA therapy, and confetti-like lesions of tuberous sclerosis. In the neoplastic category, the differential diagnosis includes hypopigmented mycosis fungoides, disseminated hypopigmented keratoses following PUVA therapy, and achromic verruca plana with the latter two entities forming papules to help distinguish them from IGH [5, 8].

4.6 Treatment

IGH does not require treatment. Patients who seek the attention of a dermatologist may choose to explore therapy for aesthetic or cosmetic reasons after being reassured of the benign nature of this condition.

Multiple therapies are available all with variable success rates of achieving the patient's desired re-pigmentation. These include cryotherapy, superficial dermabrasion, topical retinoids, fractional carbon dioxide lasers, intralesional corticosteroids, and topical tacrolimus and pimecrolimus [2, 3, 6, 9].

References

1. Kim SK, Kim EH, Kang HY, Lee ES, Sohn S, Kim YC. Comprehensive understanding of idiopathic guttate hypomelanosis: clinical and histopathological correlation. Int J Dermatol. 2010;49(2):162–6.

2. Shin J, Kim M, Park SH, Oh SH. The effect of fractional carbon dioxide lasers on idiopathic guttate hypomelanosis: a preliminary study. J Eur Acad Dermatol Venereol. 2013;27(2):e243–6.
3. Rerknimitr P, Disphanurat W, Achariyakul M. Topical tacrolimus significantly promotes repigmentation in idiopathic guttate hypomelanosis: a double-blind, randomized, placebo-controlled study. J Eur Acad Dermatol Venereol. 2013;27(4):460–4.
4. Falabella R, Escobar C, Giraldo N, et al. On the pathogenesis of idiopathic guttate hypomelanosis. J Am Acad Dermatol. 1987;16(1 Pt 1):35–44.
5. Ortonne J-P. Vitiligo and other disorders of hypopigmentation. In: Bolognia JL, Jorizzo JL, Rapini RP, editors. Dermatology, vol. 1. 2nd ed. St. Louis: Mosby; 2008. p. 935.
6. Hexsel DM. Treatment of idiopathic guttate hypomelanosis by localized superficial dermabrasion. Dermatol Surg. 1999;25(11):917–8.
7. Friedland R, David M, Feinmesser M, Fenig-Nakar S, Hodak E. Idiopathic guttate hypomelanosis-like lesions in patients with mycosis fungoides: a new adverse effect of phototherapy. J Eur Acad Dermatol Venereol. 2010;24(9):1026–30.
8. Calonje E, Brenn T, Lazar A, McKee PH. Disorders of pigmentation. In: Calonje E, Brenn T, Lazar A, McKee PH, editors. McKee's pathology of the skin with clinical correlations, vol. 2. Printed in China. Edinburgh: Elsevier/Saunders, 2012. http://www.ncbi.nlm.nih.gov/nlmcatalog/101584719.
9. Ploysangam T, Dee-Ananlap S, Suvanprakorn P. Treatment of idiopathic guttate hypomelanosis with liquid nitrogen: light and electron microscopic studies. J Am Acad Dermatol. 1990; 23(4 Pt 1):681–4.

Post-inflammatory Hyperpigmentation

5

Stephanie Alexandra Savory and Amit G. Pandya

Contents

5.1 Introduction

Post-inflammatory hyperpigmentation is an unfortunate consequence of many dermatologic processes (especially those resulting in inflammation or trauma to the skin). It arises without gender predilection and in all skin types but is particularly prominent and longer lasting in patients with skin of color (Fitzpatrick skin type IV–VI) including, but not limited to, African-Americans, Asians, Native Americans, and Hispanics.

Post-inflammatory hyperpigmentation has two major etiologies. When inflammation damages the basal keratinocytes, a large amount of melanin is released into the dermis and engulfed by macrophages, creating a characteristic blue-gray color at the site of injury that may be long lasting. An epidermal response orchestrated by inflammatory mediators such as prostaglandins and leukotrienes causes an increase in synthesis of melanin by melanocytes and subsequent transfer to keratinocytes [1].

Epidemiological studies show that post-inflammatory hyperpigmentation is the third most common reason for which African-Americans present to a dermatologist [2]. In comparison, dyschromia is a much less frequent cause for dermatologic visits by Caucasian patients [3]. Post-inflammatory hyperpigmentation can be a cause of significant, lingering concern in patients with skin of color. When managing such patients, dermatologists should focus on treating the inciting inflammatory condition but also address the resulting pigment alteration; otherwise, the patient will likely consider the treatment to be inadequate [4, 5].

Post-inflammatory hyperpigmentation may be the end result of many inflammatory conditions, including allergic reactions, papulosquamous diseases, infections, and burns [6]. In patients with skin of color, however, acne is the most common cause of post-inflammatory pigmentation [7, 8].

S.A. Savory, MD • A.G. Pandya, MD (✉)
Department of Dermatology, University of Texas Southwestern Medical Center, 5323 Harry Hines Boulevard, Dallas, TX 75390, USA
e-mail: stephanie.savory@utsouthwestern.edu; amit.pandya@utsouthwestern.edu

D. Jackson-Richards, A.G. Pandya (eds.), *Dermatology Atlas for Skin of Color*,
DOI 10.1007/978-3-642-54446-0_5, © Springer-Verlag Berlin Heidelberg 2014

5.2 Clinical Features

Post-inflammatory hyperpigmentation appears as macules or patches in the distribution of the original inflammatory dermatosis or injury. Superficial deposition of melanin within the epidermis produces a well-circumscribed tan or light brown appearance while deeper deposition of melanin within the dermis will create macules or patches that appear poorly circumscribed and dark brown to blue-gray (Figs. 5.1, 5.2, 5.3, 5.4, 5.5, 5.6, 5.7, 5.8, and 5.9) [1]. Wood's lamp examination may accentuate the borders of hyperpigmentation in the epidermal variant while the borders of dermal hyperpigmentation remain vague [9]. Post-inflammatory hyperpigmentation typically lacks associated symptoms or systemic findings aside from cosmetic or psychosocial concern.

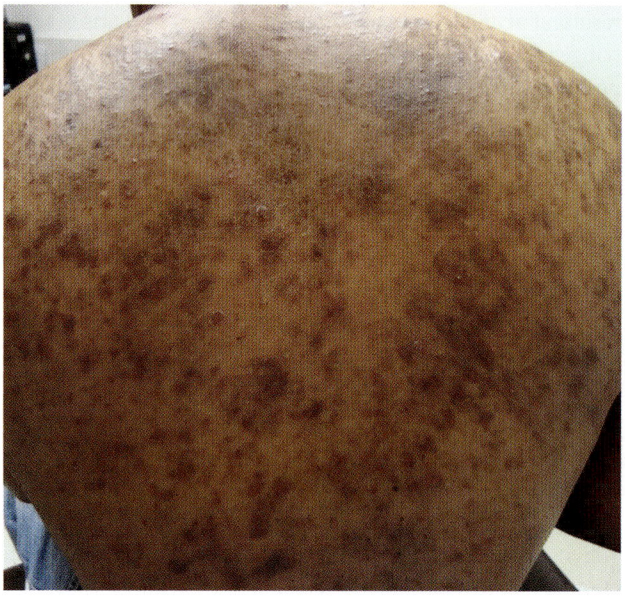

Fig. 5.1 PIH of the back from acne vulgaris in an AA male

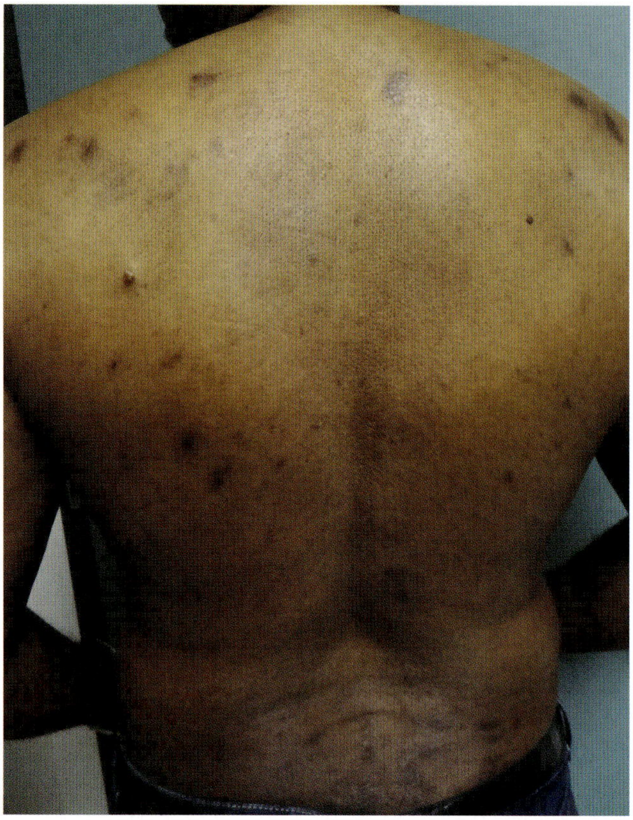

Fig. 5.2 PIH from lesions of pemphigus vulgaris in an AA male

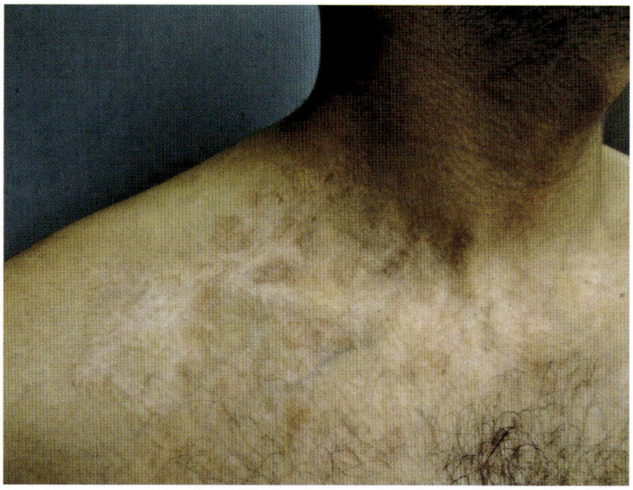

Fig. 5.3 Post-inflammatory hyper- and hypopigmentation from lesions of pemphigus vulgaris in a Hispanic male

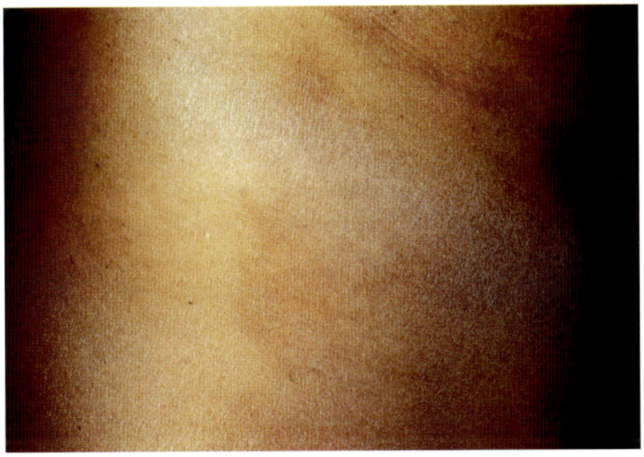

Fig. 5.4 PIH after urticarial vasculitis on the trunk of an AA female

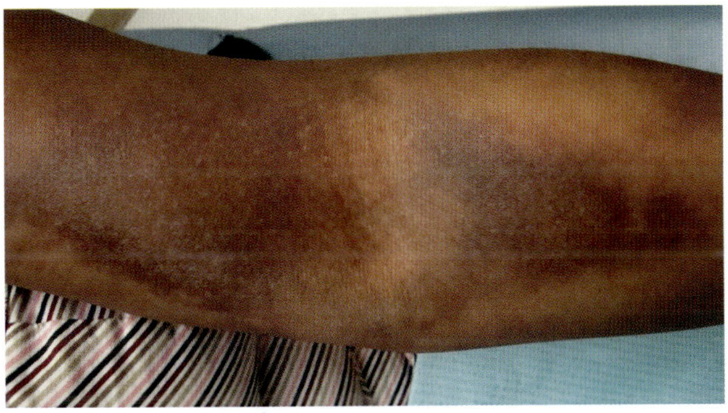

Fig. 5.5 PIH after a drug eruption in an AA female

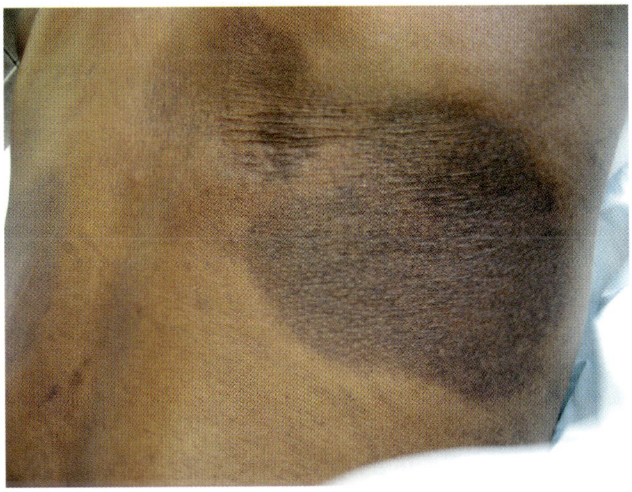

Fig. 5.6 PIH from lesions of mycosis fungoides in an AA male

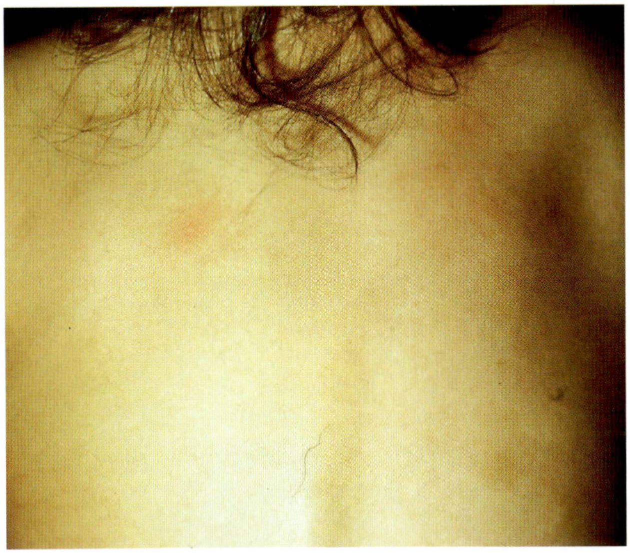

Fig. 5.7 PIH from EKG leads in a Hispanic girl

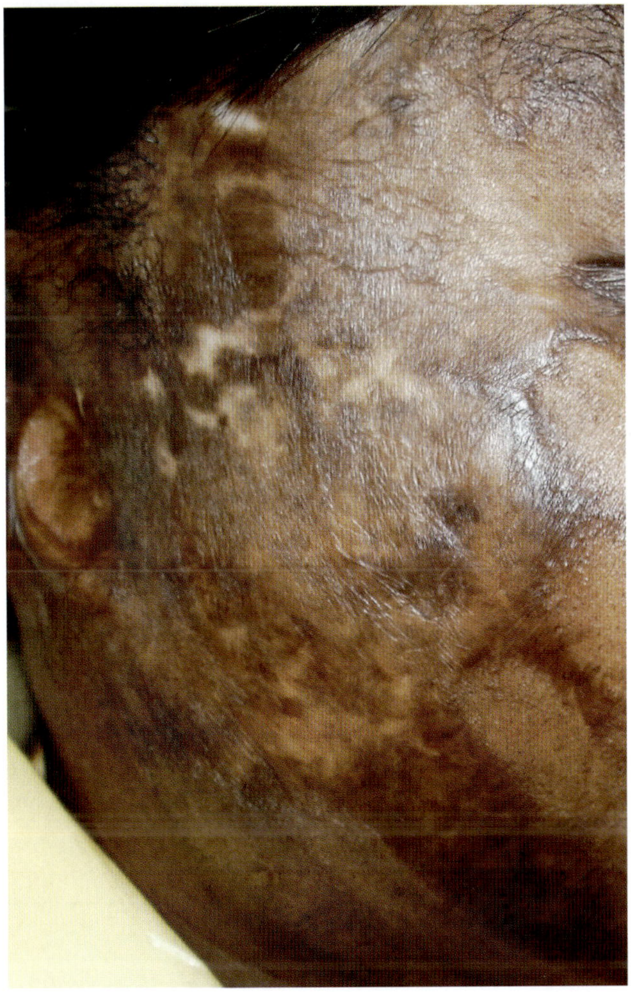

Fig. 5.8 PIH after a burn in an AA female

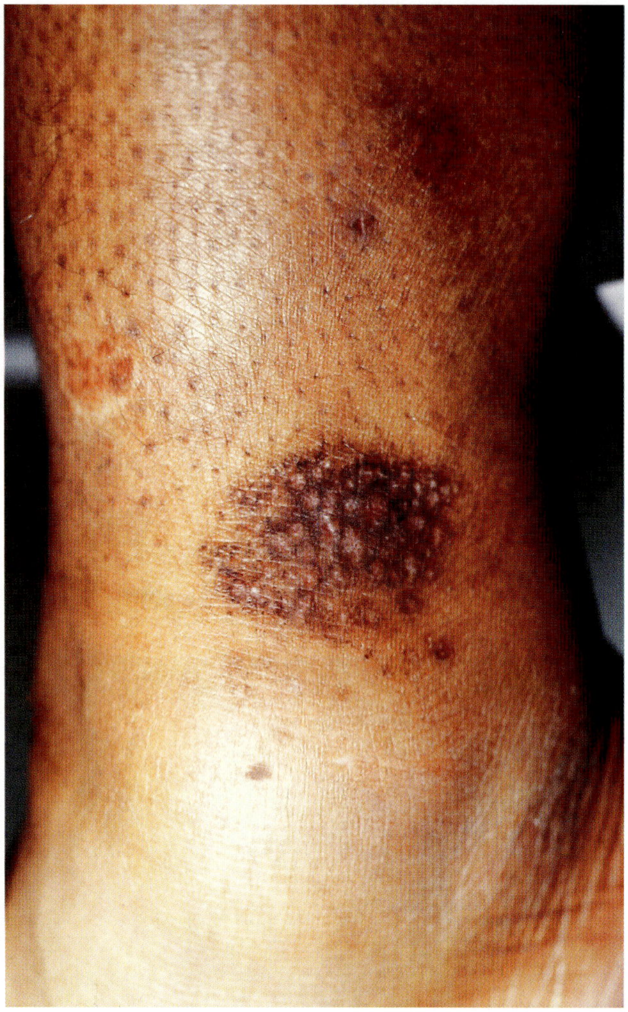

Fig. 5.9 PIH of the leg from lichen simplex chronicus in an AA female

5.3 Natural History and Prognosis

Post-inflammatory hyperpigmentation appears after an inflammatory process or trauma to the skin. Dermal hyperpigmentation may take years to fade, whereas epidermal hyperpigmentation fades in weeks to months. Post-inflammatory hyperpigmentation is not life threatening, but patients may have significant psychosocial distress from the cosmetic disfigurement [1]. Finally, the underlying disorder must be treated to prevent new areas of hyperpigmentation from developing [1].

5.4 Histopathological Features

Post-inflammatory hyperpigmentation is characterized histologically by increased epidermal melanin [10]. A sparse superficial perivascular infiltrate with melanophages may be seen in the dermis. Staining with Fontana-Masson may help identify melanin in the dermis or epidermis [1]. Basal cell vacuolization and band-like deposition of mucin have also been observed [1, 10].

5.5 Diagnosis and Differential Diagnosis

Diagnosis of post-inflammatory hyperpigmentation is fairly straightforward, especially if there is a history of a prior inflammatory dermatosis or injury to the affected area. Diagnosis may be obscured if the cause was so transient or mild that it was unnoticed by the patient [9]. Thorough history and physical exam of the skin aided by Wood's lamp or skin biopsy may be beneficial in confirming the diagnosis. The differential diagnosis includes melasma, fixed drug eruption, macular amyloid, tinea versicolor, drug-induced hyperpigmentation, and bruising [1, 9, 10]. Hyperpigmentation from medications such as tetracycline, antimalarials, bleomycin, arsenic, and doxorubicin should also be considered [10].

5.6 Treatment

Treatment of post-inflammatory hyperpigmentation can be challenging. Control of the underlying injurious process is critical to prevent new areas of hyperpigmentation. Daily photoprotection with a broad-spectrum sunscreen with sun protection factor (SPF) of 30 or greater as well as appropriate sun avoidance and use of sun protective clothing should be emphasized to help fade hyperpigmentation and prevent UV-induced darkening.

Topical agents are most useful for patients with an epidermal component to their hypermelanosis [9]. Hydroquinone in concentrations ranging from 2 to 4 % is a helpful initial treatment and may be more effective when used in combination with a mild corticosteroid and/or keratolytic such as tretinoin. Daily use of such combination creams may be irritating to the skin, leading to further pigmentation [9]. Additionally, photoprotection is critical to prevent repigmentation. Other reported treatments for post-inflammatory hyperpigmentation include azelaic acid, kojic acid, vitamin E, vitamin C, arbutin, bearberry extract, benzoquinone, chemical peels, laser, and various combinations of these interventions [1, 7, 10].

Unfortunately, while many treatment modalities may be helpful in diminishing the appearance of epidermal hyperpigmentation, they are often ineffective in dermal hypermelanosis. While the passage of time usually helps the appearance of dermal pigmentation, camouflage cosmetics may be of some use to these patients [1].

References

1. Lacz NL, Vafaie J, Kihiczak NI, et al. Post inflammatory hyperpigmentation: a common but troubling condition. Int J Dermatol. 2004;43(5):362–5.
2. Halder RM. The role of retinoids in the management of cutaneous conditions in blacks. J Am Acad Dermatol. 1998;39(2 Pt 3):S98–103.
3. Alexis AF, Sergay AB, Taylor SC. Common dermatologic disorders in skin of color: a comparative practice survey. Cutis. 2007;80(5):387–94.
4. Stratigos AJ, Katsambas AD. Optimal management of recalcitrant disorders of hyperpigmentation in dark-skinned patients. Am J Clin Dermatol. 2004;5(3):161–8.
5. Halder RM, Nootheti PK. Ethnic skin disorders overview. J Am Acad Dermatol. 2003;48(6 Suppl):S143–8.
6. Taylor SC, Grimes PE, Lim J, et al. Postinflammatory hyperpigmentation. J Cutan Med Surg. 2009;13:183–91.
7. Taylor SC, Cook-Bolden F, Rahman Z, et al. Acne vulgaris in skin of color. J Am Acad Dermatol. 2002;46(2 Suppl):S98–106.
8. Child FJ, Fuller LC, Higgens EM, et al. A study of the spectrum of skin disease occurring in a black population in southeast London. Br J Dermatol. 1999;141:512–7.
9. Ruiz-Maldonado R, Orozco-Covarrubias ML. Postinflammatory hypopigmentation and hyperpigmentation. Semin Cutan Med Surg. 1997;16(1):36–43.
10. Soriano T, Grimes PE. Post-inflammatory hyperpigmentation. In: Tosti A, Grimes PE, De Padova MP, editors. Color atlas of chemical peels. Berlin/Heidelberg: Springer; 2006. p. 177–83.

Melasma

6

Tiffany J. Lieu and Amit G. Pandya

Contents

T.J. Lieu, MD • A.G. Pandya, MD (✉)
Department of Dermatology,
University of Texas Southwestern
Medical Center, 5323 Harry Hines Boulevard,
Dallas, TX 75390-9190, USA
e-mail: tiffanylieumd@gmail.com;
amit.pandya@utsouthwestern.edu

6.1 Introduction

Melasma, also known as chloasma or mask of pregnancy, is a common acquired disorder of symmetrical hyperpigmentation. It affects both genders but appears most commonly in females, especially Fitzpatrick skin phototypes III and IV residing in areas with significant ultraviolet light exposure [1]. Melasma affects all types of skin, especially skin of color, and has been described in individuals of Latino, Arab, Southeast Asian, Ethiopian, Lebanese, African-American, South African, East Asian, South Asian, Egyptian, Iranian, Turkish, and French descent [1–8]. Though melasma is usually asymptomatic, cosmetic disfigurement caused by this disorder significantly affects quality of life.

The prevalence of melasma in the general population is not well known. Studies have reported a prevalence of 8.8 % in Hispanic females in Texas [1]. A study from Guerrero, Mexico, reported a prevalence of 6 % among women in rural areas and 4 % in urban areas [9].

The exact etiology of melasma is unknown, but it is thought to be caused by an increase in biological activity of melanocytes rather than an increase in melanocyte number [1]. Resulting hypermelanosis can be due to increased epidermal melanin or both increased epidermal melanin and deposition of melanin in the dermis [1]. Established risk factors include darker skin phototypes, genetic predisposition, exposure to ultraviolet light, pregnancy, and exogenous hormones such as hormone replacement therapy or oral contraceptives [1]. Ultraviolet light exacerbates melasma, likely due to upregulation of melanocyte-stimulating cytokines like interleukin-1, endothelin-1, alpha-melanocyte-stimulating hormone, and adrenocorticotropic hormone [1]. The effects of hormones on melasma are unclear, though pregnancy and oral contraceptive use have both been associated with the onset or worsening of melasma.

D. Jackson-Richards, A.G. Pandya (eds.), *Dermatology Atlas for Skin of Color*,
DOI 10.1007/978-3-642-54446-0_6, © Springer-Verlag Berlin Heidelberg 2014

6.2 Clinical Features

Melasma presents as light brown to dark muddy brown or gray-brown macules and patches on sun-exposed areas of the face, particularly the forehead, malar regions, upper lip, and chin (Figs. 6.1, 6.2, 6.3, 6.4, 6.5, 6.6, and 6.7). The color may be uniform or inhomogeneous. Lesions have irregular borders and are limited to sun-exposed skin. Melasma can be divided into centrofacial, malar, and mandibular types, based on the distribution of lesions. The centrofacial pattern is the most common, observed in about two-thirds of affected individuals, and manifests as lesions on the forehead, nose, upper lip, chin, and medial cheeks [1]. The malar pattern consists of lesions on the cheeks and nose, and the mandibular pattern is characterized by lesions on the ramus of the mandible (Fig. 6.8) [1]. Individuals often exhibit a mixed pattern of distribution. Melasma has also been described on the neck and arms [1]. Melasma typically lacks associated symptoms or systemic findings.

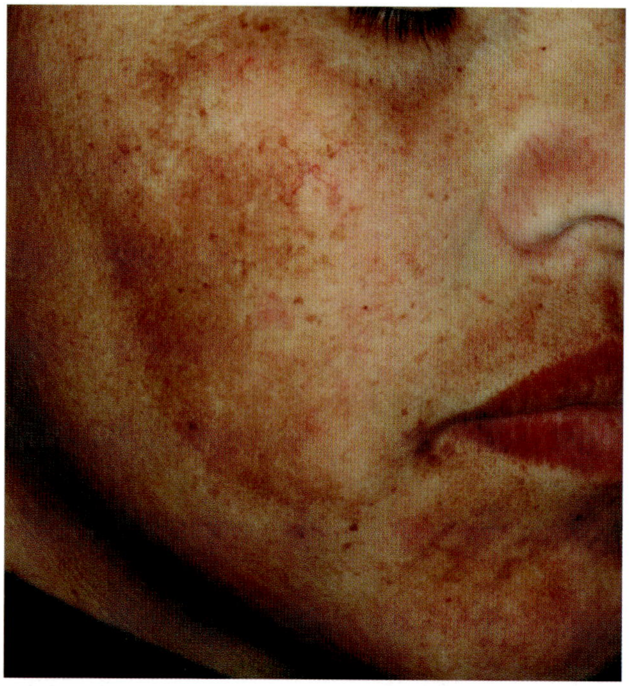

Fig. 6.1 Melasma of the cheek in a Hispanic female

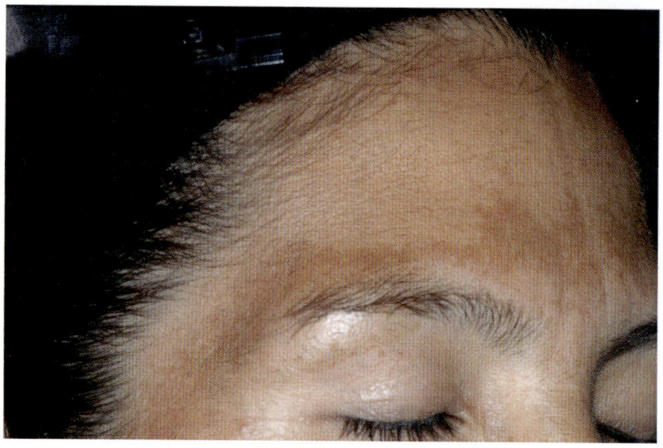

Fig. 6.2 Melasma of the forehead in a Hispanic female

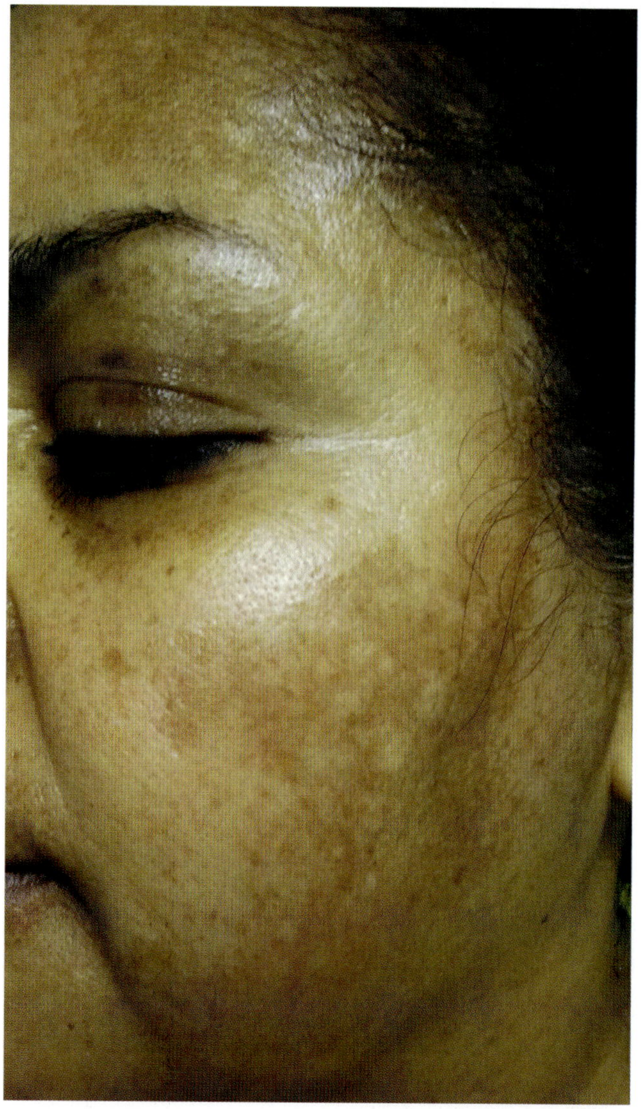

Fig. 6.3 Melasma of the cheek in a Hispanic female

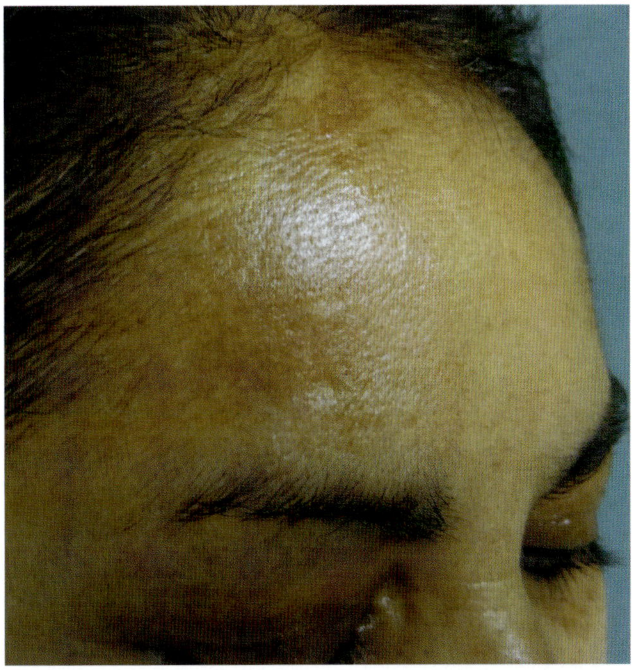

Fig. 6.4 Melasma of the forehead in a Hispanic female

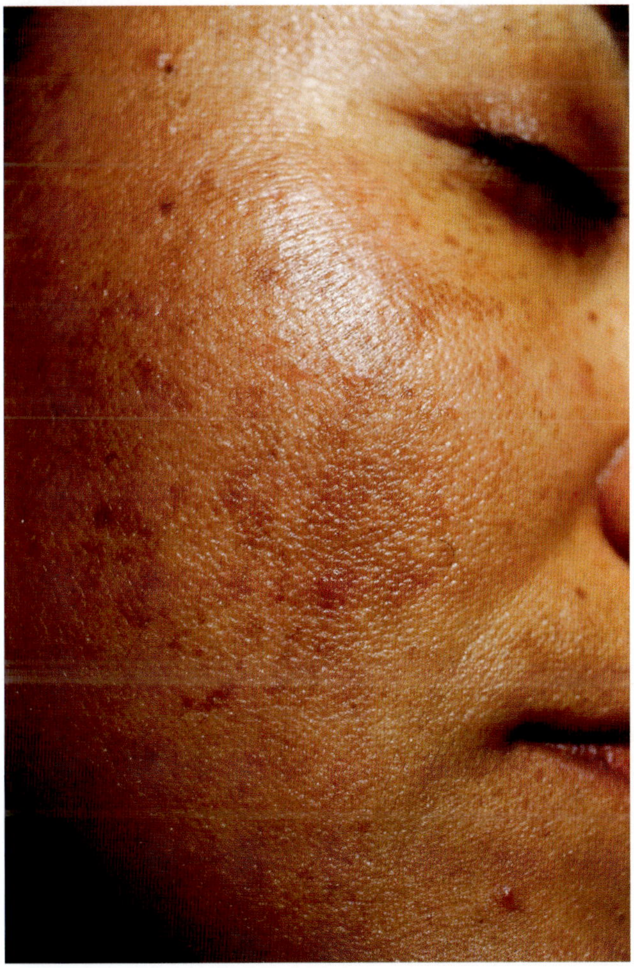

Fig. 6.5 Melasma of the right cheek in a Hispanic female

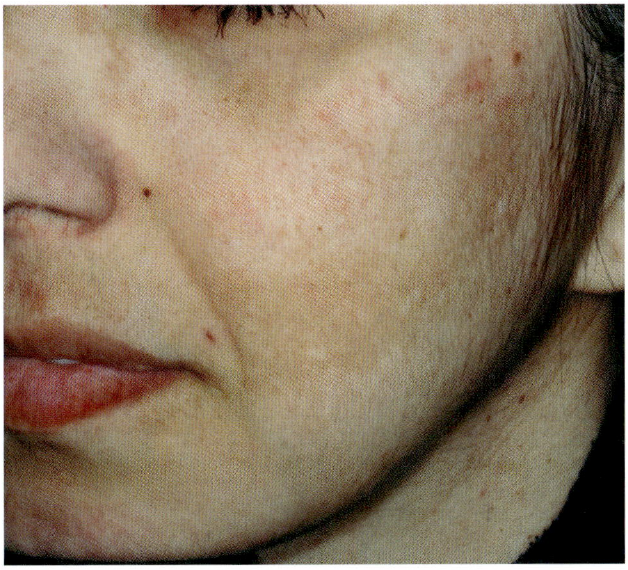

Fig. 6.6 Mild melasma of the cheek and upper lip in a Hispanic female

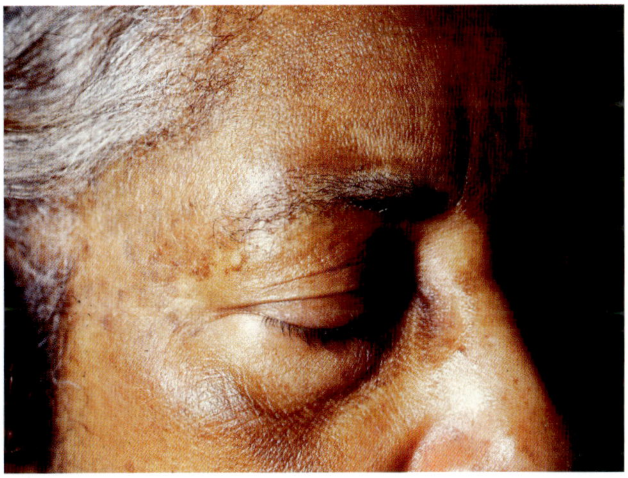

Fig. 6.7 Severe melasma of the cheek and forehead in a Hispanic female

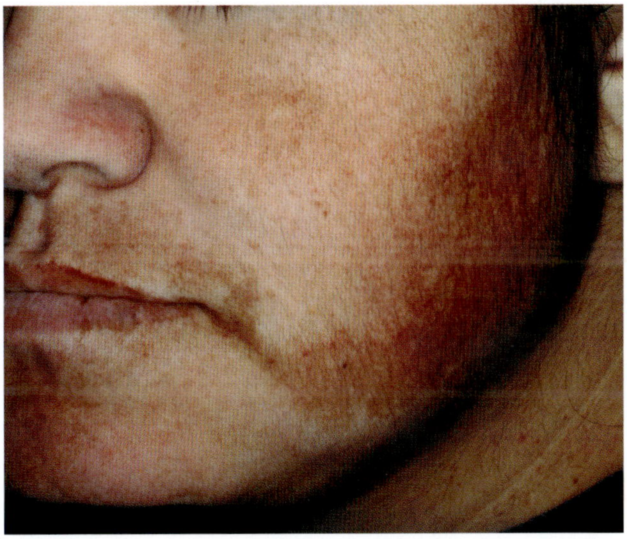

Fig. 6.8 Melasma of the upper lip and mandibular region in a Hispanic female

6.3 Natural History and Prognosis

Melasma develops gradually but can evolve rapidly over weeks, particularly after exposure to sunlight, during pregnancy, or after initiation of hormone therapy [1]. Lesions can resolve spontaneously over months, after delivery, or after cessation of exogenous hormones, depending on the circumstance. However, melasma often lasts for many years, long after pregnancy is over. This disorder can recur with subsequent pregnancies [1].

6.4 Histopathological Features

Melasma has two histopathological patterns. The epidermal form is characterized by melanin deposition in the basal and suprabasal layers and highly dendritic melanocytes full of pigment [1]. The dermal form consists of superficial and perivascular melanophages in the dermis with less prominent epidermal pigmentation [1]. Electron microscopy demonstrates highly melanized stage IV melanocytes [1]. Wood's lamp examination may show marked accentuation of hyperpigmented lesions, correlating with the epidermal histopathological pattern. More recent studies have shown that apparent epidermal melasma identified by Wood's lamp examination often demonstrates significant dermal melanin on histopathology, helping to explain the recalcitrant nature of this disorder [1].

6.5 Diagnosis and Differential Diagnosis

A careful medical history and examination of the skin including Wood's lamp examination are helpful in making the diagnosis of melasma. Skin biopsy can be utilized in difficult cases. The differential diagnosis of melasma includes post-inflammatory hyperpigmentation, solar lentigines, ephelides, drug-induced hyperpigmentation, actinic lichen planus, facial acanthosis nigricans (Fig. 6.9), frictional melanosis, acquired bilateral nevus of Ota-like macules (Hori's nevus), nevus of Ota, poikiloderma of Civatte, cutaneous lupus erythematosus, photosensitivity reaction, skin infection, and atopic dermatitis [1]. Unlike most of these diagnoses, melasma is not usually associated with inflammation.

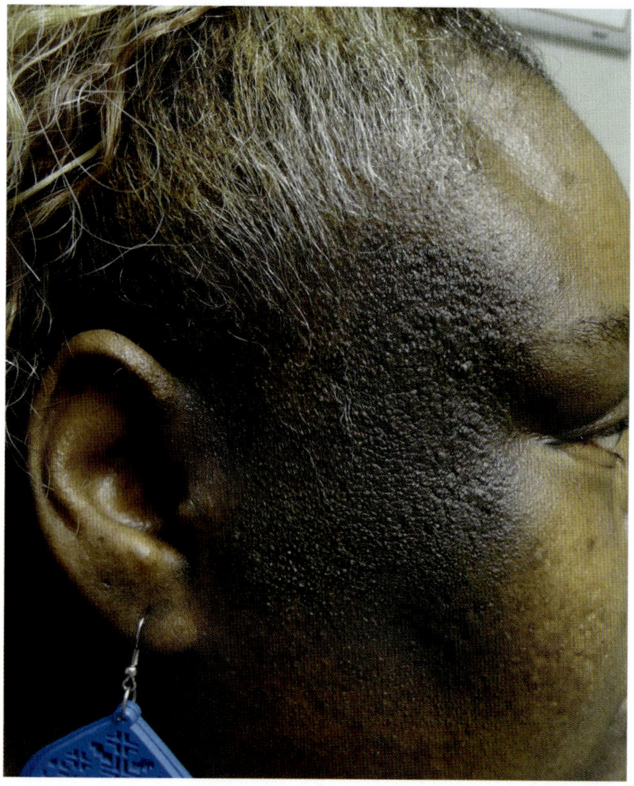

Fig. 6.9 Acanthosis nigricans mimicking melasma in an AA female

6.6 Treatment

Although melasma is asymptomatic, treatment is important, as this disorder has been shown by the Melasma Quality of Life scale (MELASQOL) to have profoundly negative psychological and emotional effects [1, 7]. Treatment options for melasma include depigmenting agents, topical retinoids, topical steroids, chemical peels, laser, and light therapies [8, 10]. Topical combination therapies have been found to be more effective than monotherapy, particularly triple combination therapy consisting of hydroquinone, tretinoin, and fluocinolone acetonide [8, 10]. Side effects are usually mild and include irritation, dryness, burning, and erythema of the skin. Kojic acid, isopropylcatechol, N-acetyl-4-cysteaminylphenol, and flavonoid extracts have been investigated as hypopigmenting agents but have not been shown to be superior to creams containing hydroquinone [8, 10]. Chemical peels, laser therapy, and intense pulsed light have been used but yield unpredictable results and also an increased risk of irritation and post-inflammatory hyperpigmentation [8, 10]. Risk of post-inflammatory hyperpigmentation is especially high in skin of color. Most importantly in the treatment of melasma, all patients should be encouraged to avoid the sun as much as possible and use broad-spectrum sunscreen regularly, as ultraviolet and visible light can exacerbate melasma. Furthermore, sunscreen enhances the effect of hydroquinone therapy [8]. In general, melasma treatment is determined on an individual basis, and long-term remission can be difficult to achieve.

References

1. Sheth VM, Pandya AG. Melasma: a comprehensive update: part I. J Am Acad Dermatol. 2011;65(4):689–97; quiz 698.
2. Kimbrough-Green CK, Griffiths CE, Finkel LJ, Hamilton TA, Bulengo-Ransby SM, Ellis CN, Voorhees JJ. Topical retinoic acid (tretinoin) for melasma in black patients. Arch Dermatol. 1994;130(6):727–33.
3. Chan R, Park KC, Lee MH, Lee ES, Chang SE, Leow YH, Tay YK, Legarda-Montinola F, Tsai RY, Tsai TH, Shek S, Kerrouche N, Thomas G, Verallo-Rowell V. A randomized controlled trial of the efficacy and safety of a fixed triple combination (fluocinolone acetonide 0.01 %, hydroquinone 4 %, tretinoin 0.05 %) compared with hydroquinone 4 % cream in Asian patients with moderate to severe melasma. Br J Dermatol. 2008;159(3):697–703.
4. Bansal C, Naik H, Kar HK, Chauhan A. A comparison of low-fluence 1064-nm Q-switched Nd: YAG laser with topical 20 % azelaic acid cream and their combination in melasma in Indian patients. J Cutan Aesthet Surg. 2012;5(4):266–72.
5. Salem A, Gamil H, Ramadan A, Harras M, Amer A. Melasma: treatment evaluation. J Cosmet Laser Ther. 2009;11(3):146–50.
6. Farshi S. Comparative study of therapeutic effects of 20 % azelaic acid and hydroquinone 4 % cream in the treatment of melasma. J Cosmet Dermatol. 2011;10(4):282–7.
7. Lieu TJ, Pandya AG. Melasma quality of life measures. Dermatol Clin. 2012;30(2):269–80. viii.
8. Sheth VM, Pandya AG. Melasma: a comprehensive update: part II. J Am Acad Dermatol. 2011;65(4):699–714; quiz 715.
9. Estrada Castañón R, Andersson N. Community dermatology and the management of skin diseases in developing countries. Trop Doct. 1992;22 Suppl 1:3–6.
10. Rivas S, Pandya AG. Treatment of melasma with topical agents, peels and lasers: an evidence-based review. Am J Clin Dermatol. 2013;14(5):359–76.

Ashy Dermatosis (Erythema Dyschromicum Perstans)

7

Alfred Wang and Amit G. Pandya

Contents

7.1 Introduction

Ashy dermatosis, also known as erythema dyschromicum perstans (EDP), is a rare dermatosis that was first described in El Salvador by Ramirez in 1957 [1]. It typically presents as asymptomatic, chronic, slowly progressive ashy-gray hyperpigmented macules on the trunk and proximal extremities.

7.1.1 Epidemiology

EDP affects males and females equally in a wide range of age groups and has been reported around the world. Adult EDP more commonly occurs in the second and third decades of life, especially in dark-skinned individuals with a Hispanic background, whereas prepubertal EDP occurs more often in Caucasians [2].

7.1.2 Etiology

There is no clearly defined etiology for ashy dermatosis; however, there have been reports of association with intravenous X-ray contrast media, exposure to pesticides, and whipworm infection in HIV patients. Oral ingestion of ammonium nitrate, ethambutol, penicillins, and benzodiazepines and contact with chlorothalonil, a fungicide, have also been associated with EDP [3, 4]. One possible pathomechanism is an abnormal immune response to MHC class II molecules (HLA-DR) and intercellular adhesion molecules; however, further research into this potential etiology is needed [5].

A. Wang, BS • A.G. Pandya, MD (✉)
Department of Dermatology,
University of Texas Southwestern Medical Center,
5323 Harry Hines Boulevard, Dallas, TX 75390, USA
e-mail: ryan.thorpe@utsouthwestern.edu;
amit.pandya@utsouthwestern.edu

D. Jackson-Richards, A.G. Pandya (eds.), *Dermatology Atlas for Skin of Color*,
DOI 10.1007/978-3-642-54446-0_7, © Springer-Verlag Berlin Heidelberg 2014

7.2 Clinical Features

7.2.1 Distribution and Arrangement

EDP can present as blue-gray macules with an active erythematous border, most commonly located on the trunk and proximal extremities and less commonly on the neck and face. Over time, the patches progressively increase in number and lose their active borders, presenting as symmetrically distributed ashy-gray to blue-brown patches with ill-defined borders (Figs. 7.1, 7.2, 7.3, 7.4, and 7.5). The patches often present as circular, oval, or polycyclic lesions that spare the palms, soles, scalp, nails, and mucous membranes. EDP is occasionally pruritic but is usually asymptomatic [1, 4, 6, 7] (Figs. 7.6, 7.7, 7.8, and 7.9).

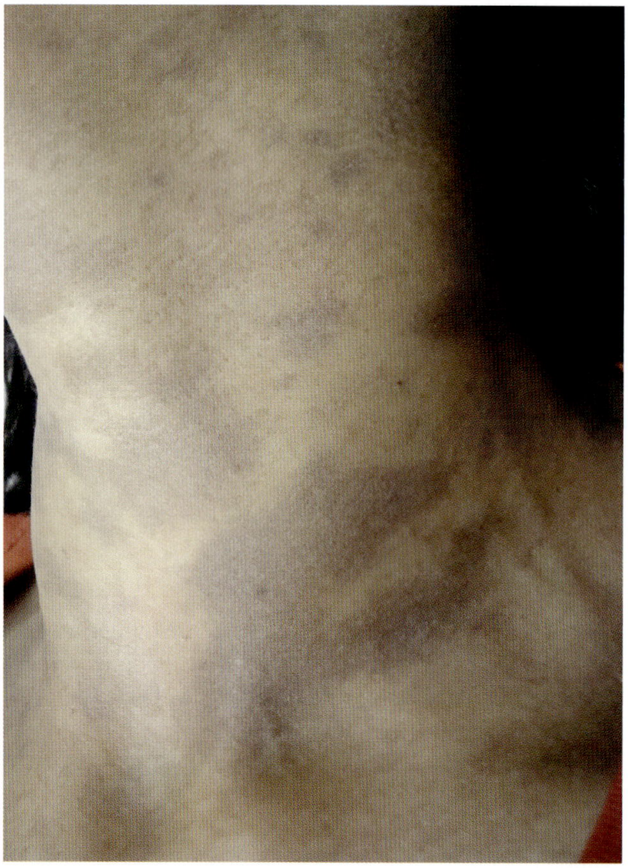

Fig. 7.1 Erythema dyschromicum perstans on the neck of a South Asian female

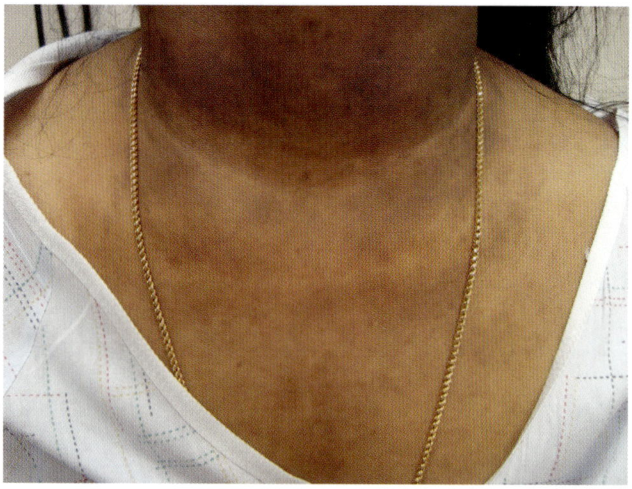

Fig. 7.2 Erythema dyschromicum perstans on the neck and chest of a South Asian female

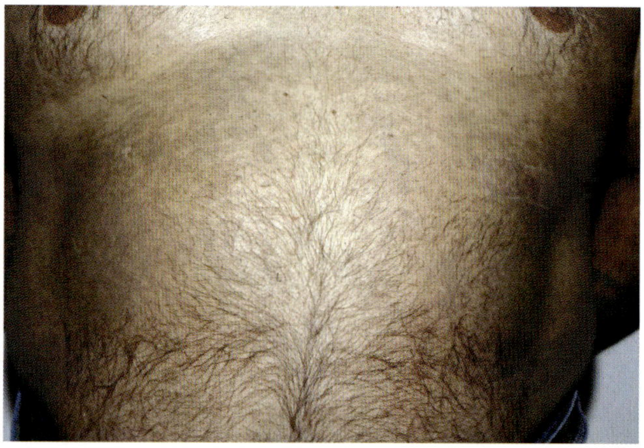

Fig. 7.3 Erythema dyschromicum perstans on the abdomen of a Hispanic male

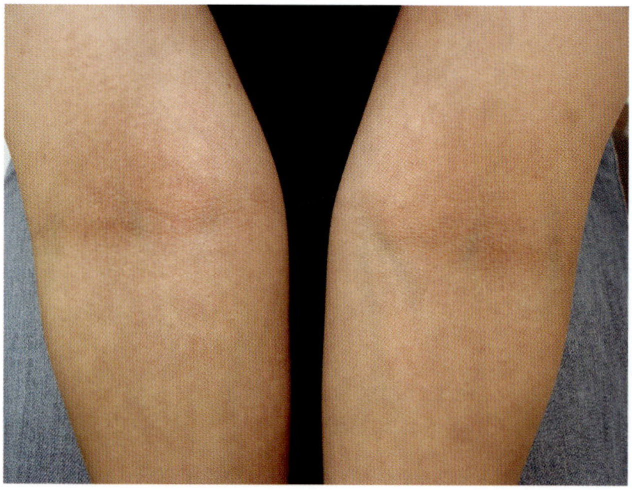

Fig. 7.4 Mild erythema dyschromicum perstans on the arms of a South Asian female

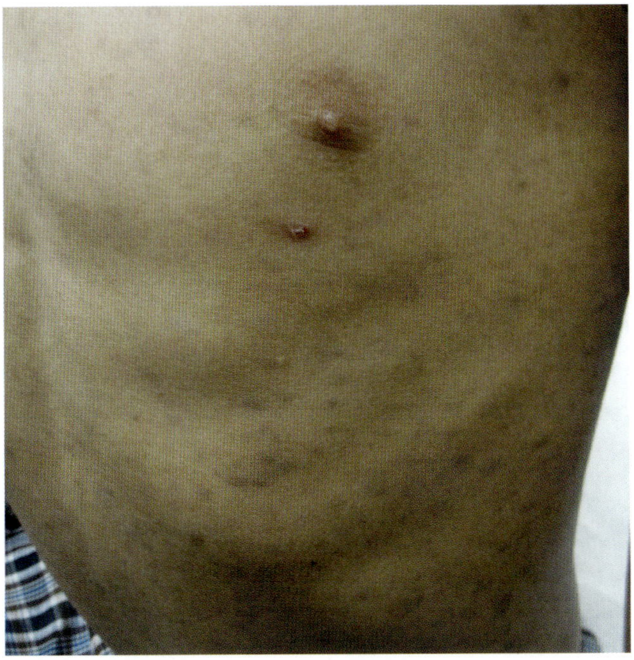

Fig. 7.5 Erythema dyschromicum perstans on the trunk of a Hispanic boy (Courtesy Dr. Nnenna Agim)

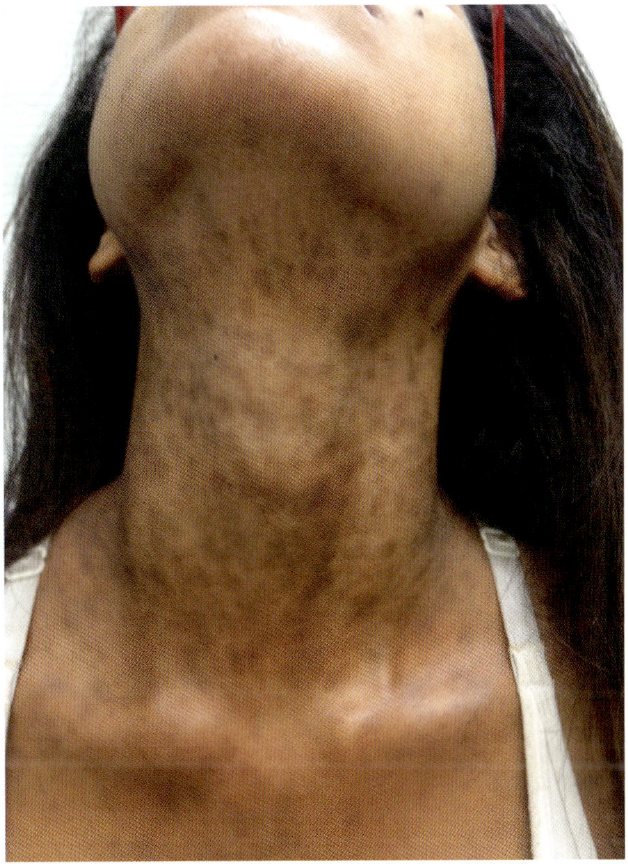

Fig. 7.7 Erythema dyschromicum perstans on the neck of a Hispanic female (Courtesy Dr. Lu Le)

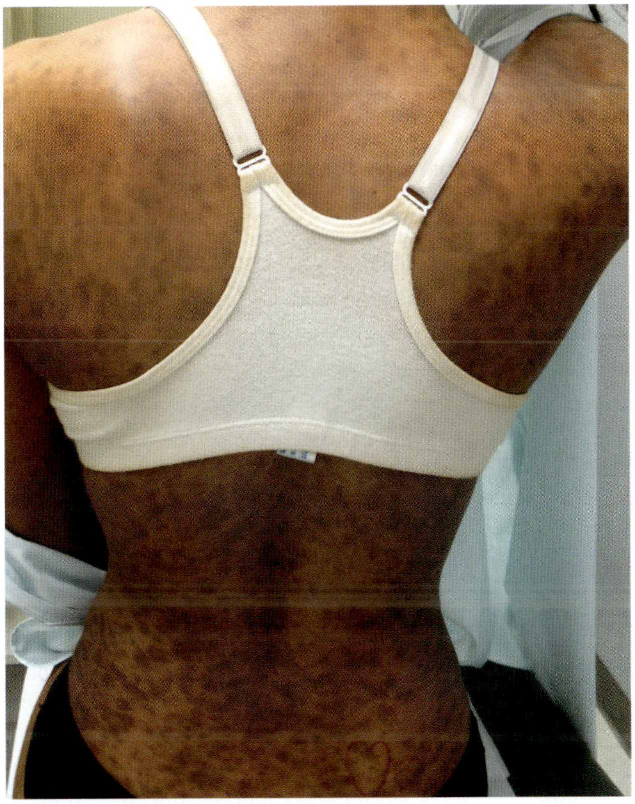

Fig. 7.6 Erythema dyschromicum perstans on the trunk of a Hispanic female (Courtesy Dr. Lu Le)

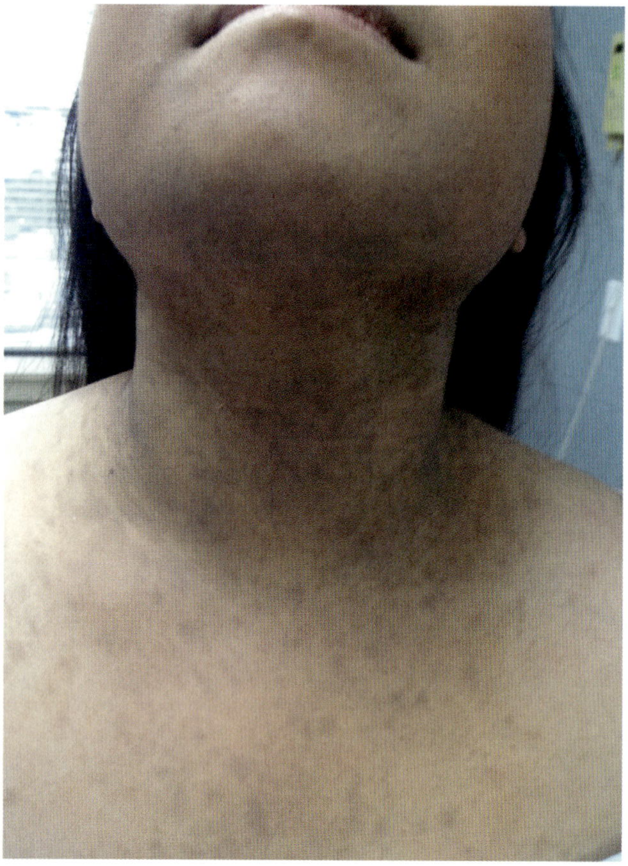

Fig. 7.8 Erythema dyschromicum perstans on the neck and chest of an Asian female (Courtesy Dr. Lu Le)

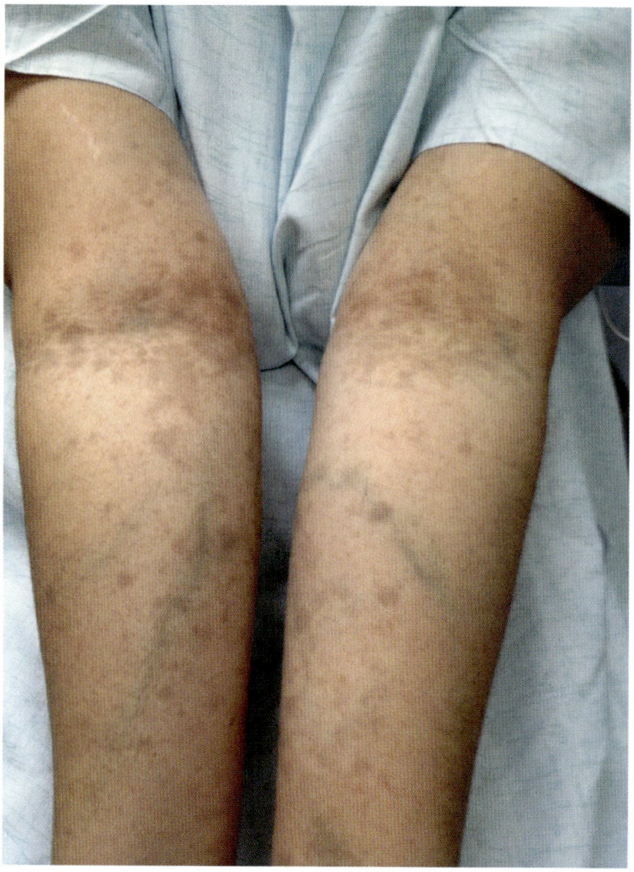

Fig. 7.9 Erythema dyschromicum perstans on the arms of an Asian female (Courtesy Dr. Lu Le)

7.3 Natural History and Prognosis

EDP is a chronic disorder with insidious onset. Often it starts as small pigmented macules with a diameter of a few millimeters, gradually increasing in number and size over a period of a few weeks extending peripherally to form converging patches. In children, these hyperpigmented patches are more likely to resolve over time compared to their adult counterparts [7].

7.4 Histopathological Features

The most common histopathological features of active EDP lesions are a noticeable mononuclear cellular infiltrate and melanophages in the upper dermis, basal layer vacuolization, necrotic keratinocytes in the basal layer, edema of dermal papillae, pigment incontinence, and a dermal perivascular lymphocytic infiltrate. Chronic lesions that have lost their erythematous border have more pronounced pigment incontinence, more melanophages, and a variable amount of cellular infiltrate and vacuolization of the basal cell layer [6, 8].

7.5 Diagnosis and Differential Diagnosis

A detailed history and physical exam is crucial for the diagnosis of EDP as it is often a diagnosis of exclusion. A characteristic pattern and timeline of lesions as well as typical lesions in an asymptomatic patient combined with a lack of clear cause points to a diagnosis of EDP. A biopsy should be done to confirm the diagnosis. Although the histopathology of EDP is not pathognomonic, it helps differentiate EDP from other similar skin dermatoses.

The most frequent disorder which can be confused with EDP is lichen planus pigmentosus (LPP), which can also mimic EDP histologically. However, LPP presents as brownish-black macules or patches without active borders in flexural folds and exposed skin, whereas EDP has erythematous borders in early lesions and prefers sun-protected areas [4].

EDP can also resemble a lichenoid drug eruption, late pinta, Addison's disease, melasma, confluent and reticulate papillomatosis, hemochromatosis, and macular amyloidosis, all of which have characteristic findings distinguishing them from EDP [4, 6, 9].

7.6 Treatment

There is no established therapy for EDP. Many treatments have been attempted, including hydroquinone, topical steroids, antibiotics, griseofulvin, and tretinoin; however, few have been effective. The use of lasers has also been suggested but not proven [4, 6, 9].

Clofazimine and dapsone may have a beneficial effect on EDP. Clofazimine's clinical efficacy may be attributed to its tendency to pigment the skin overall, thus obscuring the lesions of EDP. It may also work through its anti-inflammatory actions, which have been reported to cause a noticeable decline in the expression of an inflammatory adhesion antigen and major histocompatibility complex class II molecules (HLA-DR) [4]. Dapsone's efficacy may be due to its ability to suppress neutrophilic and lymphocytic inflammation and regulate immune responses, although its efficacy is still disputed [4, 6].

References

1. Ramirez CO. Los cenicientos: problema clinico. In: Proceedings of the First Central American Congress of Dermatology, San Salvador, December 5–8. 1957;122–30.
2. Silverberg NB, Herz J, et al. Erythema dyschromicum perstans in prepubertal children. Pediatr Dermatol. 2003;20:398–402.
3. Tlougan BE, Gonzalez ME, et al. Erythema dyschromicum perstans. Dermatol Online J. 2010;16(11):17.
4. Schwartz RA. Erythema dyschromicum perstans: the continuing enigma of Cinderella or ashy dermatosis. Int J Dermatol. 2004;43:230–2.
5. Baranda L, Torres-Alvarez B, et al. Involvement of cell adhesion and activation molecules in the pathogenesis of erythema dyschromicum perstans (ashy dermatitis): the effect of clofazimine therapy. Arch Dermatol. 1997;133:325–9.
6. Bahadir S, Cobanoglu U, et al. Erythema dyschromicum perstans: response to dapsone therapy. Int J Dermatol. 2004;43:220–2.
7. Torrelo A, Zaballos P, et al. Erythema dyschromicum perstans in children: a report of 14 cases. J Eur Acad Dermatol Venereol. 2005;19(4):422–6.
8. Vasquez-Ochoa LA, Isaza-Guzman DM, et al. Immunopathologic study of erythema dyschromicum perstans (ashy dermatosis). Int J Dermatol. 2006;45:937–41.
9. Pandya AG, Guevara I. Disorders of hyperpigmentation. Dermatol Clin. 2000;18(1):91–8.

Drug-Induced Pigmentary Changes

8

Lauren A. Baker and Amit G. Pandya

Contents

8.1 Introduction

Exposure to a variety of pharmacologic agents can result in pigmentary changes involving the skin, nails, hair, and mucous membranes. Although typically benign, the hyperpigmentation, hypopigmentation, or dyspigmentation that results can have a profound psychological impact on those affected, particularly in individuals with darker skin [1].

8.1.1 Epidemiology

The incidence of drug-induced pigmentation is dependent on the inciting agent. It is estimated that medications account for 10–20 % of all cases of acquired hyperpigmentation. While these changes may occur in individuals of any ethnic background, hypomelanosis and hyperpigmentation are seen more commonly in those with darker skin [1]. There are no reported differences in the prevalence of drug-induced dyschromia between males and females, and it occurs in persons of all ages.

8.1.2 Etiology

The main causes of drug-induced dyschromia are cytotoxic drugs, antimalarials, amiodarone, tetracyclines, psychotropic drugs, nonsteroidal anti-inflammatory drugs, and heavy metals [2].

L.A. Baker, BS • A.G. Pandya, MD (✉)
Department of Dermatology,
University of Texas Southwestern Medical Center,
5323 Harry Hines Boulevard, Dallas, TX 75390, USA
e-mail: lauren.banker@utsouthwestern.edu;
amit.pandya@utsouthwester.edu

D. Jackson-Richards, A.G. Pandya (eds.), *Dermatology Atlas for Skin of Color*,
DOI 10.1007/978-3-642-54446-0_8, © Springer-Verlag Berlin Heidelberg (outside the USA) 2014

Several mechanisms are responsible for the pathogenesis of drug-induced pigmentation, and these vary depending on the offending agent. Often, the cause of drug-induced dyschromia is the accumulation of melanin after nonspecific cutaneous inflammation, with or without an accompanying increase in melanocytes. Other mechanisms include drug or drug metabolite deposition in the epidermis and dermis, drug-induced synthesis of special pigments, and iron deposits following damage to vessels in the dermis [2]. Sun exposure is often an exacerbating factor in drug-induced pigmentation via the stimulation of melanin production or transformation of the offending drug into more visible particles [2].

8.2 Clinical Features

8.2.1 Distribution and Arrangement

Each offending drug typically induces pigmentation in a characteristic distribution and arrangement:

1. NSAIDs typically cause dyspigmentation on the extremities, trunk, and mucous membranes that may or may not be exacerbated by sun exposure (Figs. 8.1 and 8.2) [2].
2. The lesions caused by antimalarials initially appear as oval macules that progressively coalesce into large patches, with pigmentation of the nails; lower extremities, particularly the pre-tibial areas; and head, and, rarely, the mucous membranes.
3. Drugs such as amiodarone, daunorubicin, gold, methotrexate, psoralens, and 5-fluorouracil tend to result in a patchy dyspigmentation in sun-exposed areas such as the face, neck, chest, upper back, and distal extremities.
4. Amiodarone tends to cause a blue-gray or purple coloration of sun-exposed skin.
5. Zidovudine may cause a diffuse blue pigmentation of the nail with transverse or longitudinal banding that begins in the proximal nail bed.
6. Four patterns of minocycline-induced dyspigmentation exist: (1) blue-black macules localized to scars and postinflammatory sites; (2) blue-gray macules on the lower extremities, particularly the anterior shins; (3) a generalized brown hyperpigmentation most prominent on sun-exposed areas; and (4) hyperpigmentation of the vermilion border of the lower lip [2].
7. While tetracycline-induced pigmentation is also seen in sun-exposed areas, it is also found in acne scars, sites of previous inflammation, mucous membranes, and internal organs.
8. Chemotherapeutic agents cause pigmentation that is photosensitive and may be generalized or diffuse and may include the hair, nails, and mucous membranes:
   (a) Nail changes caused by cyclophosphamide, cisplatin, doxorubicin, idarubicin, fluorouracil, bleomycin, docetaxel, dacarbazine, and hydroxyurea manifest as transverse or longitudinal pigmented bands or diffuse pigmentation (Fig. 8.3).
   (b) Bleomycin characteristically results in a specific flagellated pigmentation (Fig. 8.4).
   (c) Imatinib, a tyrosine kinase inhibitor, may cause reversible, dose-related, generalized or localized hypopigmentation and, rarely, hyperpigmentation. In addition to causing repigmentation of gray hair, imatinib has recently been reported to result in the development of gray hair in an African-American patient [3].
9. Dyschromia induced by psychotropic drugs typically occurs on sun-exposed areas, sparing the mucous membranes, and may involve the nail beds. In particular, chlorpromazine and tricyclic antidepressants cause a violet, metallic discoloration and a blue-gray slate pigmentation on sun-exposed areas, respectively.
10. Gold salts result in a blue-gray color change on sun-exposed areas that spares the mucous membranes and is most prominent in the periorbital region.
11. If absorbed systemically, silver, commonly used in the treatment of extensive burns, causes diffuse slate-gray pigmentation of the skin, with sparing of the skin folds, as well as the nails and mucous membranes [2].
12. Topical and injected corticosteroids may cause depigmentation of treated skin (Fig. 8.5).
13. Miscellaneous drugs can cause pigmentation in both sun-exposed and sun-protected locations (Fig. 8.6).
14. Fixed drug eruptions may occur from a variety of medications, leaving hyperpigmentation which may last for months (Figs. 8.7 and 8.8).

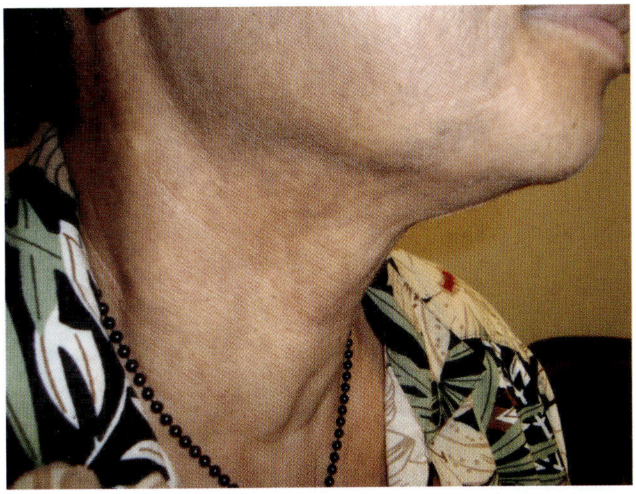

Fig. 8.1 Hyperpigmentation due to etodolac in an African-American female

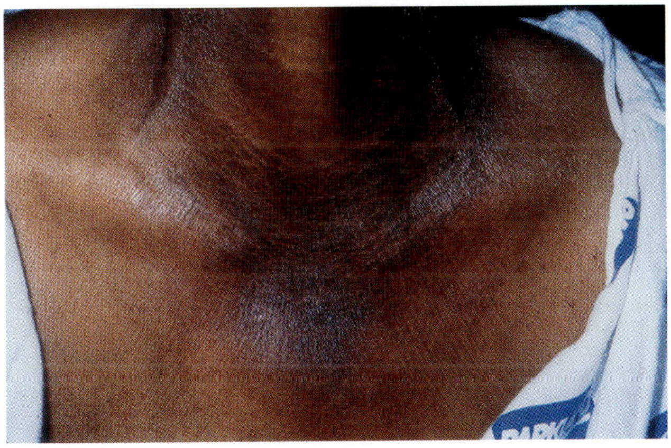

Fig. 8.2 Hyperpigmentation in sun-exposed skin due to piroxicam in an African-American female

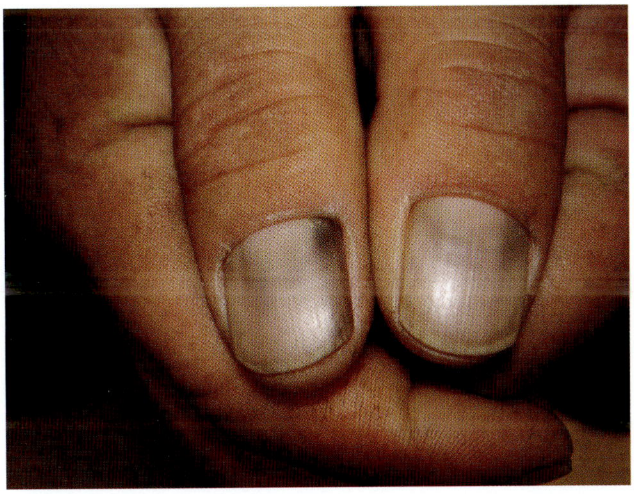

Fig. 8.3 Hyperpigmentation of the nails due to cyclophosphamide in a Hispanic male

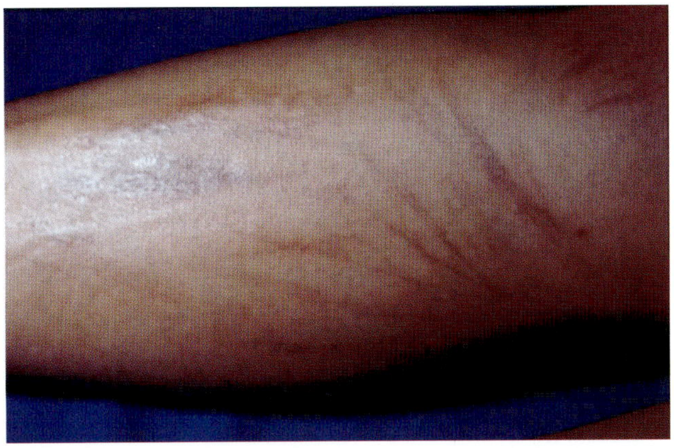

Fig. 8.4 Flagellate hyperpigmentation of the leg due to bleomycin in an African-American female

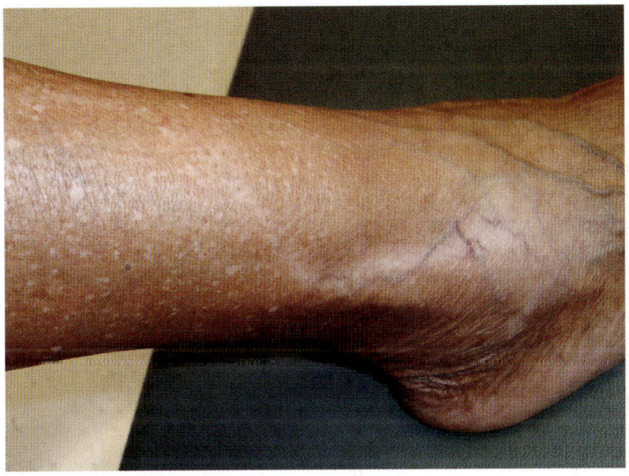

Fig. 8.5 Depigmentation of the foot and ankle after joint injection with steroid in an African-American female. The patient also has telangiectasias due to skin atrophy and migration of depigmentation along lymphatics. Incidental lesions of idiopathic guttate hypomelanosis on calf

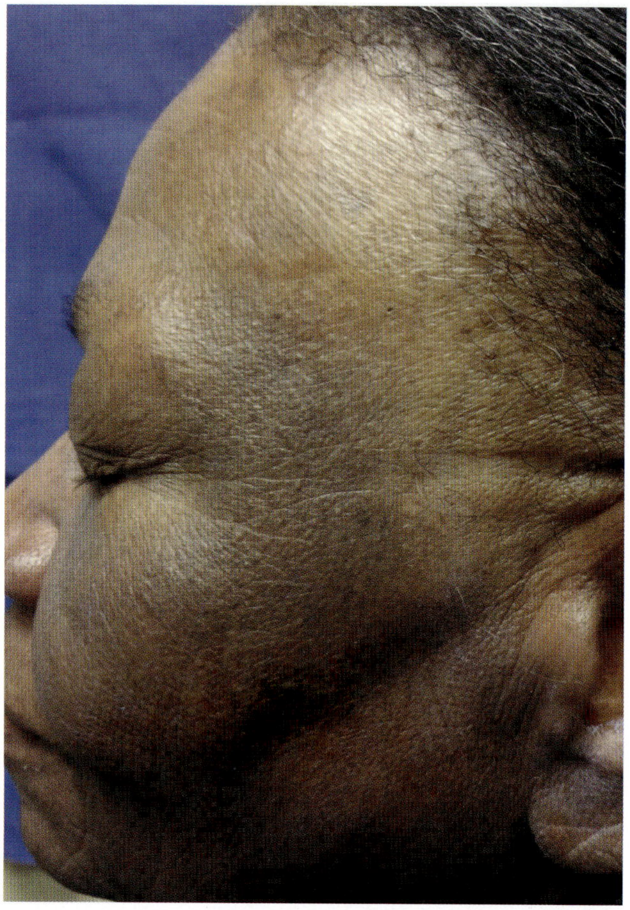

Fig. 8.6 Hyperpigmentation due to diltiazem in an African-American female

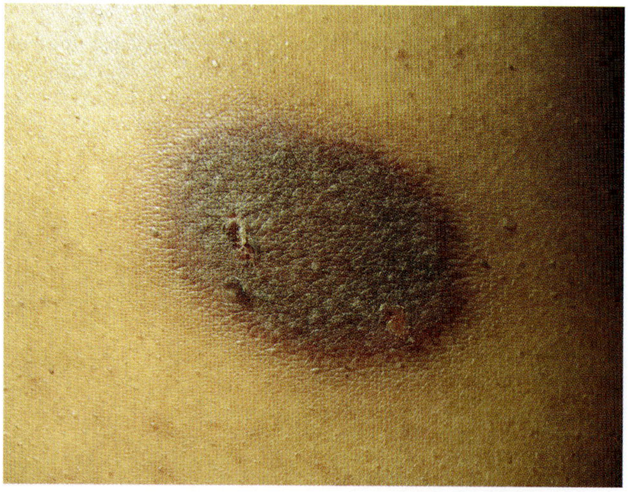

Fig. 8.7 Hyperpigmentation due to fixed drug eruption from ibuprofen in an African-American male (Courtesy Dr. Henry Lim)

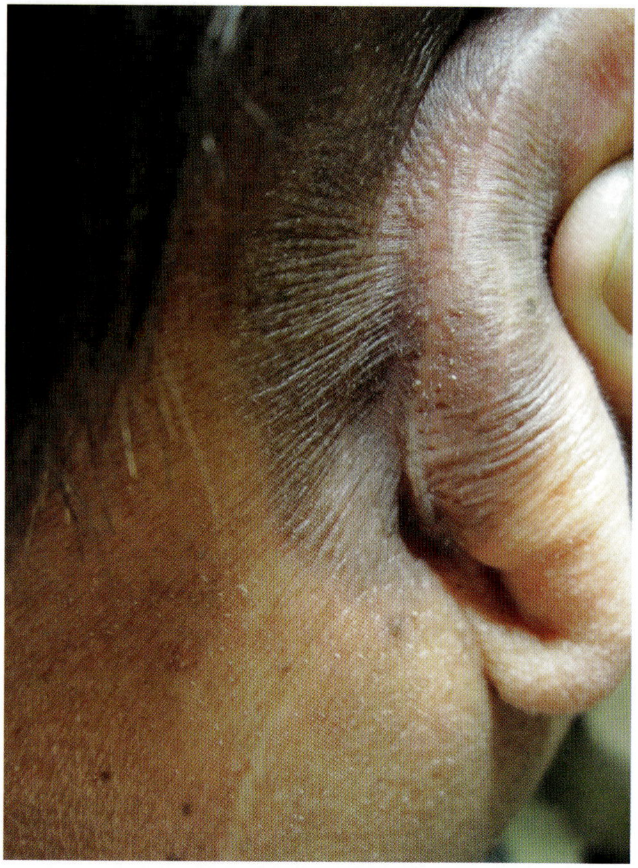

Fig. 8.8 Hyperpigmentation due to fixed drug eruption from antimalarial in an African-American female (Courtesy Dr. Henry Lim)

8.3 Natural History and Prognosis

Drug-induced pigmentation usually has an insidious onset with progressive worsening over months or years following treatment initiation. While the skin changes typically fade once use of the offending drug has been discontinued, recovery back to a normal appearance of the skin is slow and, at many times, incomplete [2].

8.4 Histopathological Features

In the majority of acquired pigmentation disorders, histological examination reveals an increase in melanin. Contingent on the offending drug, the histological findings may also show characteristic patterns of melanin accumulation, distinctive collections of pigment-laden macrophages in the dermis and neighboring vessels and glands, or the presence of metal deposition or unusual pigments within the dermis [2].

8.5 Diagnosis and Differential Diagnosis

Individuals presenting with acquired pigmentation should raise suspicion for a drug-related etiology, especially when the lesions are observed in sun-exposed skin and/or exhibit atypical shades such as blue, gray, and purple. A patient history should reveal intake of a drug known to cause skin changes with the onset of pigmentation coinciding with its use. In addition, a physical exam demonstrating characteristic distributions, patterns, and/or dyschromias and the lack of an alternative interpretation of the findings point to a diagnosis of drug-induced pigmentation. Moreover, histological examination may reveal characteristic findings consistent with certain drugs, particularly in the case of heavy-metal dyschromia. However, only improvement of the pigmentation once the suspected drug has been discontinued will confirm the diagnosis. A definitive diagnosis may prove daunting as the pigmentation may persist after treatment termination or cessation of treatment may not be an option [2].

Several conditions can mimic drug-induced pigmentation, the majority being endocrine or metabolic in origin. The cutaneous changes of Addison's disease manifest as a diffuse, gray pigmentation of the skin, mucosa, skin folds, and scar tissue. However, patients with this condition have associated electrolyte abnormalities such as hyponatremia and hyperkalemia as well as low serum cortisol levels and an inappropriate response to a corticotrophin stimulation test. Individuals afflicted with hemochromatosis or Wilson's disease may have a generalized, blue-gray, metallic pigmentation, typically with an accompanying positive family history and abnormal iron (elevated ferritin and trans-ferritin saturation levels) or copper (low serum copper or low ceruloplasmin) studies, respectively. Vitamin deficiencies such as in nicotinic acid, a condition known as pellagra, and vitamin B12 may generate pigmentation aggravated by sun exposure [2]. Acanthosis nigricans, a marker of insulin resistance, appears as dark velvety patches and plaques in intertriginous areas and the neck and may be misdiagnosed as hyperpigmentation. Melasma, an acquired hypermelanosis of sun-exposed areas, presents as hyperpigmented macules, particularly on the face in women with darker skin [2].

8.6 Treatment

The most important element in the treatment of drug-induced pigmentation is the identification and discontinuation of the offending drug. However, this may not be an option as many of these medications are part of a life-saving regimen, and the pigmentation may be permanent or may not resolve completely. Since the majority of drug-induced dyschromia is photosensitive, avoidance of sun exposure, wearing protective clothing, and the diligent application of sunscreen may aid in avoiding or ameliorating skin changes. This is especially applicable to individuals of color, as having naturally pigmented skin increases the risk of generating a melanin-mediated pigmentation [2]. The utilization of depigmenting agents, such as hydroquinone, has not proven to be very efficacious due to the typical deposition of the pigment in the dermis [4]. Recent case reports have demonstrated that oral isotretinoin resulted in a dramatic improvement in minocycline-induced hyperpigmentation in persons of color [5]. Also, the use of vitamin C may prove beneficial as a prophylactic measure against dyspigmentation [5]. Pigmentation induced by certain drugs, such as minocycline and amiodarone, has shown promising results when treated with short-pulsed, pigment-specific Q-switched lasers [4]. In general, these lasers are the best types of lasers to treat patients with skin of color [6].

References

1. Halder RM, Nandedkar MA, Neal KW. Pigmentary disorders in ethnic skin. Dermatol Clin. 2003;21(4):617–28.
2. Dereure O. Drug-induced skin pigmentation: epidemiology, diagnosis, and treatment. Am J Clin Dermatol. 2001;2(4):253–62.
3. Balagula Y, Pulitzer MP, Maki RG, Myskowski PL. Pigmentary changes in a patient treated with imatinib. J Drugs Dermatol. 2011; 10(9):1062–6.
4. Stratigos AJ, Katsambas AD. Optimal management of recalcitrant disorders of hyperpigmentation in dark-skinned patients. Am J Clin Dermatol. 2004;5(3):161–8.
5. Soung J, Cohen J, Phelps R, Cohen SR. Minocycline-induced hyperpigmentation resolves during oral isotretinoin therapy. J Drugs Dermatol. 2007;6(12):1232–6.
6. Hobbs L. The use of lasers for treatment of skin of color patients. In: Kelly AP, Taylor SC, editors. Dermatology for skin of color. New York: McGraw Hill; 2009. p. 555–70.

9 Confluent and Reticulated Papillomatosis

Diane Jackson-Richards

Contents

9.1 Epidemiology and Etiology

Gougerot and Carteaud described confluent and reticulated papillomatosis (CRP) in 1927. The onset of CRP is soon after puberty with the average age of those affected being 18–25. Females are affected almost twice as often as males. Although studies and unofficial reports suggest it is twice as common in darker-skinned persons, other studies have found no racial predilection.

The etiology of CRP is unknown, but theories include a defect of keratinization, *Pityrosporum* colonization, or bacterial infection by the *Dietzia* strain of actinomycete [1]. The evidence is most compelling for this being a disorder of keratinization, supported by the finding of increased transition cell layer and increased lamellar granules in the stratum granulosum. CRP has been reported to respond to treatment with topical and oral retinoids as well as vitamin D derivatives, further supporting the keratinization disorder hypothesis [2]. However, this would not explain the fact that various antibiotics, most notably minocycline, have been found to be the best treatment for CRP. Although *Pityrosporum* has been implicated in the pathogenesis of CRP, potassium hydroxide preparations and PAS stains on biopsies have not consistently supported this hypothesis [3]. The yeast may be a coincidental finding, or perhaps cases of tinea versicolor are being confused with CRP. Although there are reports of topical antifungals being used successfully for CRP, there are an equal number reporting the ineffectiveness of antifungals. Natarajan et al. isolated the *Dietzia* bacteria in a patient with CRP that was successfully treated with minocycline, however, CRP recurred after minocycline was discontinued and the *Dietzia* organism could not be re-isolated [1, 2]. Again, the exact etiology of CRP is unknown and remains controversial.

D. Jackson-Richards, MD
Department of Dermatology, Multicultural Dermatology Center,
Henry Ford Hospital, 3031 West Grand Blvd.,
Detroit, MI 48202, USA
e-mail: djackso1@hfhs.org

D. Jackson-Richards, A.G. Pandya (eds.), *Dermatology Atlas for Skin of Color*,
DOI 10.1007/978-3-642-54446-0_9, © Springer-Verlag Berlin Heidelberg 2014

9.2 Clinical Features

CRP presents as 1–2 mm hyperkeratotic, hyperpigmented papules that coalesce into confluent thin plaques with a reticular pattern at the periphery of the plaques. Classic locations are the inframammary or epigastric skin as well as the sternal and interscapular skin (Figs. 9.1 and 9.2). Other areas which may be involved include the upper back and nape of the neck. Although much less common, lesions in the pubic area have been reported. Increased skin line markings can be seen within plaques, giving CRP a velvety appearance similar to that of acanthosis nigricans. CRP is usually asymptomatic [2].

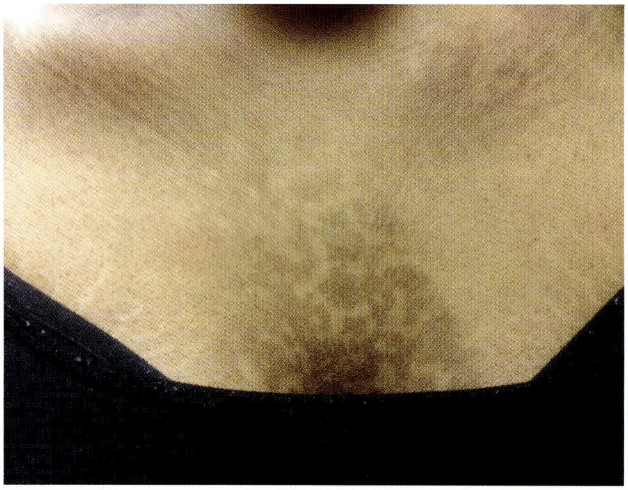

Fig. 9.1 Confluent and reticulated papillomatosis on the chest of an African-American female

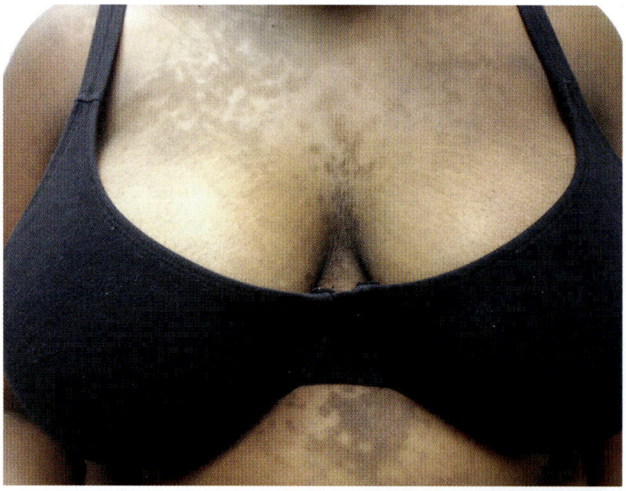

Fig. 9.2 Confluent and reticulated papillomatosis on the chest and abdomen of an African-American female

9.3 Histopathologic Features

Histopathology shows undulating hyperkeratosis and papillomatosis, with acanthotic downgrowths between the papillomatous areas [4]. Mild dilatation of superficial dermal vessels is also seen. Electron microscopy has shown increased transitional cells between the stratum granulosum and stratum corneum, hypermelanosis of the basal layer, and increased melanosomes in the horny layer.

9.4 Diagnosis and Differential Diagnosis

CRP is usually diagnosed clinically and does not require a biopsy in most cases. It is often confused with acanthosis nigricans, but this entity is not reticulate and usually involves intertriginous areas beyond the neck. The hyperpigmentation might lead one to think of tinea versicolor, but CRP has no scaling and fungal scrapings and stains are usually negative. CRP lesions in the inframammary areas might resemble Darier's disease, but unlike Darier's, involvement of the scalp, hands, feet, and intertriginous areas is not typical of CRP. The differential diagnosis also includes macular amyloidosis, but this condition is usually not reticulate and is limited to the upper back. Dermatopathia pigmentosa reticularis may resemble CRP, but it is very rare and usually has associated alopecia and nail changes.

9.5 Treatment

The most widely used treatment, oral minocycline 100 mg twice daily for 1–3 months, has been shown to provide excellent clearing of lesions (Figs. 9.3 and 9.4), but recurrences are common [3]. Azithromycin 500 mg daily, three times a week for 3 weeks, has also been used successfully. Since the exact etiology of CRP is unknown and specific pathogenic bacteria have not been universally proven, it is unclear why antibiotics are successful. Antibiotics are known to have anti-inflammatory properties and have been successfully used for this reason in many dermatologic conditions. Supporting the theory of abnormal keratinization is the fact that there are reported cases of excellent response to oral isotretinoin and etretinate. Oral retinoids have more adverse effects than topical therapies and antibiotics that must be considered. Topical tazarotene and tretinoin have reported effectiveness as well. There are few reports of positive responses to topical antifungals.

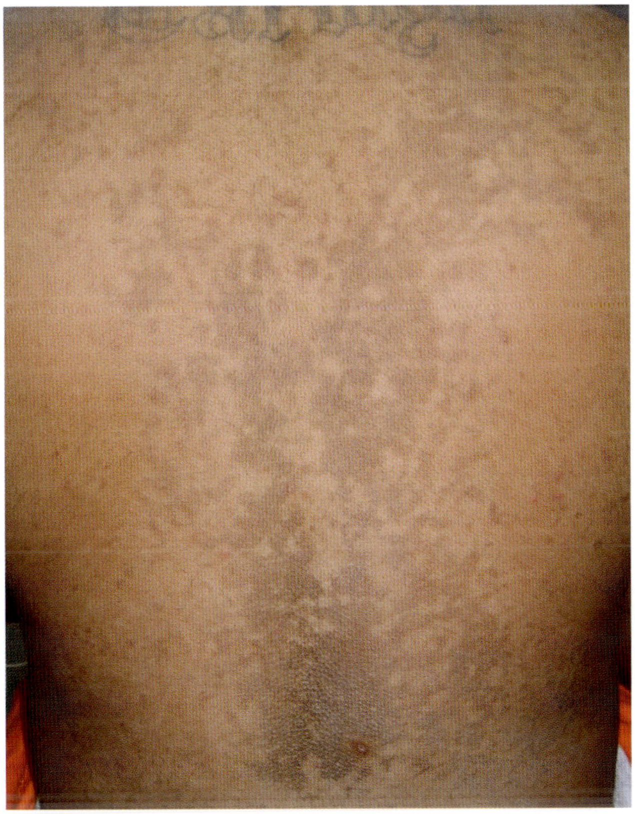

Fig. 9.3 Confluent and reticulated papillomatosis on the back of an African-American male (Courtesy Dr. Chauncey McHargue)

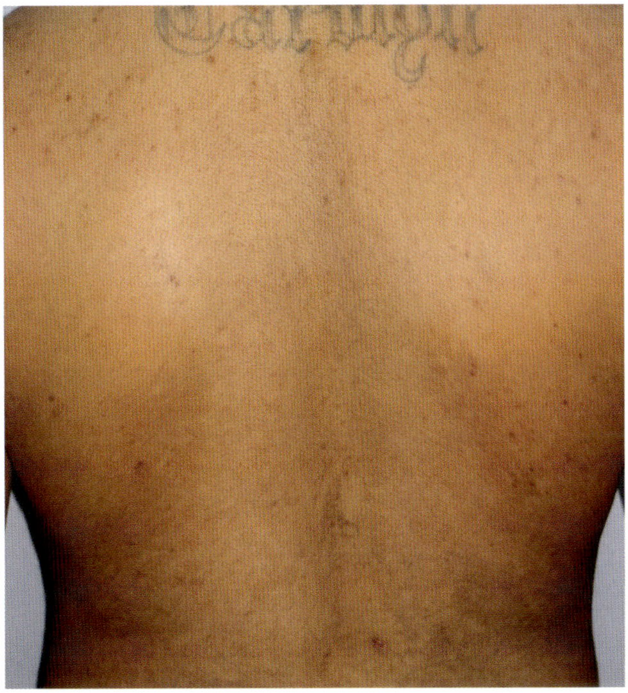

Fig. 9.4 Confluent and reticulated papillomatosis on the back of an African-American male after 1 month of minocycline 100 mg twice daily (Courtesy Dr. Chauncey McHargue)

References

1. Natarajan S, Milne D, Jones AL, et al. Dietzia strain X: a newly described Actinomycete isolated from confluent and reticulated papillomatosis. Br J Dermatol. 2005;153:825.
2. Scheinfeld N. Confluent and reticulated papillomatosis: a review of the literature. Am J Clin Dermatol. 2006;7:305–13.
3. Davis MDP, Weenig RH, Camilleri MJ. Confluent and reticulate papillomatosis: a minocycline-responsive dermatosis without evidence for yeast in pathogenesis. A study of 39 patients and a proposal of diagnostic criteria. Br J Dermatol. 2006;154:287–93.
4. Griffiths CE. Gougerot-Carteaud still an enigma after all these years. J Dermatolog Treat. 2002;13(1):27–30.

Dark Circles of the Eyes

10

Tara Rao

Contents

10.1 Introduction

Dark circles of the eyes have been noted to make people look, "tired, sad, or hungover" [1]. The Japanese word *Kuma* was coined to describe darkness of the lower eyelid and is used in daily conversation to describe a person as appearing exhausted [2]. While there is no cited estimate of the incidence or prevalence of this problem, several authors have suggested that dark circles are more pronounced in certain ethnic groups and research of the problem has focused on Indians, Koreans, and Japanese. While dark circles are commonly associated with transient episodes of fatigue, illness, or dehydration, when dark circles persist despite good health and rest, other etiologies should be considered.

T. Rao, MD
Department of Dermatology, General Dermatology Clinic,
UTSW Medical Center, 5939 Harry Hines Blvd.,
POB II, Dallas, TX 75235, USA
e-mail: tara.rao@utsouthwestern.edu

D. Jackson-Richards, A.G. Pandya (eds.), *Dermatology Atlas for Skin of Color*,
DOI 10.1007/978-3-642-54446-0_10, © Springer-Verlag Berlin Heidelberg 2014

10.2 Clinical Features

Dark circles have a range of clinical appearances but generally can be defined as bilateral and symmetric darkening of the lower and often upper eyelids. They can present as hyperpigmented, erythematous, or violaceous patches and plaques (Figs. 10.1, 10.2, 10.3, 10.4, 10.5, and 10.6).

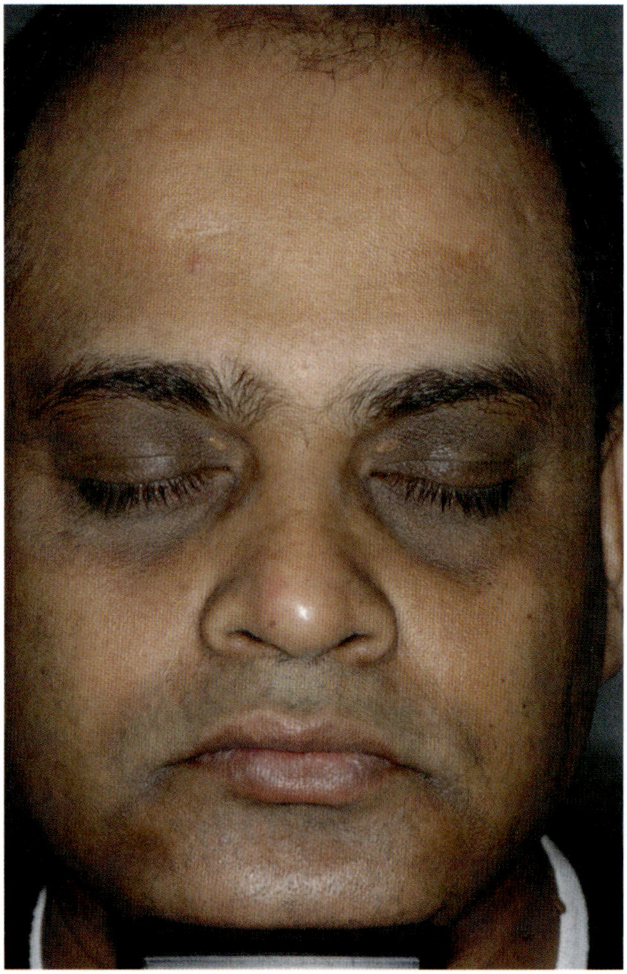

Fig. 10.1 Pakistani male with gray-brown, hyperlinear thin plaques that are confluent around the upper and lower eyelid as well as tear trough. There is some erythema at the inferior border of the dark circle

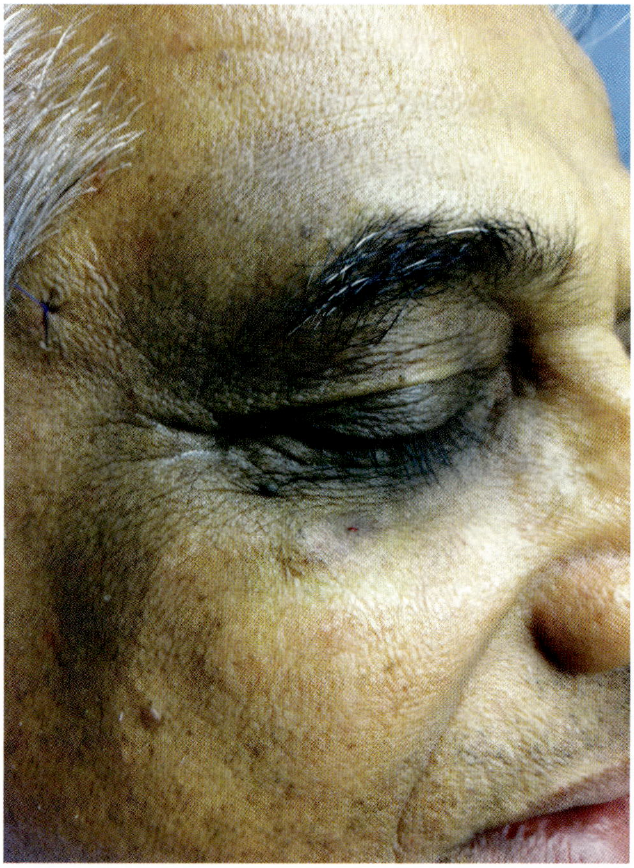

Fig. 10.2 Asian Indian male with a dark circle under eye. The upper and lower eyelids as well as the tear trough are notable for gray-black darkening. Notice confluence of eyelid darkening with a vertically oriented band of darkened skin of the temple area of the face known as a pigmentary demarcation line. The small scar is due to a recent skin biopsy

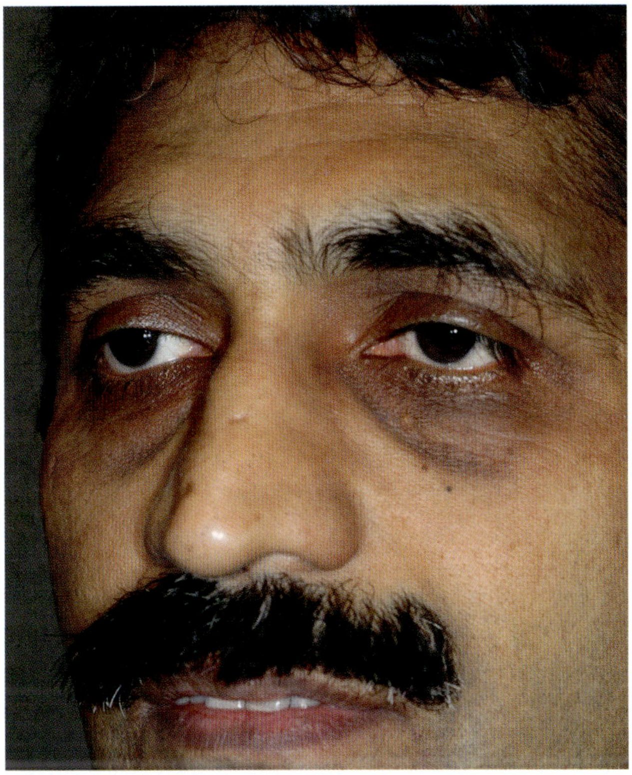

Fig. 10.3 Asian Indian male with red-brown darkening of the skin of the lower eyelid. There is some erythema of the bilateral upper eyelids as well

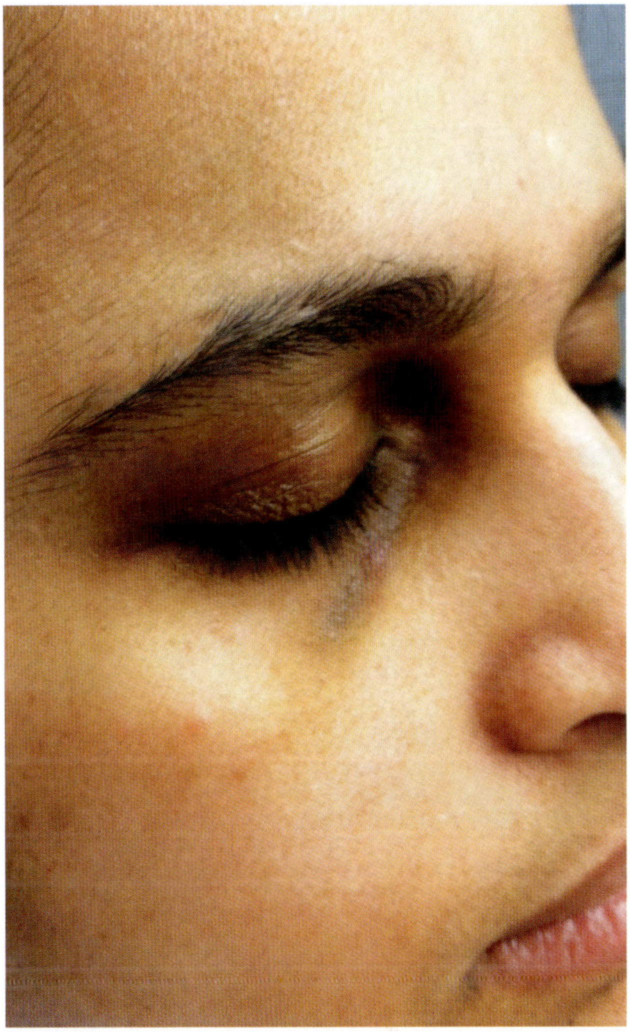

Fig. 10.4 Asian Indian female with a well-defined violaceous thin plaque below the right eye. The upper eyelid is also notable for tan to dark brown darkening of the skin

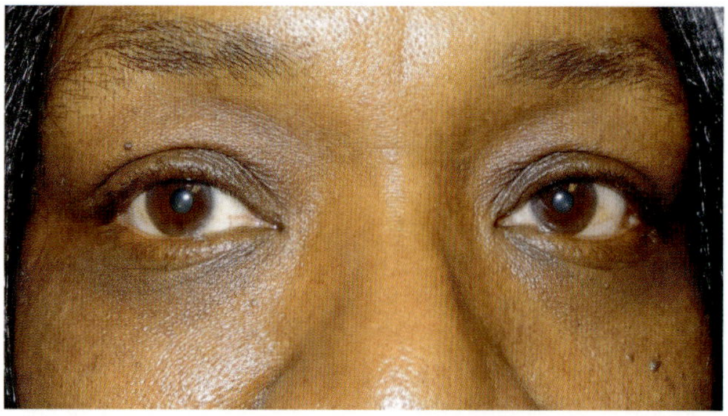

Fig. 10.5 African American female with dark macules under eyes

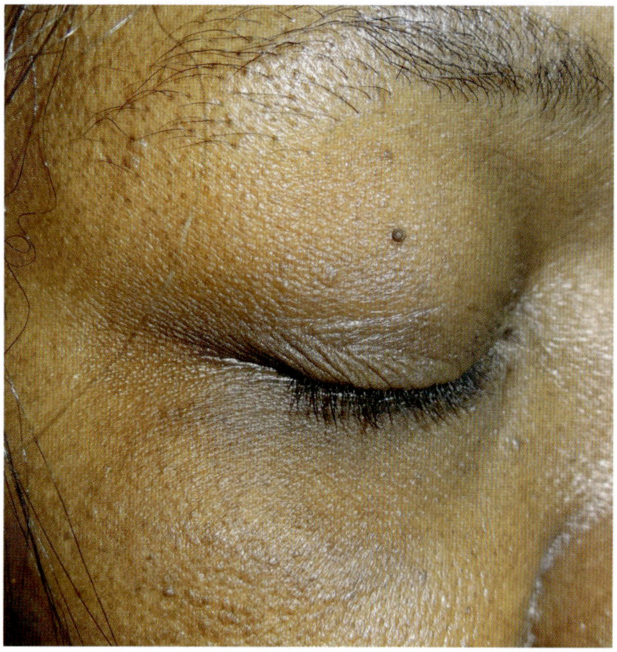

Fig. 10.6 African American female with dark macule under right eye

10.3 Natural History and Prognosis

This is a fixed problem that usually becomes worse over time. There is often a family history of the problem and sunscreen use has been found to be of limited use in a study of South Asians [3].

10.4 Histopathological Features

In South Asians, dark circles have more melanin and more melanocytes in the epidermis as compared to nearby uninvolved skin [3]. One study in Japanese patients showed evidence of dermal melanocytosis [4], while another showed epidermal and dermal melanophages [2].

10.5 Diagnosis and Differential Diagnosis

Tear trough depression, pseudoherniation of orbital fat, and translucent lower eyelid skin are nonpigmentary causes of dark circles which have been reported. Shadowing within the tear trough is also thought to contribute to dark circles. The tear trough deepens with loss of fat and cheek descent, normally occurring with age [5]. Pseudoherniation of fat occurs with weakening of the overlying septum and/or surrounding muscles [6]. Translucent skin overlying the orbicularis oculi muscle is also another cause for dark circles. Thin skin allows visibility of the subcutaneous vascular plexus or vasculature contained within the underlying muscle producing a dark, violaceous color [1]. However, dark circles in skin of color patients cannot be entirely or consistently explained by any of the nonpigmentary conditions described above.

Pigmentary causes of dark circles include postinflammatory hyperpigmentation due to atopic dermatitis and contact dermatitis, erythema dyschromicum perstans, and drug or heavy metal deposition [1, 7, 8]. Additionally, in a study of 100 Indian patients, age 11–22 years with dark circles, 92 % of patients were found to have periorbital dark circles that were continuous with the ipsilateral facial pigmentary demarcation line on the affected side of the face [9]. Chrysiasis, the deposition of gold in the skin, is the only side effect of a drug specifically associated with periorbital dark circles. This tends to occur in patients who have received gold therapy and are exposed to UV light [7].

10.6 Treatment

Without a clear understanding of the pathology of periorbital dark circles, treatment methods are likewise unsatisfactory. The range of treatments include autologous fat transplantation, CO_2 laser surgery, depigmenting creams, chemical peels, lasers, fillers, herbs, and supplements, the latter two being the most often mentioned in broad literature searches.

The first step in evaluating the etiology of the dark circles is to examine clean periorbital skin. The clinician should pay special attention to remove all traces of eye makeup. Gentle spreading or stretching of the upper and lower eye lid along with infraorbital skin helps to eliminate the shadowing effects created by the patient's anatomy. If stretching of the skin reveals prominent blood vessels, the clinician may recommend treatment with fat transplantiation or hyaluronic-acid based fillers placed inject in the area can help treat the problem.

In a study by Epstein et al., transconjunctival blepharoplasty (TCB) with a phenol peel improved dark circles, suggesting that periorbital dark circles are due to both anatomical and pigmentary abnormalities [10]. In South Asians, treatments often include bleaching creams and such home remedies as application of turmeric powder and use of neti pots. Both are cumbersome and largely ineffective treatments. However, if a clinician notes obvious hyperpigmentation when the skin is stretched, a gentle depigmenting cream may be effective.

References

1. Roh MR, Chung KY. Infraorbital dark circles: definition, causes, and treatment options. Dermatol Surg. 2009;35:1163–71.
2. Momosawa A, Kurita M, Ozaki M, Miyamoto S, Kobayashi Y, Ban I, Harii K. Combined therapy using Q-switched ruby laser and bleaching treatment with tretinoin and hydroquinone for periorbital skin hyperpigmentation in Asians. Plastic Reconst Surg. 2007;121: 282–8.
3. Rao T, Bhawan J, Polyak I, Pandya AG. Dark circles in South Asians. (Manuscript in progress).
4. Watanabe S, Nakai K, Ohnishi T. Condition known as "dark rings under the eyes" in the Japanese population is a kind of dermal melanocytosis which can be successfully treated by Q-switched ruby laser. Dermatol Surg. 2006;32:785–9.
5. Freitag F, Cestari T. What causes dark circles under the eyes? J Cosmet Dermatol. 2007;6:211–5.
6. Goldberg R, McCann J, Fiaschetti D, Ben Simon GJ. What causes eyelid bags? Analysis of 114 consecutive patients. Plast Reconstr Surg. 2005;115(5):1395–402.
7. Granstein R, Sober A. CME, drug and heavy metal induced hyperpigmentation. J Am Acad Dermatol. 1981;5:1–18.
8. Sardana K, et al. Periorbital hyperpigmentation mimicking fixed drug eruption: a rare presentation of erythema dyschromicum perstans in a paediatric patient. J Eur Acad Dermatol Venereol. 2006; 20:1328–99.
9. Malakar S, Lahiri K, Banerjee U, Mondal S, Sarangi S. Periorbital melanosis is an extension of pigmentary demarcation line-F on the face. Indian J Dermatol Venereol Leprol. 2007;73:323–5.
10. Epstein J. Management of infraorbital dark circles. Arch Facial Plast Surg. 1999;1:303–7.

Lentigines

11

Nan Guo and Amit G. Pandya

Contents

11.1 Introduction

Lentigines are common benign hyperpigmented lesions induced by chronic ultraviolet (UV) radiation exposure [1]. The prevalence varies with lesion type, patient age, and skin tone. Facial lesions are most abundant in older Caucasian and Asian females with skin types I–III, while increased melanin production in darker-toned patients inhibits sun damage and subsequent development of lentigines [2]. However, patients with skin of color develop more visually pronounced lentigines at an earlier age, as well as a greater number of acral lesions. Interestingly, UV radiation-induced dyspigmentation is the primary sign of aging in Asian skin, with wrinkling appearing 10–20 years later, unlike Caucasian skin, in which wrinkling appears much earlier [3]. African-Americans are relatively protected from solar lentigines, but they have the highest prevalence of inherited patterned lentiginosis [4].

The hyperpigmentation of lentigines is a result of UV irradiation, which increases melanocyte proliferation and melanin production. Photodamage stimulates the release of proinflammatory mediators, including tumor necrosis factor-alpha (TNF-α), interleukin-1 (IL-1), IL-6, nitric oxide, and prostaglandin E2 [5]. These mediators induce keratinocytes to increase the production of paracrine melanogenic factors, which lead neighboring melanocytes to upregulate melanin synthesis. An additional proposed mechanism is a decrease in Langerhans cells, which normally help to remove excess melanin [6]. With chronic UV radiation exposure, the distribution of melanocytes and melanin becomes more uneven across the epidermis, and areas of damage become more prominent. Interestingly, histologic reviews have found that in Caucasians, the density of activated melanocytes decreases with age in both sun-exposed and sun-protected skin [7]. However in Asians, the density of melanocytes increases with age in sun-exposed skin only, with the resulting melanin sometimes extending to the upper spinous layer [7]. These findings may help to explain why Asians develop more visually pronounced facial lentigines lesions in response to chronic photodamage.

N. Guo, BS • A.G. Pandya, MD (✉)
Department of Dermatology, University of Texas Southwestern Medical Center, 5323 Harry Hines Boulevard, Dallas, TX 75390, USA
e-mail: nan.guo@utsouthwestern.edu; amit.pandya@utsouthwestern.edu

D. Jackson-Richards, A.G. Pandya (eds.), *Dermatology Atlas for Skin of Color*,
DOI 10.1007/978-3-642-54446-0_11, © Springer-Verlag Berlin Heidelberg 2014

11.2 Clinical Features

Lentigines usually present as multiple hyperpigmented lesions on sun-exposed skin. Common sites are the face, hands, forearms, chest, back, and shins [1]. Each lesion is macular and has an irregular but well-defined border (Figs. 11.1, 11.2, 11.3, 11.4, 11.5, and 11.6). Within the same individual, lesions vary in size and color, and they are arranged in a nonuniform manner.

Though rare, lentigines can present in specific patterns that reflect underlying genetic abnormalities. For example, Peutz-Jeghers syndrome causes hamartomatous gastrointestinal polyps and an increased risk of internal malignancies, and it classically presents with small mucocutaneous lentigines on the lips, buccal mucosa, and labia [4]. LEOPARD syndrome is an autosomal dominant condition characterized by generalized lentigines sparing the mucous membranes, in addition to cardiac conduction abnormalities, ocular hypertelorism, pulmonary stenosis, genital abnormalities, growth retardation, and deafness [4]. On the other hand, inherited patterned lentiginosis of Blacks, also inherited in an autosomal dominant fashion, is not associated with systemic findings and presents exclusively in patients of African descent [4]. Noonan syndrome is an autosomal dominant disorder in which some patients have multiple lentigines scattered over the body (Fig. 11.7). Note that in these familial cases of lentigines, the lesions are likely due to inherited defects in either melanocyte hyperplasia or melanization.

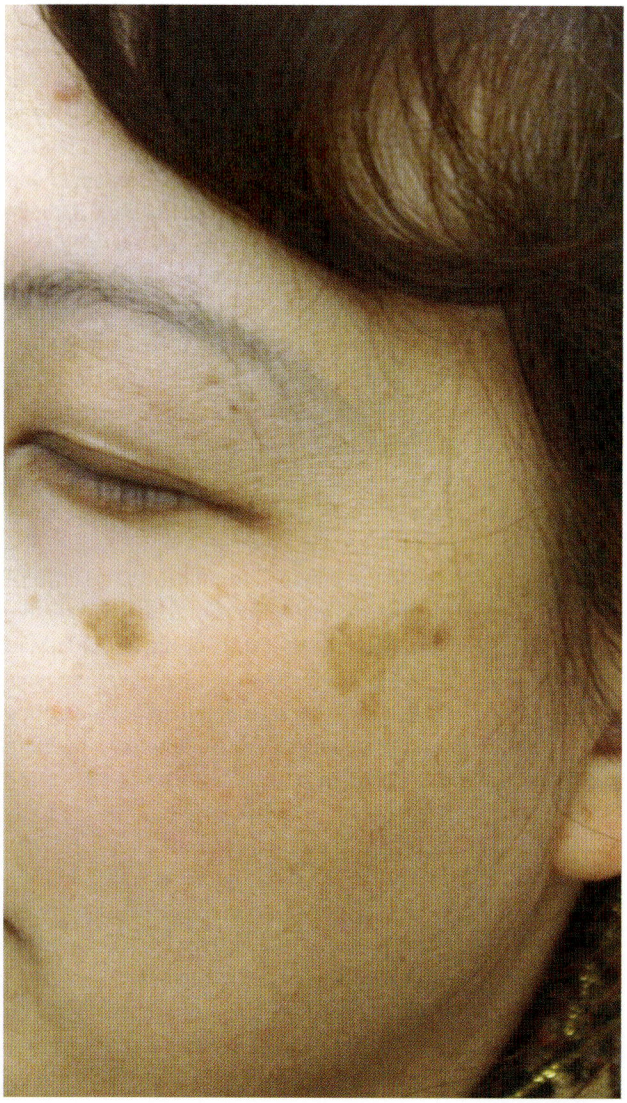

Fig. 11.1 Lentigines of the face in an Asian female

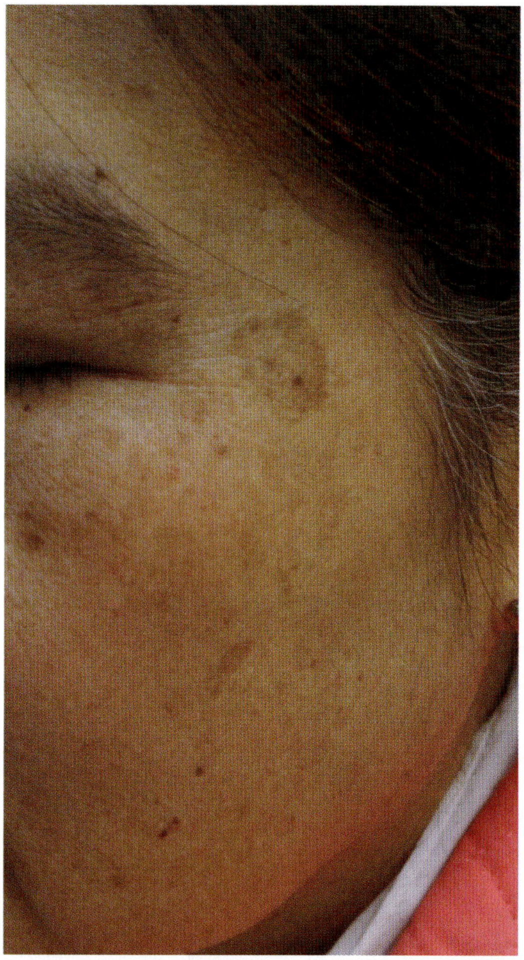

Fig. 11.2 Large lentigo on the temple of an Asian female

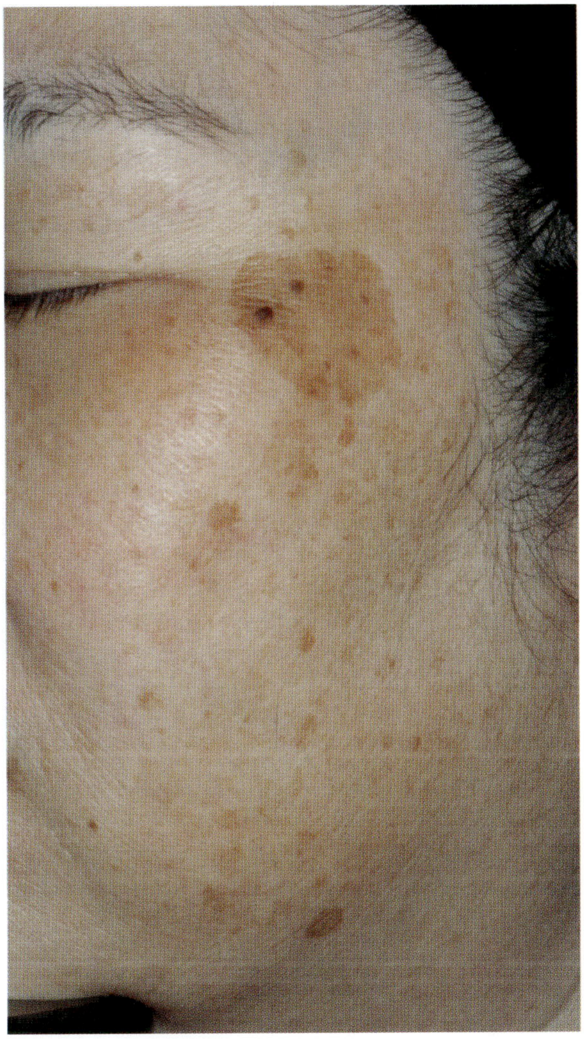

Fig. 11.3 Multiple lentigines on the left cheek of an Asian female

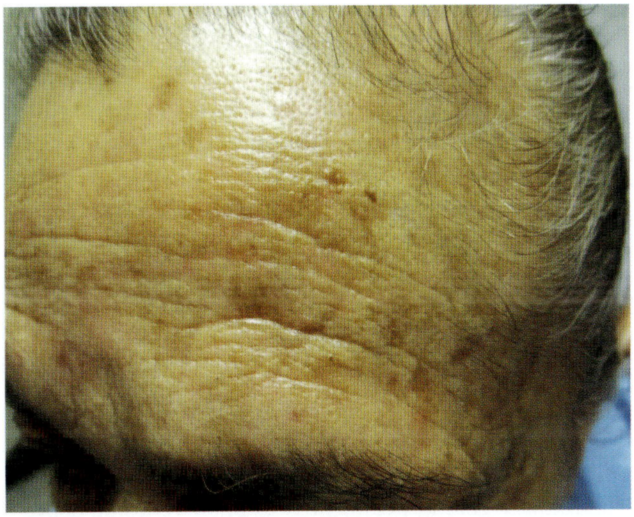

Fig. 11.4 Multiple lentigines on the forehead of a Hispanic female

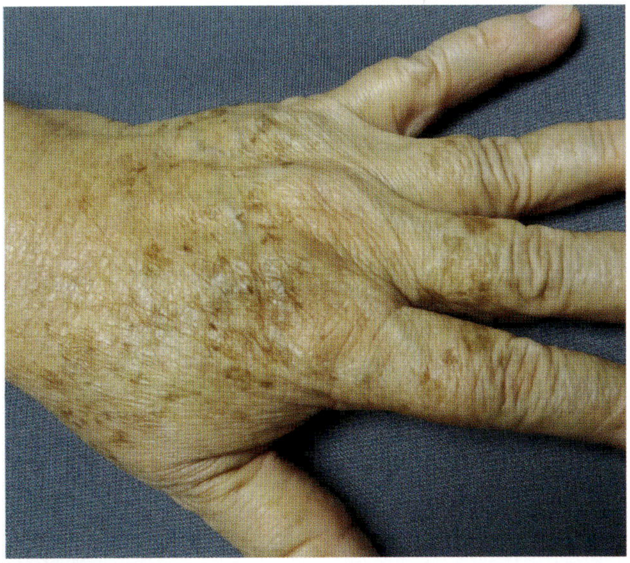

Fig. 11.5 Multiple lentigines on the dorsal hand and fingers of a Hispanic female

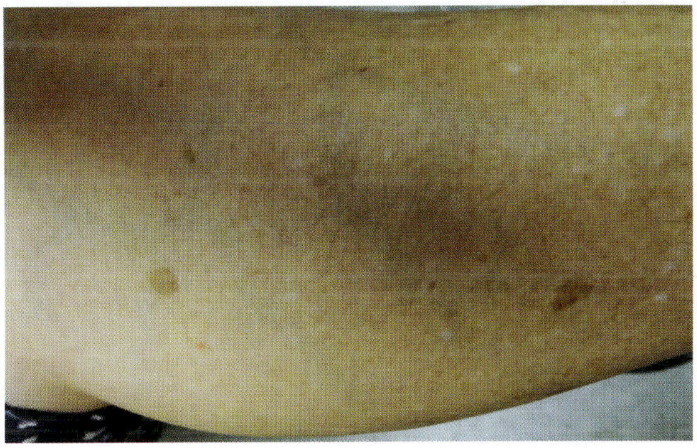

Fig. 11.6 Lentigines on the calf of a Hispanic female

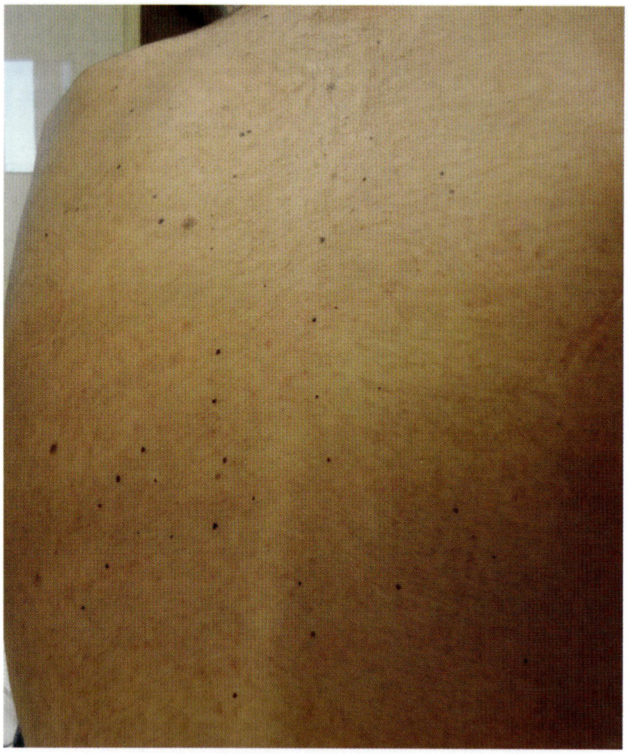

Fig. 11.7 Multiple lentigines on the back of a Hispanic male with Noonan syndrome

11.3 Natural History and Prognosis

The lesions of lentigines are benign, and prognosis is good in the absence of any patterns suggestive of systemic disease. When underlying diseases exist, the prognosis depends on the severity of associated conditions. Without treatment and with further sun exposure, lesions tend to enlarge and darken with time. When appropriate gentle treatments are applied, the appearance of most lesions can improve significantly over the course of several months.

11.4 Histopathologic Features

Lentigines have several classic findings on biopsy. They include an increased density of melanocytes in the basal layer, hypermelanosis with melanin extending to portions of the spinous layer, and elongated epidermal rete ridges [1]. Recent studies further divide these lesions into two groups with distinct patterns, termed the "budding" group and the "flattened epidermis" group [6]. The "budding group" has epidermal hyperplasia with a deeply pigmented basal layer atop elongated rete ridges, while the "flattened epidermis" group has a thin epidermis, basal melanosis, and a lower density of Langerhans cells. The latter pattern occurs on a background of severe solar elastosis and likely reflects a later stage of lentigines with more severe photodamage.

11.5 Diagnosis and Differential Diagnosis

The diagnosis of lentigines relies mostly on clinical exam, with a history of sun exposure and similar lesions in family members increasing the strength of the diagnosis. When the diagnosis is uncertain, biopsy can be confirmatory. Lentigines are most commonly confused with ephelides (freckles). Unlike lentigines, ephelides present most commonly in adolescents, and the lesions are uniform in distribution, size, and color [1]. Histologically, ephelides demonstrate increased melanin in the epidermis but no increase in the density of melanocytes. Another particularly worrisome look-alike is melanoma in situ (lentigo maligna), which can be differentiated from lentigines by biopsy [1].

Other diseases on the differential diagnosis are pigmented actinic keratosis, lichenoid-type seborrheic keratoses, acquired nevus of Ota-like macules, postinflammatory hyperpigmentation (PIH), and melasma.

11.6 Treatment

The primary goal in treatment is to improve lesion appearance without inciting PIH, for which patients with skin of color are predisposed. Q-switched lasers are commonly used to treat hyperpigmented skin, but this method has a 25 % risk of inciting PIH in darker skin types [8]. To reduce the risk of PIH without compromising efficacy, recent studies have demonstrated that mild, sequential laser treatments causing slight immediate whitening are preferable to aggressive treatments that cause obvious immediate whitening [8]. Laser treatments are often followed in the short term by a betamethasone/antibiotic combination cream and chronically by topical hydroquinone [8]. Broad spectrum sunscreen with SPF >30 must be applied before and after treatments for both primary and secondary prevention [1]. As an alternative to laser therapy, topical agents can be used alone. A combination cream of 2 % 4-hydroxyanisol (mequinol) and 0.01 % tretinoin has shown a response in >80 % of patients with skin types II–V; however, the lesions often do not disappear completely [9]. Other more experimental modalities include intense pulsed light for photorejuvenation and lotions containing *Glechoma hederacea* extract, a widely used method of lentigo treatment in Asia [5].

References

1. Plensdorf S, Martinez J. Common pigmentation disorders. Am Fam Physician. 2009;79(2):109–16.
2. Coleman WP, Gately LE, Krementz AB, et al. Nevi, lentigines, and melanomas in Blacks. Arch Dermatol. 1980;116:548–51.
3. Ho GY, Chan HL. The Asian dermatologic patient: review of common pigmentary disorders and cutaneous diseases. Am J Clin Dermatol. 2009;10(3):153–68.
4. O'Neill JF, James WD. Inherited patterned lentiginosis in Blacks. Arch Dermatol. 1989;125:1231–5.
5. Ha JH, Kang WH, Lee JO, et al. Clinical evaluation of the depigmenting effect of Glechoma Hederacea extract by topical treatment for 8 weeks on UV-induced pigmentation in Asian skin. Eur J Dermatol. 2011;21(2):218–22.
6. Yonei N, Kaminaka C, Kimura A, et al. Two patterns of solar lentigines: a histopathological analysis of 40 Japanese women. J Dermatol. 2012;39(10):829–32.
7. Chung JH. Photoaging in Asians. Photodermatol Photoimmunol Photomed. 2003;19:109–21.
8. Negishi K, Akita H, Tanaka S, et al. Comparative study of treatment efficacy and the incidence of post-inflammatory hyperpigmentation with different degrees of irradiation using two different quality-switched lasers for removing solar lentigines on Asian skin. J Eur Acad Dermatol Venereol. 2013;27(3):307–12.
9. Draelos ZD. The combination of 2 % 4-hydroxyanisole (mequinol) and 0.01 % tretinoin effectively improves the appearance of solar lentigines in ethnic groups. J Cosmet Dermatol. 2006;5(3):239–44.

Melanonychia Striata

12

Padma Nallamothu

Contents

P. Nallamothu, MD
Department of Dermatology, Henry Ford Hospital/
Wayne State University Program,
3031 West Grand Blvd, Suite 800, Detroit, MI 48202, USA
e-mail: pnallam1@hfhs.org

12.1 Introduction

Melanonychia striata, or longitudinal melanonychia, are brown to black pigmented bands caused by melanin-derived pigment in the nail plate (Fig. 12.1) [1]. These bands are seen most commonly in African Americans and other dark skin races with reports of up to 90–100 % of African Americans having at least one nail affected by the age of 50 [2, 3]. Melanonychia occur in other races as well with reports of about 20 % of Asians and 10 % of Hispanics also having these nail findings [4, 5]. It is seen much less frequently in Caucasians, about 1 %; however, the incidence is increasing. The higher incidence of melanonychia striata in darker-skinned individuals demonstrates the close relationship of nail melanogenesis and skin color [2]. The incidence of melanonychia also increases with age and is most likely associated with trauma (Fig. 12.2).

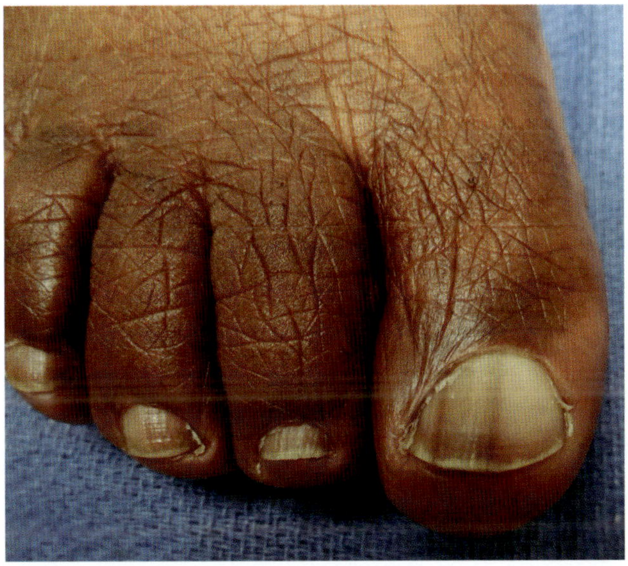

Fig. 12.1 Melanonychia of the great toe in an African American female

D. Jackson-Richards, A.G. Pandya (eds.), *Dermatology Atlas for Skin of Color*,
DOI 10.1007/978-3-642-54446-0_12, © Springer-Verlag Berlin Heidelberg 2014

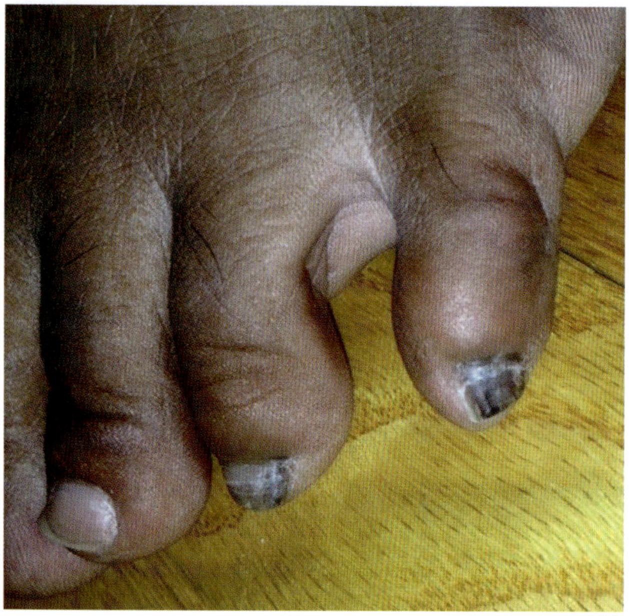

Fig. 12.2 Trauma-induced melanonychia on the fifth toe of a South Asian male

12.2 Clinical Features

Melanonychia presents as one or more longitudinally pigmented bands extending from the proximal nail fold to the distal end of the nail plate [6]. The band can vary in color from light brown to black (Figs. 12.3 and 12.4). In darker-skinned individuals, nail streaks can be heavily pigmented and there can be variegations of color (Figs. 12.5 and 12.6). The width can also range from less than 1 mm to the entire width of the nail plate. Single or multiple nails can be involved. Multiple bands are often seen as a result of melanocyte activation and single bands may be due to a subungual tumor or melanocyte hyperplasia. Dermoscopy features have been described for benign versus malignant lesions although with some limitations. End-on nail plate dermoscopy is helpful to determine if the pigment is within the nail plate or not.

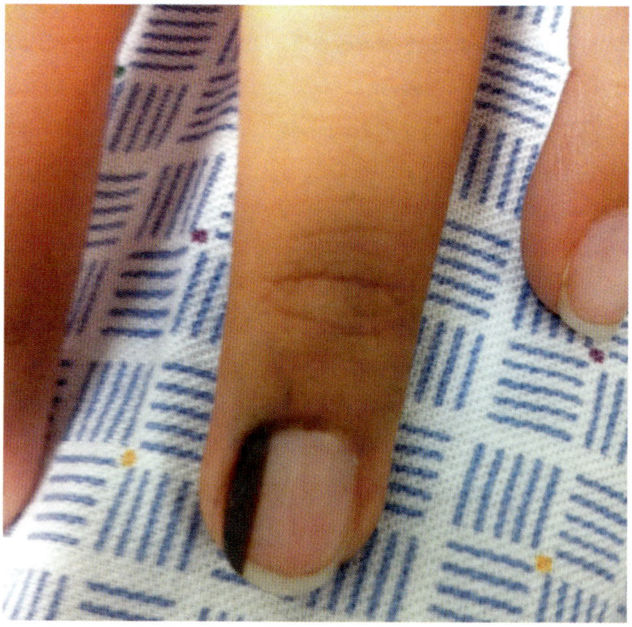

Fig. 12.3 Darkly pigmented band in a Filipino boy – representing severe atypical melanocyte hyperplasia

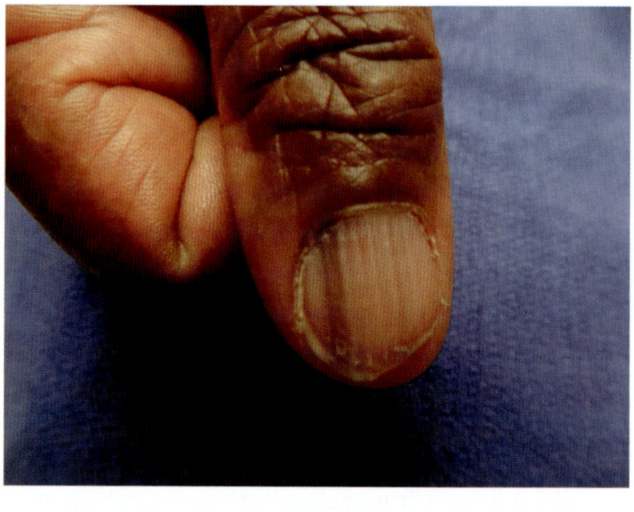

Fig. 12.4 Melanonychia in an African American male, benign racial variant, with associated onychorrhexis and onychoschizia

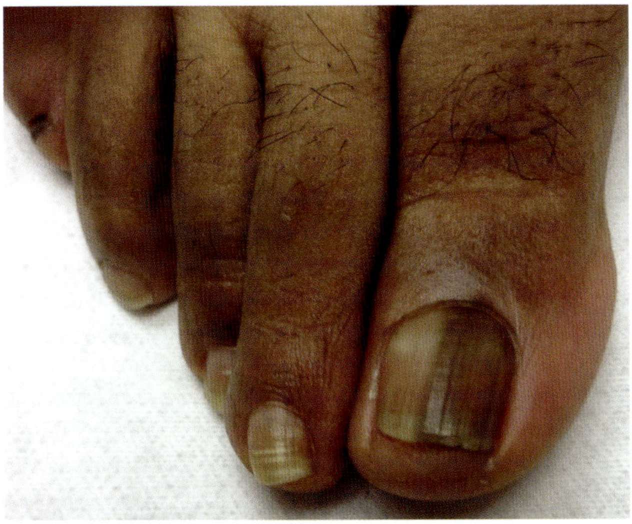

Fig. 12.5 Wide light brown pigmented band in an African American male with associated thickened nail plate

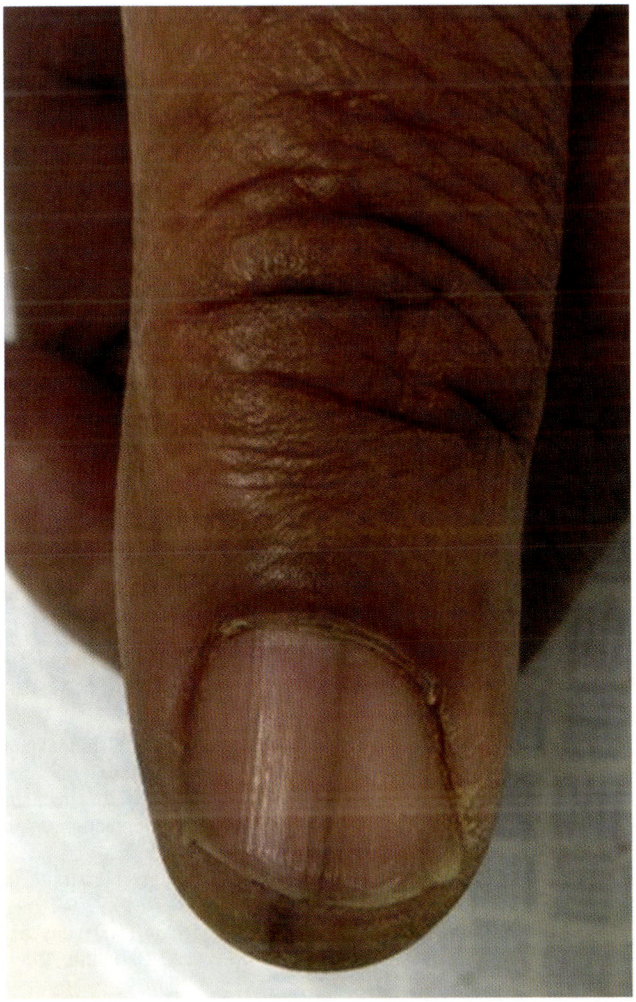

Fig. 12.6 Variegated pigmented band in an African American female with associated pigmented macule on the tip of the finger

12.3 Histopathologic Features

Pathologic features correlate to the cause of the melanonychia. In cases of melanocyte activation, there is an increase in melanin pigmentation of the nail plate epithelium and nail matrix without a concurrent increase in the number of melanocytes. In cases of melanocyte hyperplasia, there is an increase in the number of matrix melanocytes. Nail matrix nevi present with at least one melanocytic nest, whereas lentigines would be devoid of melanocytic nests [7]. Features suggesting malignant melanoma are similar to those seen with melanoma in non-nail locations.

12.4 Differential Diagnosis

There are two broad categories of causes of melanonychia: melanocyte activation and melanocyte hyperplasia (Tables 12.1 and 12.2). Melanonychia present a diagnostic challenge for many clinicians. Features of melanonychia striata and subungual melanoma are interestingly similar. Both predominantly occur on the thumb, index finger, or first toe, have a disproportionately greater incidence in dark-skinned individuals, and have a relationship to trauma [2].

Table 12.1 Causes of melanonychia due to melanocyte activation

Melanocyte activation	
Physical	Race, pregnancy
Trauma	Poor footwear, onychotillomania, nail biting
Dermatologic causes	Onychomycosis, paronychia, psoriasis, lichen planus, amyloid, chronic radiodermatitis
Non-melanocytic tumors	Bowen's, verrucae, basal cell carcinoma, subungual keratosis, myxoid cysts
Systemic causes	Infections, HIV, Addison's disease, porphyria, nutritional disorders
Iatrogenic	Phototherapy, X-ray exposure, EBT, drugs
Syndromes	Laugier-Hunziker, Peutz-Jegher, Touraine

Table 12.2 Causes of melanonychia due to melanocyte hyperplasia

Melanocyte hyperplasia	
Benign	Lentigines
	Nevi – congenital or acquired
Malignant	Melanoma in situ
	Melanoma

12.5 Natural History and Prognosis

Melanonychia due to melanocyte activation often persist. If the cause is due to an inflammatory nail condition (Fig. 12.7) or tumor, once the underlying condition is treated, the pigment may lighten. Any change in a pigmented band should alert the clinician that further monitoring or workup is necessary. One can utilize the ABCDEF guidelines to identify key clinical features that raise the suspicion of a possible subungual melanoma (Table 12.3) [7].

Nail unit melanoma is most commonly observed in the great toes, index fingers, and thumbs of patients with a mean age of 60–70 years old. They are more prevalent in darker-skinned individuals compared to Caucasians. Regrettably, patients with nail unit melanomas are often misdiagnosed and with an average diagnostic delay of 2 years; this diagnosis carries a poor prognosis [4]. The incidence of melanoma is lower in general in individuals with darker skin; however, the percent of those that are nail unit melanomas is disproportionately higher in certain racial groups (Table 12.4) [7].

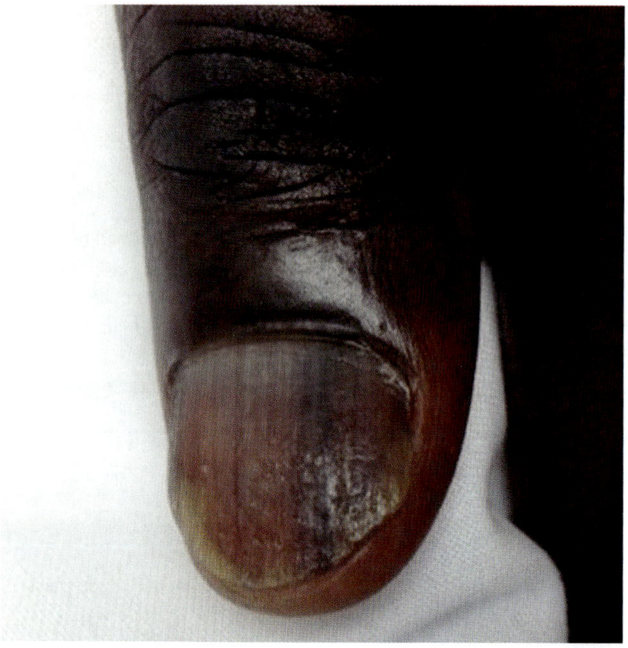

Fig. 12.7 Melanonychia in an African American male with associated psoriatic nail changes

Table 12.3 ABCDEF guidelines for subungual melanoma

A	Age of patient	Most commonly presents in fifth to seventh decade of life (but has been reported from age 1 to 90)
B	Band features	Variegated shades of *brown* to *black* pigment, *breadth* of >3 mm, or irregular or *blurred borders*
C	Change	Sudden, recent, or rapid increase in the size of the pigmented band or change in nail plate morphology
D	Digit	Thumb, great toe, or index finger involved
E	Extension	Extension of pigment into perionychium or Hutchinson's sign
F	Family history	Family or personal history of melanoma or atypical nevus syndrome

Table 12.4 Percent of melanoma that occur in the nail unit by race

Caucasians	1–3 %
Blacks	15–20 %
Mexicans	16 %
Japanese	10–30 %
Chinese	17 %
American-Indians	33 %

12.6 Treatment

The course of treatment depends on the cause of the melanonychia striata.

If the melanonychia is due to racial variation, no treatment is warranted. There is no available treatment to remove the pigment from the nail plate. Nail polish is recommended for those who do not like the cosmetic appearance of the melanonychia.

If other causes are suspected, such as tumors, melanocyte activation, or melanoma, then a nail unit biopsy including the matrix is recommended.

References

1. Bolognia JL et al. Dermatology. St. Louis: Mosby Elsevier; 2008.
2. Krull EA et al. Nail surgery. A text and atlas. Philadelphia: Lippincott Williams & Williams; 2001.
3. Leyden JJ, Sport DA, Goldschmidt H. Diffuse and banded melanin pigmentation in nails. Arch Dermatol. 1972;105:548–50.
4. Dominguez-Cherit J, Roldan-Marin R, et al. Melanonychia, melanocytic hyperplasia, and nail melanoma in a Hispanic population. J Am Acad Dermatol. 2008;59(5):785–91.
5. Leung AK, Robson WL, Liu EK, et al. Melanonychia striata in Chinese children and adults. Int J Dermatol. 2007;46(9):920–2.
6. Baran R, Kechijian P. Longitudinal melanonychia (melanonychia striata): diagnosis and management. J Am Acad Dermatol. 1989; 21(6):1165–75.
7. Jefferson J, Rich P. Melanonychia. Dermatol Res Pract. 2012; 2012:952186.

Part II

Follicular Disorders

Acne Vulgaris

13

Diane Jackson-Richards

Contents

13.1 Epidemiology

Acne is a multifactorial disorder of the pilosebaceous unit. It is one of the most common disorders that individuals seek dermatologic treatment for and is felt to affect 85 % of persons 12–24 years old. Although it starts during adolescence, many adults are affected by acne even in the fourth decade of life [1]. Acne affects all races and has been found to be the leading cause for visits to dermatologists by African Americans, Asians, and Hispanics [2–4].

13.2 Pathophysiology

The pathogenesis of acne begins with androgens stimulating sebaceous glands to increase sebum production. Hyperkeratosis of the follicular infundibulum along with increased sebum production leads to microcomedone formation. Rupture of microcomedones leads to an inflammatory response with influx of neutrophils and lymphocytes. There are increased levels of *Propionibacterium acnes* bacteria within the follicles. *P. acnes* also releases inflammatory mediators, IL-1, IL-8, and TNF-alpha [1]. More severe cases of nodulocystic acne may be familial [5].

D. Jackson-Richards, MD
Department of Dermatology, Multicultural Dermatology Center, Henry Ford Hospital, 3031 West Grand Blvd., Detroit, MI 48202, USA
e-mail: djackso1@hfhs.org

D. Jackson-Richards, A.G. Pandya (eds.), *Dermatology Atlas for Skin of Color*, DOI 10.1007/978-3-642-54446-0_13, © Springer-Verlag Berlin Heidelberg 2014

13.3 Clinical Features

Acne affects the face, upper chest, and upper back, corresponding to the distribution of sebaceous glands. Lesions include comedones, inflammatory papules, and pustules (Figs. 13.1, 13.2, 13.3, 13.4, 13.5, and 13.6). In more severe acne there are tender nodules and cysts. Postinflammatory hyperpigmented macules, often lasting for months, are extremely common in darker-skinned individuals. The resultant postinflammatory hyperpigmentation (PIH) is often more distressing to the individual than the acne itself [7, 10]. Taylor et al. reported PIH occurring in 65 % of blacks, 52 % of Hispanics, and 47 % of Asians [7]. Pitted scarring is a common sequelae of acne as well as hypertrophic or keloidal scars. Keloidal scarring is more common in patients with darker skin. Nodulocystic acne is felt to be less common in the African American population, but when nodules and cysts occur, they more often heal with hypertrophic scarring and keloids [6]. Acne conglobata (Figs. 13.7 and 13.8) is a severe form of nodulocystic acne and can be part of the follicular occlusion tetrad when associated with hidradenitis suppurativa, pilonidal cysts, and dissecting cellulitis of the scalp. Hormonal influence can cause neonatal acne at 2 weeks to 3 months of age and infantile acne at 3–6 mos. of age. Fortunately, neonatal acne resolves spontaneously [1]. Women with resistant acne and hirsutism should be evaluated for polycystic ovarian syndrome. Drug-induced acne can be associated with systemic or topical corticosteroids (Fig. 13.9), anabolic steroids, lithium, phenytoin, iodides, and bromides.

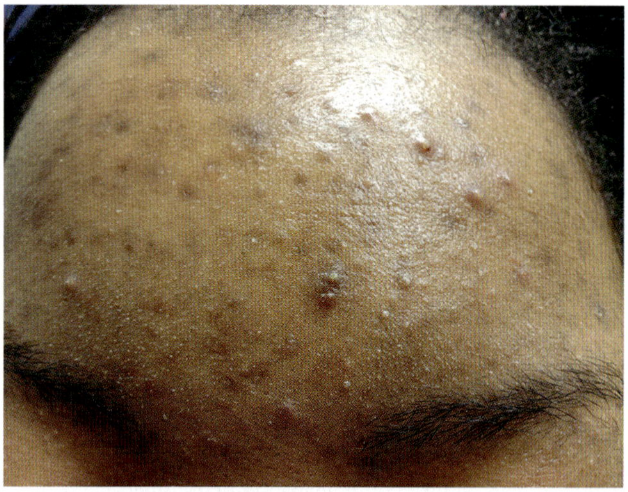

Fig. 13.1 Pustules, papules, comedones, and postinflammatory hyperpigmentation of the forehead in an African American female with acne

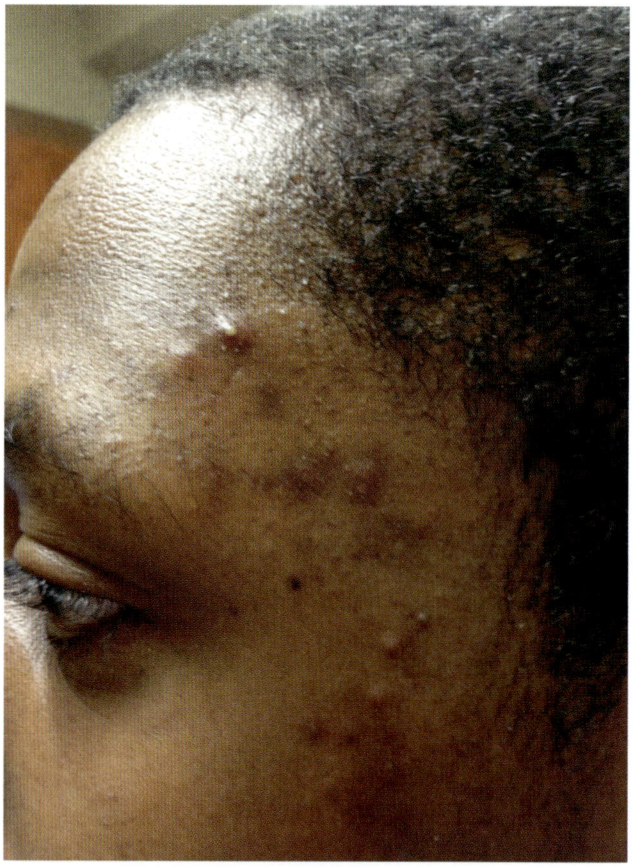

Fig. 13.2 Pustules, papules, comedones, and postinflammatory hyperpigmentation of the face in an African American male with acne

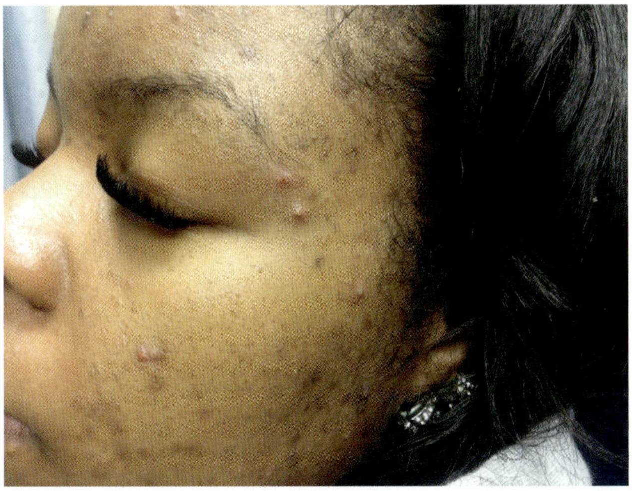

Fig. 13.3 Pustules, papules, comedones, and postinflammatory hyperpigmentation of the face in an African American female with acne

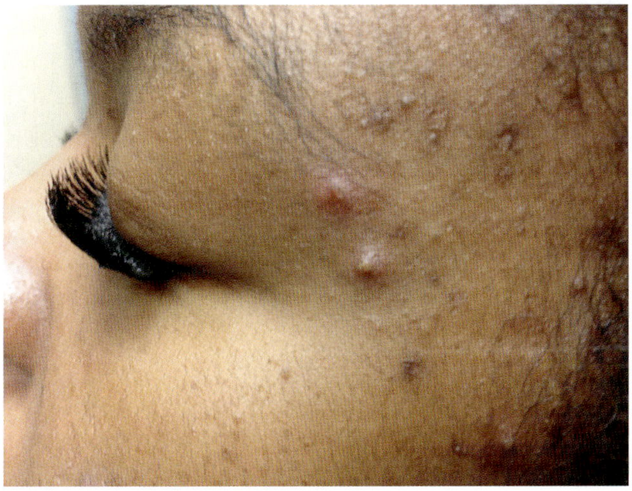

Fig. 13.4 Pustules, papules, comedones, and postinflammatory hyperpigmentation of the temple in an African American female with acne

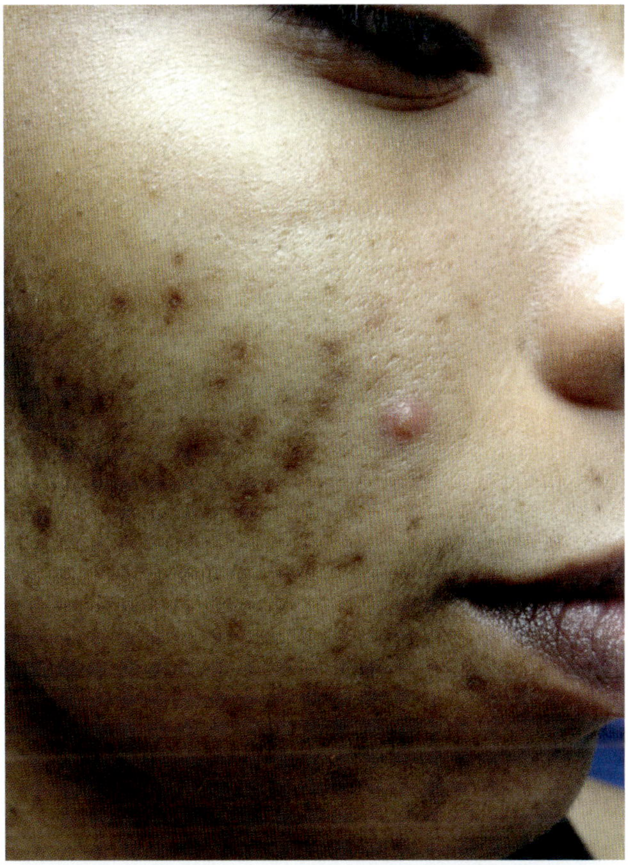

Fig. 13.5 Pustules and postinflammatory hyperpigmentation of the cheek and chin in an African American female with acne

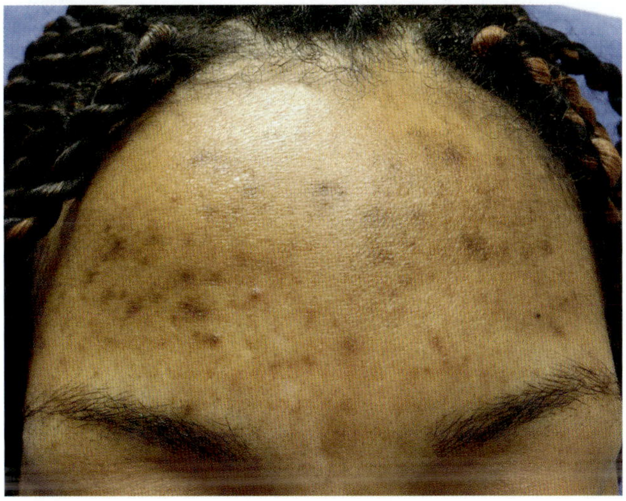

Fig. 13.6 Postinflammatory hyperpigmentation of forehead from acne in an African American female

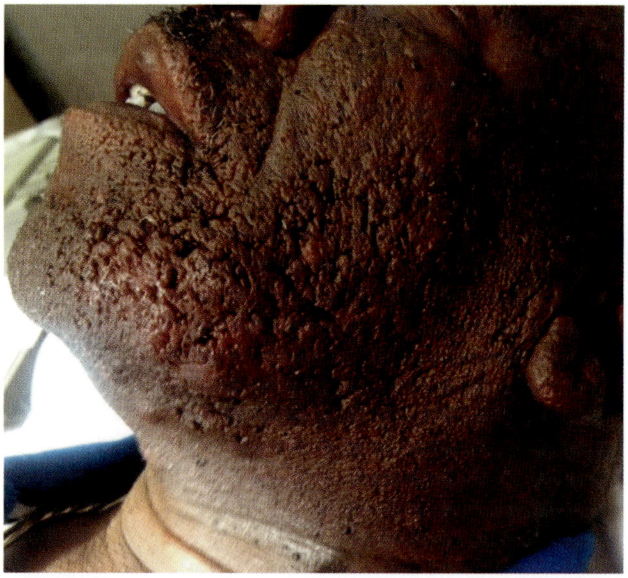

Fig. 13.7 Acne conglobata of the face in an African American male with SAPHO syndrome

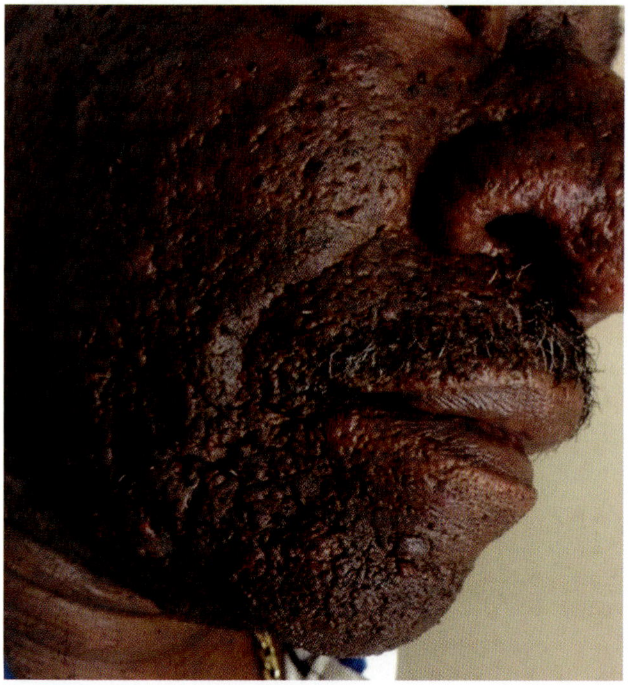

Fig. 13.8 Close-up of acne conglobata of the face in an African American male with SAPHO syndrome

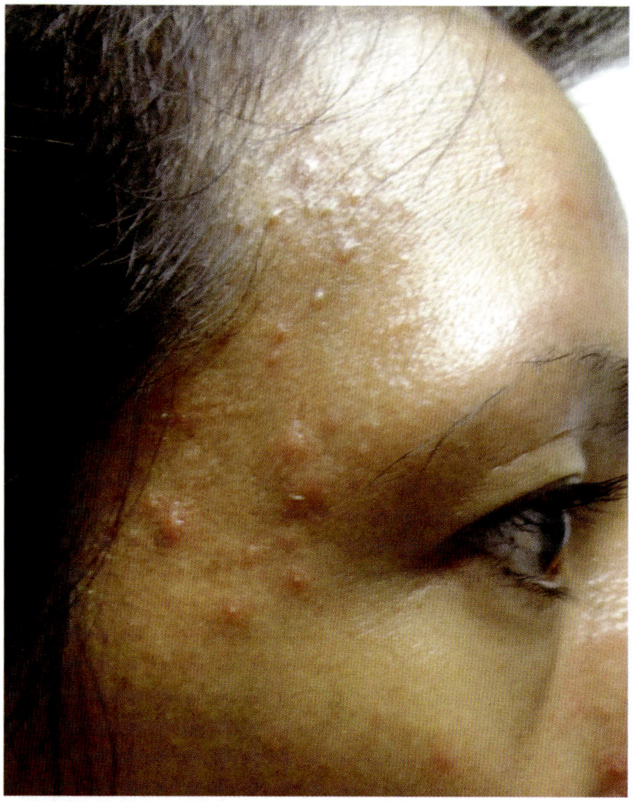

Fig. 13.9 Acne from systemic steroids in a Hispanic female

13.4 Histopathologic Features

Histopathology shows a distended follicle impacted with keratinocytes, hair, and bacteria. Early on there is a mononuclear cell infiltrate around the follicle. Once the follicle ruptures into the dermis, a neutrophilic inflammatory infiltrate develops. A foreign body granulomatous reaction ensues, commonly followed by perifollicular scarring. A study by Halder et al. examined biopsies of African American females and found marked inflammation surrounding comedonal acne lesions that did not appear to be inflamed on clinical exam [9]. This could explain why patients with skin of color develop PIH even when affected by mild to moderate acne.

13.5 Differential Diagnosis

Differential diagnosis of acne in infants includes miliaria and sebaceous hyperplasia. Overuse of topical corticosteroids may lead to perioral dermatitis. Oral corticosteroid treatment often leads to numerous monomorphic papules and pustules on the face and trunk, referred to as "steroid acne." Monomorphic papules associated with pruritus and history of HIV might indicate eosinophilic folliculitis.

13.6 Treatment

The treatment of acne must be tailored to the severity of the disease. Signs of possible hyperandrogenic conditions in females should be investigated with a thorough history, free testosterone, and DHEAS levels. The history should include questions regarding the use of any occlusive or petrolatum-based products, as these often exacerbate acne. Topical retinoids are commonly used to treat mild to moderate acne. Retinoids normalize the keratinization of the follicle and thus are comedolytic. In addition to being comedolytic, retinoids are anti-inflammatory and have been shown to improve the PIH that is so common in darker-skinned patients. Although topical retinoids are very beneficial, they can cause irritation which can in turn lead to further hyperpigmentation. Starting with a lower concentration of retinoids and gradually titrating up allows topical retinoids to be used in ethnic skin with less risk of irritation. The concomitant use of noncomedogenic moisturizers is also helpful in reducing irritation. Tretinoin, adapalene, and tazarotene are the most commonly used topical retinoids. Topical antibiotics, erythromycin and clindamycin, reduce *P. acnes* levels in the follicles and also inhibit release of proinflammatory mediators. Topical benzoyl peroxides are bacteriostatic by oxidizing bacterial proteins. Use of benzoyl peroxide also decreases bacterial resistance that can occur with use of topical and oral antibiotics. Benzoyl peroxides can be drying to the skin and cause irritation and PIH if not used carefully in skin of color [8]. Starting with lower concentrations of benzoyl peroxide and the use of moisturizers is recommended for initial therapy [11]. Treatment is more successful when multiple agents, including topical antibiotics, benzoyl peroxides, and retinoids, are used in combination.

Topical treatment alone is often not adequate for moderate to severe acne. Oral antibiotics inhibit *P. acnes* but are also anti-inflammatory. Oral antibiotics that have long been used for acne include tetracycline, doxycycline, minocycline, and trimethoprim/sulfamethoxazole. When oral antibiotics are used, patients must be warned of possible side effects, including GI upset, *Candida* infections, hyperpigmentation with minocycline, and hypersensitivity syndrome. Oral contraceptives and spironolactone as an androgen receptor blocker are helpful in women with hormone-induced acne. Estrogen is also known to decrease sebum production.

Oral isotretinoin is the best treatment for nodulocystic acne that is resulting in scarring. This drug normalizes follicular keratinization but also causes atrophy of sebaceous glands and reduces sebum production. Teratogenicity is the most serious side effect and childbearing age females must be on two forms of birth control during and for 2 months after completion of isotretinoin therapy. Other side effects include xerosis, elevation of triglycerides, and liver enzymes. Arthralgias, myalgias, pseudotumor cerebri, and depression can also occur. Intralesional triamcinolone acetonide 2.5–5.0 mg/cc can quickly reduce the inflammation of larger nodules and cysts. Other adjuvant therapies include glycolic acid and salicylic acid peels, photodynamic therapy, and laser resurfacing [12, 13]. These treatments have increased risk of pigmentary complications in darker skin and must be used with extreme caution and care. Skin lightening agents such as hydroquinone, azelaic acid, and kojic are useful in reducing PIH. Early treatment of acne in patients with skin of color is important in reducing the PIH that is particularly problematic for this group of patients.

References

1. Zaenglein AL, Thiboutot DM. Acne vulgaris. In: Jorizzo JL, Rapini JL, Bolognia RP, editors. Dermatology. 2nd ed. St. Louis: Elsevier Mosby; 2009.
2. Davis SA, Narahari S, Feldman SR, Huang W, Pichardo-Geisinger RO, McMichael AJ. Top dermatologic conditions in patients of color: an analysis of nationally representative data. J Drugs Dermatol. 2012;11(4):466–73.
3. El-Essawi D, Musial JL, Hammad A, Lim HW. A survey of skin disease and skin-related issues in Arab Americans. J Am Acad Dermatol. 2007;56(6):933–8.
4. Child FJ, Fuller LC, Higgins EM, Du Vivier AW. A study of the spectrum of skin disease occurring in a black population in south-east London. Br J Dermatol. 1999;14(3):512–7.

5. Goulden V, McGeown CH, Cunliffe WJ. The familial risk of adult acne: a comparison between first-degree relatives of affected and unaffected individuals. Br J Dermatol. 1999;141:297–300.
6. Halder RM. The role of retinoids in management of cutaneous conditions in blacks. J Am Acad Dermatol. 1998;39:S98–103.
7. Taylor SC, Cook-Bolden F, Rahman Z, et al. Acne vulgaris in skin of color. J Am Acad Dermatol. 2002;46:S98–106.
8. Davis EC, Callender VD. A review of acne in ethnic skin. J Clin Aesthet Dermatol. 2010;3(4):24–38.
9. Halder RM, Brooks HL, Callender VD. Acne in ethnic skin. Dermatol Clin. 2003;21(4):609–15.
10. Baldwin HE, Friedlander SF, Eichenfield LF, Mancini AJ, Yan AC. The effects of culture, skin color and other nonclinical issues on acne treatment. Semin Cutan Med Surg. 2011;30:S12–5. Elsevier.
11. Zeichner J. Strategies to minimize irritation and potential iatrogenic post-inflammatory pigmentation when treating acne patients with skin of color. J Drugs Dermatol. 2011;10(12):S25–6.
12. Alexis A. Fractional laser resurfacing for acne scarring in patients with Fitzpatrick skin types IV-VI. J Drugs Dermatol. 2011;10(12): S6–8.
13. Swindhart J. Case reports: surgical therapy of acne scars in pigmented skin. J Drugs Dermatol. 2007;6(1):74–7.

Rosacea

14

Prescilia Isedeh and Diane Jackson-Richards

Contents

14.1 Introduction

Rosacea is a chronic inflammatory disorder characterized by facial flushing, telangiectasia, papules, and pustules affecting the central face. It commonly affects the light-skinned Caucasian population with the estimated prevalence ranging from 1–10 % in those between the ages of 30 and 50 years old [1]. Although rosacea is most common in light-skinned individual, it may occur in patients from other racial and ethnic groups. The prevalence in African Americans, Latinos, and Asians is about 4 % [2]. Men and women are equally affected, although men tend to have a more progressive form of the disease, including rhinophyma and sebaceous hyperplasia [2].

The etiology of rosacea remains unknown, but both genetic and environmental factors have been thought to play a role in the pathogenesis of the disease. Factors implicated include ultraviolet (UV) light exposure, vascular abnormalities, dermal matrix degeneration, chemical and ingested agents, pilosebaceous unit abnormalities, and microbial organisms [2]. Mechanisms proposed in the development of rosacea include UV-induced apoptosis and dermal matrix changes. Microbes such as Bacillus oleronius isolated from mite Demodex folliculorum, found in sebaceous follicles, act as triggers for susceptible innate immune system in rosacea patients. Hypervascularity in rosacea patients can be triggered by emotional stress, spicy foods, hot beverages, high environmental temperatures, and menopause. UV irradiation and sun exposure causes a flushing response and worsens the clinical symptoms of rosacea [3]. Ultimately, regardless of the etiology, inflammation leads to disruption of the stratum corneum resulting in the many signs and symptoms of rosacea [2].

P. Isedeh, MD (✉) • D. Jackson-Richards, MD
Department of Dermatology, Multicultural Dermatology Center, Henry Ford Hospital, 3031 West Grand Blvd., Detroit, MI 48202, USA
e-mail: pisedeh1@hfhs.org; djacksol@hfhs.org

D. Jackson-Richards, A.G. Pandya (eds.), *Dermatology Atlas for Skin of Color*,
DOI 10.1007/978-3-642-54446-0_14, © Springer-Verlag Berlin Heidelberg 2014

14.2 Clinical Features

Rosacea is underdiagnosed and undertreated due to the fact that patients are reluctant to mention their concerns, failure to remove makeup prior to examination, failure for clinicians to recognize the disease, and difficulties in recognizing the changes in ethnic skin [4]. Rosacea primarily affects the convexities of the central face including the cheeks, chin, nose, and central forehead [2]. Signs and symptoms are often transient, occurring independent of each other. There are four classic subtypes of rosacea: erythematotelangiectatic type (ETR), papulopustular, phymatous, and ocular. Additionally, granulomatous rosacea is a well-described variant.

ETR has a predominance of flushing and persistent facial erythema. Telangiectasias are common, but are not necessary for the diagnosis. Flushing can last several seconds to greater than 10 minutes, which can be triggered by certain types of foods, particularly spicy foods, alcohol, emotional stress, vigorous activity, medications, and variations in temperature [2]. Patients with ETR tend to have the most sensitive skin; in these patients, topical products can exacerbate symptoms [2]. Patients with skin of color tend to have less ETR compared to light-skinned patients, in which telangiectasias and sun damage are more prevalent. Papulopustular rosacea is characterized by persistent central facial erythema with transient papules or pustules, or both (Figs. 14.1 and 14.2) [2]. Phymatous rosacea consists of marked thickening of the skin with irregular surface nodularities and edema. Rhinophyma is the most common form of phymatous rosacea (Figs. 14.3 and 14.4), but it may also occur on the chin (gnathophyma), forehead (metophyma), one or both ears (otophyma), and eyelids (blepharophyma) [2]. Ocular rosacea is reported in 58 % of patients with cutaneous lesions [2]. The diagnosis should be considered if one or more of the following signs or symptoms are present: watery blood shot appearance, foreign body sensation, burning or stinging, dryness, blurred vision, or telangiectasias of the conjunctiva. In addition blepharitis, conjunctivitis, keratitis, chalazia, corneal scarring or perforation, and iritis have been associated with ocular rosacea [2]. Lastly, granulomatous rosacea is characterized by periorificial, firm, yellow, brown, or red cutaneous papules or nodules which can lead to scarring in severe cases [2].

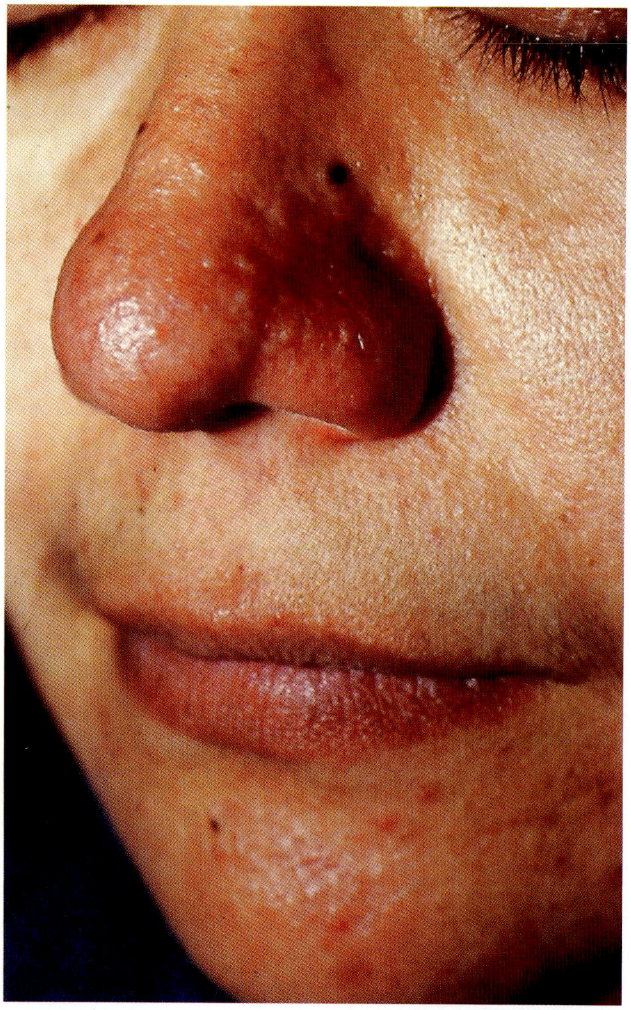

Fig. 14.1 Papulopustular rosacea in a Hispanic female

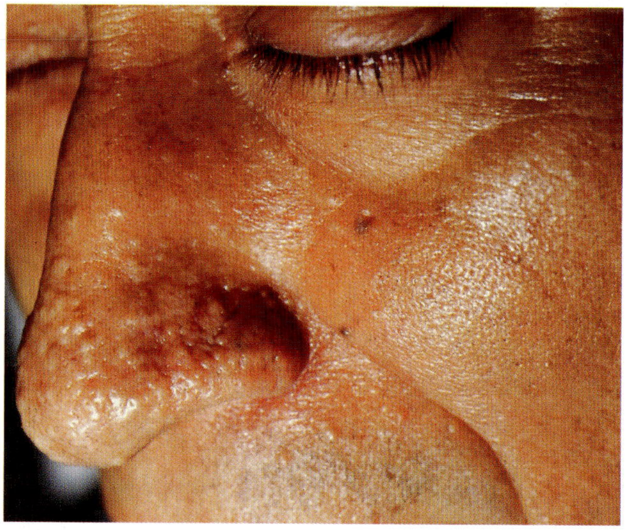

Fig. 14.2 Rosacea with papules on the nose in a Hispanic male

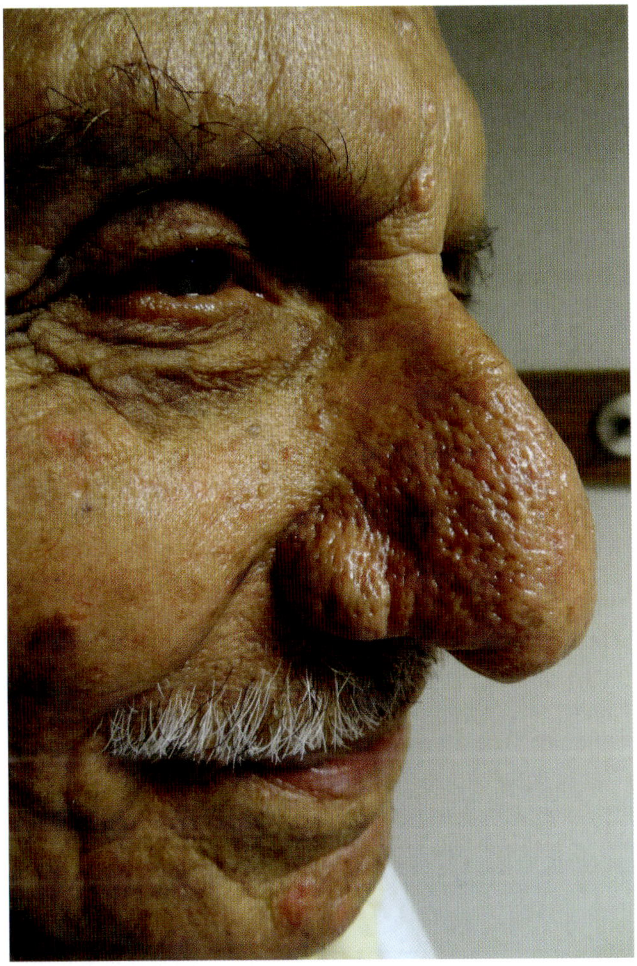

Fig. 14.3 Rhinophyma with scattered papules of sebaceous hyperplasia in a Hispanic male

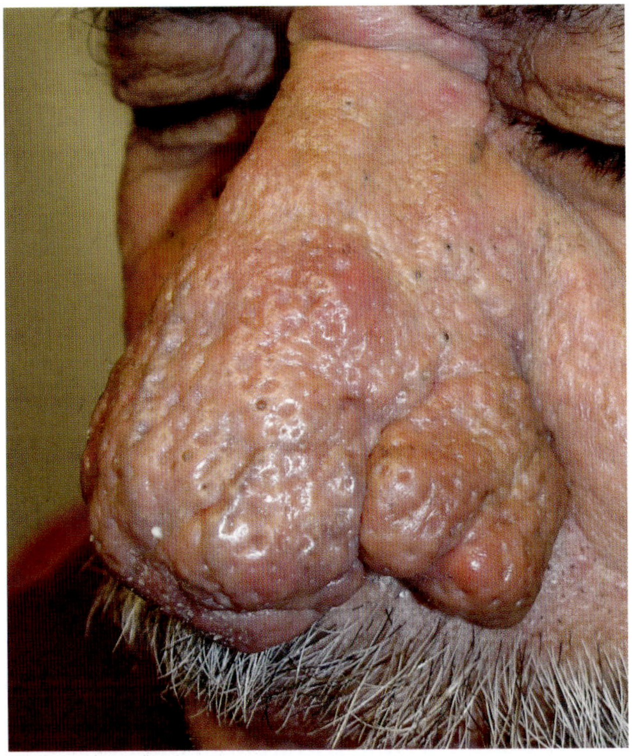

Fig. 14.4 Rhinophyma in a Hispanic male

14.3 Natural History and Prognosis

Although rosacea is usually chronic, depending on the subtype, patients often respond well to therapy. [4] Patients with the ETR subtype can have improvement in the erythematous component, while the telangiectasia remains. [4] Phymatous rosacea worsens over time and is often difficult to treat. Although the eye findings of ocular rosacea vary, the development of keratitis can be severe and may lead to visual impairment. [4]

14.4 Histopathological Features

Histologically, vascular dilatation with degenerative changes in the collagen and elastic fibers are seen in the upper dermis [4]. The papules and pustules seen in patients with rosacea resemble those in acne vulgaris histologically, although the inflammatory infiltrate of rosacea tends to have a more granulomatous component than acne vulgaris [4].

14.5 Diagnosis and Differential Diagnosis

There are no specific lab tests to make the diagnosis of rosacea, since the assessment of affected patients is mainly clinical. In order to make the diagnosis, at least one primary feature must be present: flushing, transient erythema, nontransient erythema, papules and pustules, or telangiectasia. Secondary features such as burning, stinging, plaques, dry appearance, edema, ocular manifestations, peripheral location, or phymatous changes may occur but are not necessary for the diagnosis [5]. Differential diagnoses include acne vulgaris, systemic lupus erythematosus, seborrheic dermatitis, and photodermatitis [4].

14.6 Treatment

Conservative treatment includes trigger avoidance, photoprotection, gentle skin care, and cosmetic camouflaging [2]. The most commonly used topical medications include metronidazole gel, 15 % azelaic acid, and 10 % sodium sulfacetamide with or without 5 % sulfur [2]. These agents are usually successful in the treatment of mild to moderate papulopustular rosacea. Other topical therapies include benzoyl peroxide, clindamycin, calcineurin inhibitors, retinoids, and topical corticosteriods [2]. Systemic therapy such as oral tetracyclines (used mainly for their anti-inflammatory effects) and macrolides are effective for treatment of papules, pustules, erythema, and ocular inflammation [3]. In 2006, the FDA approved an anti-inflammatory dose of doxycycline (40 mg capsule containing 30 mg immediate-release and 10 mg delayed-release beads) to be taken once daily for up to 12 months [2]. Additionally, low dose isotretinoin can be used for the treatment of granulomatous, phymatous, and severe inflammatory rosacea [2]. Rosacea associated with erythema and telangiectasia has been successfully treated with a variety of vascular lasers such as the pulsed dye laser (PDL), potassium titanyl phosphate laser, and intense pulsed light [2]. A side effect of laser therapy in patients with ethnic skin is postinflammatory hyperpigmentation [2]. Lastly, due to the underlying inflammatory etiology of rosacea, these patients may develop postinflammatory hypo- or hyperpigmentation. Therefore, the management of rosacea in patients with skin of color should include preventative and symptomatic treatment of dyschromia, including photoprotection and the use of topical depigmenting agents to treat postinflammatory hyperpigmentation [6].

References

1. Korting HC, Schollman C. Current topical and systematic approaches to treatment of rosacea. J Eur Acad Dermatol Venereol. 2009;23:876–82.
2. Kennedy Carney C, Cantrell W, Elewski BE. Rosacea: a review of current topical, systemic and light based therapies. G Ital Dermatol Venereol. 2009;144:673–88.
3. Elsaie M, Choudhary S. Updates on the pathophysiology and management of acne rosacea. Postgrad Med. 2009;121(5):178–86.
4. Marks JG, Miller JJ. Pustules. Principles of dermatology. Philadelphia, PA, China: Elsevier, Inc.; 2006. p. 171–86.
5. Baldwin H. Diagnosis and treatment of rosacea: state of the art. J Drugs Dermatol. 2012;11(6):725–30.
6. Woolery-Lloyd H, Good E. Acne and rosacea in skin of color. Cosmet Dermatol. 2011;24(4):159–62.

Hidradenitis Suppurativa

15

Pranita V. Rambhatla

Contents

P.V. Rambhatla, MD
Department of Dermatology, Henry Ford Hospital,
3031 West Grand Blvd., Detroit, MI 48202, USA
e-mail: prambha1@hfhs.org

15.1 Introduction

Hidradenitis suppurativa, also known as acne inversa, or Verneuil's disease, is a chronic, inflammatory, debilitating skin follicular disease that manifests with painful deep-seated inflamed lesions in the apocrine gland-bearing areas of the body, most commonly the axillary, inframammary, inguinal, and anogenital regions.

15.2 Epidemiology

Global epidemiological data on hidradenitis suppurativa is limited and most available statistics are based on self-reported and clinical assessment data. Population-based estimates from France, Denmark, and the United States have proposed a prevalence of 0.5–1 % [1].

15.3 Etiology

Aristide Verneuil, a French surgeon, initially proposed the pathogenesis of the disease to be a disorder of the sweat glands in 1864 [2]. It is now widely accepted that HS is a disorder of the folliculopilosebaceous unit, characterized by abnormal follicular occlusion and inflammation. It is categorized as part of the follicular occlusion tetrad alongside acne conglobata, dissecting cellulitis, and pilonidal sinus. Strong associations have been demonstrated with smoking and high body mass index [3]. A female predominance has been suggested as well as a genetic predisposition, with up to 38 % of patients reporting a positive family history [4]. Emerging research has shown that bacterial infection, particularly coagulase-negative staphylococci and anaerobe infections, may play a role in the pathogenesis of HS and may indicate a role for antibiotics in the treatment of this disease [5].

D. Jackson-Richards, A.G. Pandya (eds.), *Dermatology Atlas for Skin of Color*,
DOI 10.1007/978-3-642-54446-0_15, © Springer-Verlag Berlin Heidelberg 2014

15.4 Clinical Features

HS has a predilection for intertriginous areas and presents as erythematous papules, subcutaneous nodules and sinus tracts, most commonly in the axillae, inframammary skin, inguinal folds, gluteal and perineal areas. The lesions often cause chronic pain and patients frequently report spontaneous serous, purulent, or bloody discharge. Individual lesions may progress to form interconnecting sinus tracts or abscesses. The Hurley staging system is a convenient and useful method of classifying disease severity and can help guide management. Stage I is characterized by abscess formation (single or multiple) without sinus tracts or cicatrization (Fig. 15.1). Stage II has recurrent abscesses with tract formation and cicatrization (single or multiple widely separated lesions) (Figs. 15.2 and 15.3). Stage III disease has diffuse or near-diffuse involvement or multiple interconnected tracts and abscesses across the entire affected area [6] (Figs. 15.4, 15.5, and 15.6).

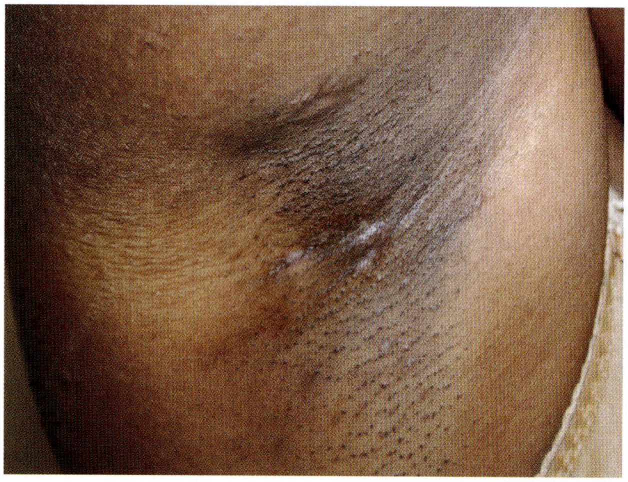

Fig. 15.1 Stage 1 HS in axilla of an African American female

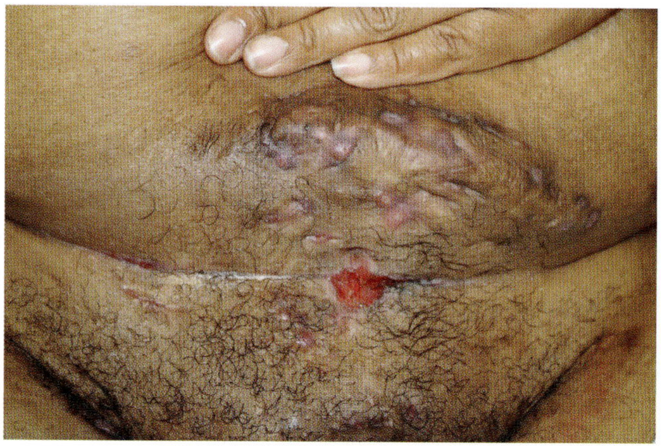

Fig. 15.3 Stage 2 HS under pannus of a Hispanic female

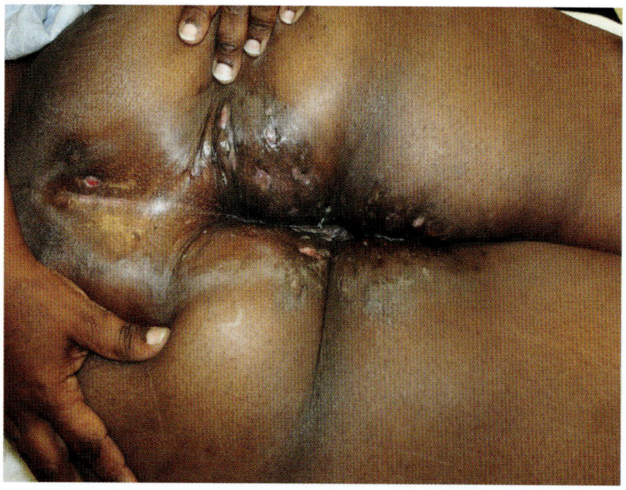

Fig. 15.2 Stage 2 HS in gluteal area of an African American female

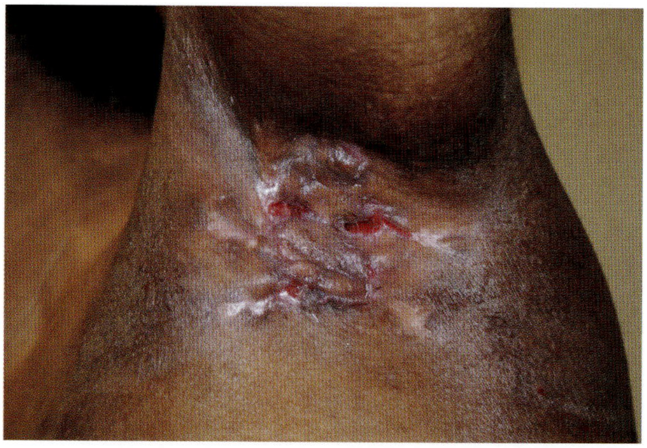

Fig. 15.4 Stage 3 HS in axilla of an African American female

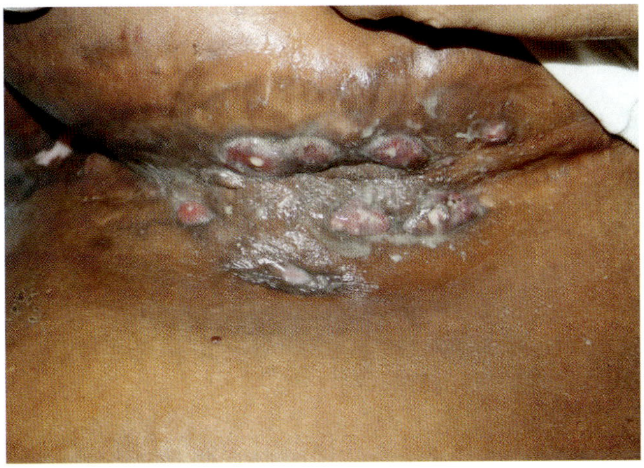

Fig. 15.5 Stage 3 HS in right inframammary area of an African American female

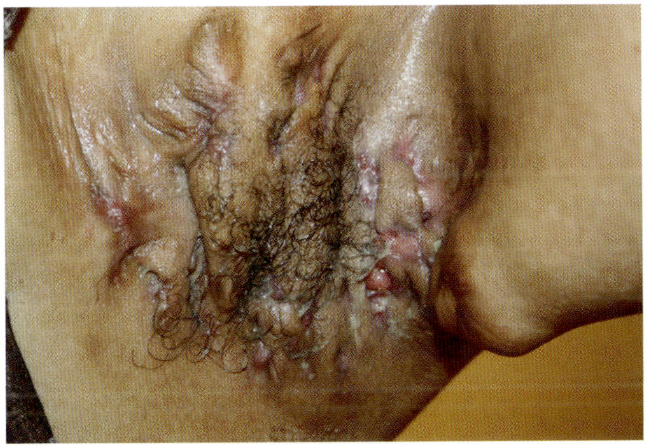

Fig. 15.6 Stage 3 HS in axilla of a Hispanic female

15.5 Diagnosis and Differential Diagnosis

Multiple sites of involvement, fragmented care by multiple specialists, and nonspecific lesions often lead to a long delay in diagnosis. Differential diagnoses include acne, folliculitis, carbuncle, furuncle, pilonidal cyst, epidermoid or dermoid cyst, erysipelas, granuloma inguinale, lymphogranuloma venereum, and Crohn's disease. The diagnostic criteria for hidradenitis suppurativa (adopted by the 2nd International Conference on HS, March 5, 2009, San Francisco CA, USA) are primarily clinical and include (1) typical lesions, i.e., deep-seated painful nodules ("blind boils" in early lesions), abscesses, draining sinus, bridged scars, and "tombstone" double-ended pseudocomedones in secondary lesions; (2) typical topography, i.e., axillae, groins, perineal and perianal region, buttocks, infra- and intermammary folds; (3) chronicity and recurrences [7]. Skin biopsy is not needed for diagnostic purposes, but histopathologic findings include follicular plugging and perifollicular mixed inflammatory infiltrate. Abscesses, sinus tracts, and fibrosis may also be present. In patients with suspected superinfection, or refractory disease, lesions may be cultured for aerobic and anaerobic bacteria. If hyperandrogen states or metabolic syndromes are suspected, it is appropriate to request a consultation with an endocrinologist.

15.6 Treatment

HS has a chronic, relapsing course and requires long-term management. A multidisciplinary approach utilizing medical and surgical treatment modalities is often required. In all patients, it is essential to stress the importance of lifestyle changes including weight loss, smoking cessation, and decreased pressure/friction of intertriginous areas. Current treatments are based on the categorization of HS as an inflammatory disease and the presence of microbes. Early stage HS lesions can be treated with topical antibiotics and benzoyl peroxide washes. More advanced disease necessitates the use of systemic therapy. Oral antibiotics and biologics are the most commonly used systemic therapies. Successful outcomes have been reported with doxycycline and combination therapy with clindamycin and rifampin. Infliximab and adalimumab are TNF alpha blockers which have been shown to have efficacy. Patients with extensive disease require referral to a general or plastic surgeon for excisional surgery. Other reported therapies include various combinations of antibiotics, retinoids, antiandrogens, CO_2 laser, Nd:Yag laser, deroofing procedures, and external beam radiation [8].

References

1. Cosmatos I, Matcho A, Weinstein R, Montgomery MO, Stang P. Analysis of patient claims data to determine the prevalence of hidradenitis suppurativa in the United States. J Am Acad Dermatol. 2013;68(3):412–9.
2. Verneuil A. De L' hidrosandenite phlegmoneuse et des abces sudoripares. Arch Gen Med Paris. 1864;114:537–57.
3. Revuz JE, Canoui-Poitrine F, Wolkenstein P, et al. Prevalence and factors associated with hidradenitis suppurativa: results from two case–control studies. J Am Acad Dermatol. 2008;59(4):596–601.
4. Von der Werth JM, Williams HC. The natural history of hidradenitis suppurativa. J Eur Acad Dermatol Venereol. 2000;14:389–92.
5. Revuz J. Antibiotic treatment of hidradenitis suppurativa. Ann Dermatol Venereol. 2012;139(8–9):532–41. doi:10.1016/j.annder.2012.05.016. Epub 2012 Jun 22. French. Erratum in: Ann Dermatol Venereol. 2012;139(11):787.
6. Hurley HJ. Axillary hyperhidrosis, apocrine bromhidrosis, hidradenitis suppurativa and familial benign pemphigus: surgical approach. In: Roenigk RK, Roenigk HH, editors. Dermatologic surgery. New York: Marcel Dekker; 1989. p. 729–39.
7. Hidradenitis Suppurativa Foundation (HSF). www.hs-foundation.org.
8. Rambhatla PV, Lim HW, Hamzavi I. A systematic review of treatments for hidradenitis suppurativa. Arch Dermatol. 2012;148(4):439–46.

Pseudofolliculitis Barbae

16

Richard H. Huggins

Contents

16.1 Introduction

Pseudofolliculitis barbae (PFB), first described in 1908 by Fox, is an inflammatory skin condition affecting hair-bearing portions of the body as a result of shaving [1].

16.2 Epidemiology

PFB primarily affects males of African descent, but individuals of all races and both sexes can develop this disorder. Between 45 and 83 % of black males are estimated to develop PFB [2]. Among males, this condition develops most frequently between the ages of 14 and 25 years [3]. The perimenopausal period, when hormonal changes can result in facial hypertrichosis, is the most common time during which females develop this condition, though hirsute women can develop PFB at any age.

R.H. Huggins, MD
Department of Dermatology, Henry Ford Hospital, 3031 West Grand Blvd., Suit 800 Dermatology, Detroit, MI 48202, USA
e-mail: rhuggin1@hfhs.org

D. Jackson-Richards, A.G. Pandya (eds.), *Dermatology Atlas for Skin of Color*,
DOI 10.1007/978-3-642-54446-0_16, © Springer-Verlag Berlin Heidelberg 2014

16.3 Clinical Features

PFB typically presents with follicular-based papules. Some patients have associated erythema, pustules, and hypertrophic and keloidal scarring. Lesions most commonly develop in the beard region. Lesions may also develop in the axillae or suprapubic regions in individuals who shave or pluck these areas. PFB may be associated with pain, pruritus, and/or irritation. Diagnosis is made solely on the basis of typical-appearing lesions (Figs. 16.1, 16.2, and 16.3).

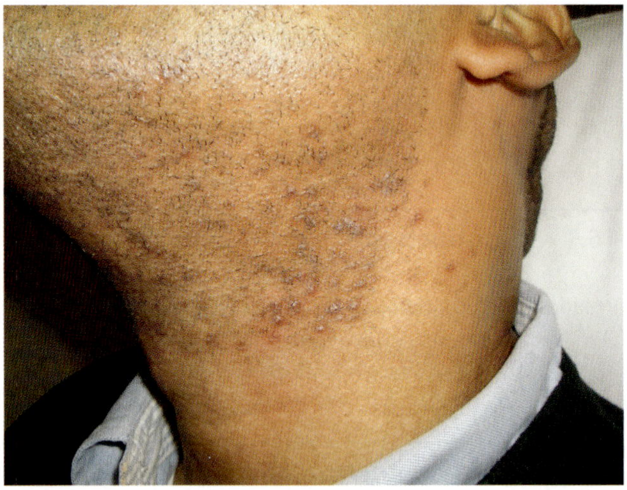

Fig. 16.1 Erythematous follicular papules on the left submental beard region of an African-American male (Courtesy of Iltefat Hamzavi, MD)

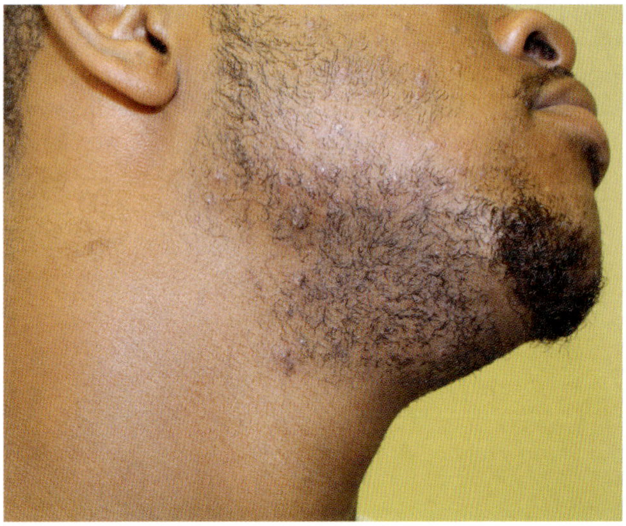

Fig. 16.2 Erythematous follicular papules on the right cheek and submental beard region of an African-American male (Courtesy of Tor Shwayder, MD)

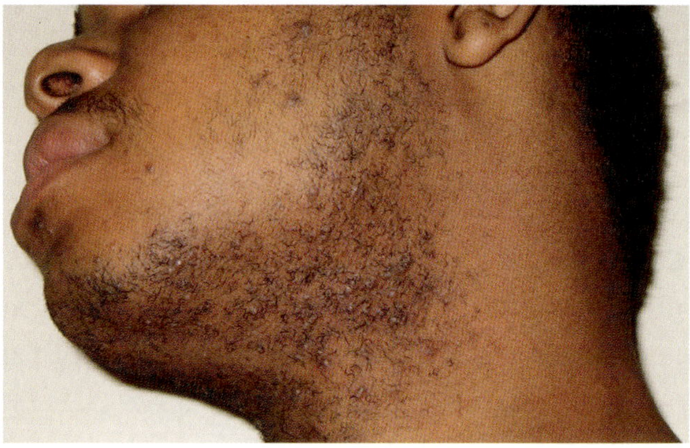

Fig. 16.3 Erythematous follicular papules on the left beard region of an African-American male (Courtesy of Tor Shwayder, MD)

16.4 Etiology

The critical phenomenon in the development of PFB is the penetration of the shaved hair shaft into the dermis or epidermis. This occurs most frequently in individuals of African descent because of the oblique orientation of the hair follicle relative to the epidermis and the coiling nature of hair growth commonly observed in this group [1]. These two characteristics of African hair predispose the hair shaft for penetration into the skin. Shaving and plucking make up another key part of this process as it turns the naturally blunt edges of hair shafts into sharp, obliquely cut edges that can more easily pierce the skin. PFB is thought to result from either penetration of the hair shaft through the follicle into the dermis below the level of the epidermis (transfollicular penetration) or secondary to the coiled hair shaft growing out of the follicular opening then curling back and reentering the epidermis at another site (extrafollicular penetration) [1]. Specific hair-grooming practices may predispose individuals, particularly those with curly hair, to PFB via one or both of these mechanisms.

The presence of the hair shaft within the skin outside the follicle triggers a foreign body reaction. The penetrating hair also provides a portal and vehicle for entry of cutaneous bacteria, which can result in localized infection. Individuals often further traumatize the primary inflammatory papules by shaving over them. In the bikini region, shaved hairs, coiled or not, may extrafollicularly penetrate the epidermis as a result of the natural folds of the area and friction from undergarments [1]. Genetics may also play a role in the development of the condition as a predisposition to the development of PFB has been associated with an unusual single-nucleotide polymorphism affecting the keratin of the hair follicle [4].

16.5 Treatment

Management of PFB should focus on interrupting the development of the hair foreign body reaction and its sequelae as far upstream in the process as possible. The most effective strategies are those which eliminate shaving and plucking altogether. Though not always practical, maintenance of a full beard without any shaving is a very effective approach, typically with resolution of PFB lesions in 2–6 weeks [1]. Use of topical depilatories, such as those containing barium sulfide and calcium thioglycolate, may also be effective. This practice is associated with risk of irritant contact dermatitis, especially with improper use. In willing patients, laser hair removal can be an extremely effective treatment and is the only treatment with long-term efficacy, with permanent results in some case. The ruby (694 nm), pulse alexandrite (755 nm), diode (800–810 nm), neodymium: yttrium aluminum garnet (Nd:YAG, 1,064 nm), and pulsed light systems can all be used for hair depilitation. Treatment carries the risks of erythema, crusting, burns with scarring and dyspigmentation, and paradoxical hypertrichosis [1]. Burns are particular concerns in skin phototypes IV–VI. In these phototypes, the diode laser and the Nd:YAG laser are the safest. The diode laser may be more effective, as the follicle absorbs three to four times as much energy at a wavelength of 800 nm compared to 1,064 nm with the Nd:YAG laser; however, the latter laser is thought to have an increased hair bulb to epidermis ratio of absorption, which may produce better results [5, 6]. Both the Alexandrite laser and intense pulsed light have been used to safely and successfully treat PFB in skin types II–IV, though the Alexandrite laser was found to work faster, result in higher efficacy, and had more durable results than intense pulsed light [7].

When shaving is necessary, strategies to avoid leaving the sharp-tipped shaved hair shaft below the level of or just above the epidermis should be employed to minimize transfollicular and extrafollicular penetration, respectively. Clippers or razors with guards which prevent unnecessarily close shaves are recommended over traditional razors. When using traditional razors, single blade razors are preferable to multiblade systems which shave too close for this condition. Shaving with traditional razors should also be performed in the direction of hair growth and without stretching the skin, which can cause the shaved hair tip to retract below the surface of the skin, a setup for transfollicular penetration [8]. Shaving frequency recommendations range from twice daily to two to three times per week, though a recent study showed significantly reduced ingrown hairs with bi- and triweekly shaving compared with daily shaving [2]. Additionally, manual extraction of the tips of clearly visible and easily accessible ingrown hairs can also be helpful, as long as the base of the hair is not plucked out.

Medical treatments for PFB include low- to mid-potency topical corticosteroids and topical retinoids. Particularly in cases where secondary infection is apparent, topical and, possibly, oral antibiotics can be helpful. Eflornithine cream causes irreversible inhibition of ornithine decarboxylase, resulting in local inhibition of hair growth. It can be used as an adjunct to any hair depilation technique and has been shown to accelerate and improve the response of PFB to laser hair removal [9]. Over-the-counter moisturizing shaving products can also help reduce the pruritus associated with PFB [2].

References

1. Bridgeman-Shah S. The medical and surgical therapy of pseudofolliculitis barbae. Dermatol Ther. 2004;17:158–63.
2. Daniel A, Gustafson CJ, Zupkosky PJ, et al. Shave frequency and regimen variation effects on the management of pseudofolliculitis barbae. J Drugs Dermatol. 2013;12:410–8.
3. Perry PK, Cook-Bolden FE, Rahman Z, et al. Defining pseudofolliculitis barbae in 2001: a review of the literature and current trends. J Am Acad Dermatol. 2002;46(2 Suppl Understanding):S113–9.
4. Winter H, Schissel D, Parry DA, et al. An unusual Ala12Thr polymorphism in the 1A alpha-helical segment of the companion layer-specific keratin K6hf: evidence for a risk factor in the etiology of the common hair disorder pseudofolliculitis barbae. J Invest Dermatol. 2004;122:652–7.
5. Smith EP, Winstanley D, Ross EV. Modified superlong pulse 810 nm diode laser in the treatment of pseudofolliculitis barbae in skin types V and VI. Dermatol Surg. 2005;31:297–301.
6. Emer JJ. Best practices and evidenced-based use of the 800 nm diode laser for the treatment of pseudofolliculitis barbae in skin of color. J Drugs Dermatol. 2011;10(12 Suppl):s20–2.
7. Leheta TM. Comparative evaluation of long pulse Alexandrite laser and intense pulsed light systems for pseudofolliculitis barbae treatment with one year of follow up. Indian J Dermatol. 2009;54:364–8.
8. Quarles FN, Brody H, Johnson BA, et al. Pseudofolliculitis barbae. Dermatol Ther. 2007;20:133–6.
9. Xia Y, Cho S, Howard RS, et al. Topical eflornithine hydrochloride improves the effectiveness of standard laser hair removal for treating pseudofolliculitis barbae: a randomized, double-blinded, placebo-controlled trial. J Am Acad Dermatol. 2012;67:694–9.

Central Centrifugal Cicatricial Alopecia

17

Diane Jackson-Richards

Contents

17.1 Epidemiology and Etiology

The term central centrifugal cicatricial alopecia or CCCA evolved to describe hair loss starting in the central crown area with symmetric expansion centrifugally. LoPresti et al. first termed this condition "hot comb alopecia." They hypothesized that the process of using a hot comb along with petrolatum-based products to straighten the hair led to inflammation and eventual hair loss. Later Sperling and Sau termed the condition "follicular degeneration syndrome" due to lack of correlation with hot comb usage. More recently the North American Hair Research Society adopted the name central centrifugal cicatricial alopecia to describe this form of scarring hair loss [1–3]. The exact etiology is unclear, but many studies have linked the condition to hair grooming practices. Some studies have reported an association with chemical relaxer use, whereas others report an association with use of cornrow braids, braids with extensions, and sew-in and glue-in hair weaves [2, 3]. Hereditary factors may play a role, but this is unclear.

Specific epidemiologic data is not available, but it is seen almost exclusively in women of African descent. Although CCCA is seen quite commonly, studies on the exact prevalence are lacking.

D. Jackson-Richards, MD
Department of Dermatology, Multicultural Dermatology Center, Henry Ford Hospital, 3031 West Grand Blvd., Detroit, MI 48202, USA
e-mail: djackso1@hfhs.org

D. Jackson-Richards, A.G. Pandya (eds.), *Dermatology Atlas for Skin of Color*, DOI 10.1007/978-3-642-54446-0_17, © Springer-Verlag Berlin Heidelberg 2014

17.2 Clinical Features

Onset of CCCA ranges from 20 to 40 years of age with average age of presentation being 36. Initially there may be insidious thinning of the hair, associated with mild pruritus and tenderness, but symptoms may be absent. Early on, follicular pustules may be present. The hair loss progresses circumferentially, revealing a shiny scalp with absent or markedly decreased follicular openings (Figs. 17.1, 17.2, 17.3, and 17.4). Although the distribution is similar to female pattern hair loss, loss of follicles (Fig. 17.5) and scarring distinguish CCCA from non-scarring alopecia. Symptoms are often absent. The condition may progress for several years before eventually stopping, leaving permanent alopecia in its wake (Figs. 17.6 and 17.7).

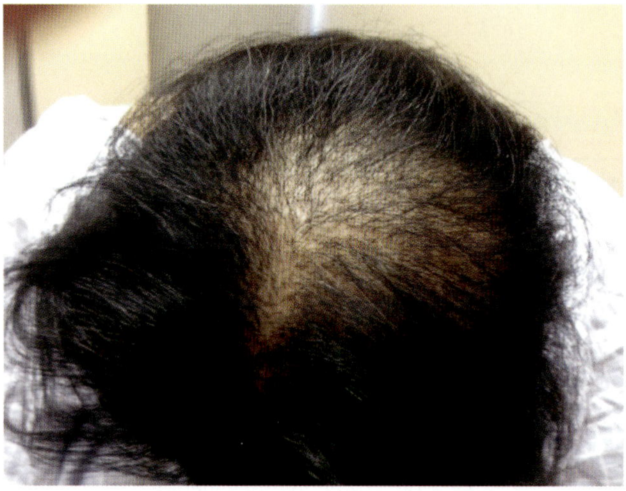

Fig. 17.1 Mild to moderate CCCA in an African American female

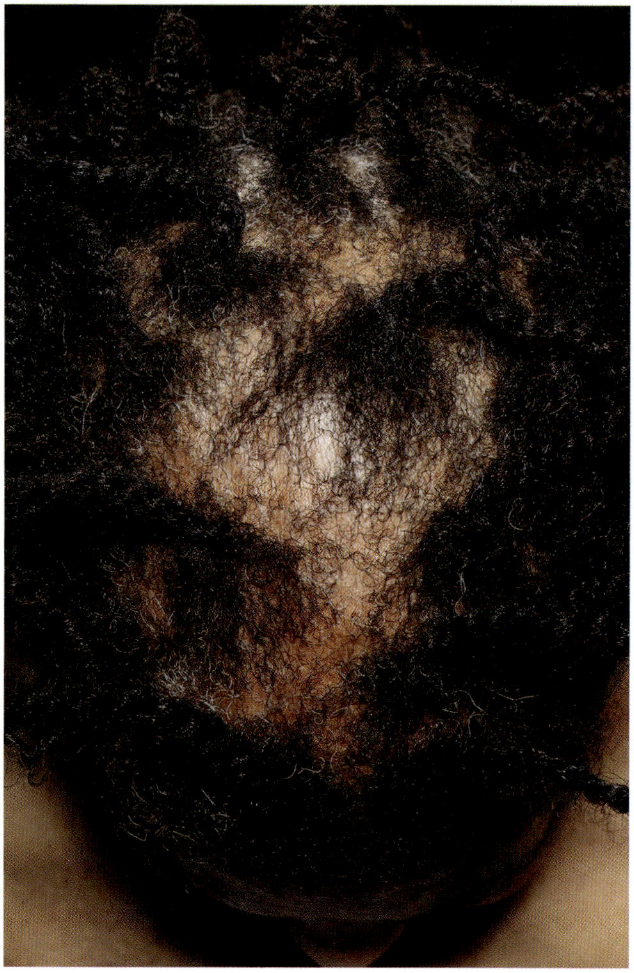

Fig. 17.2 CCCA in an African American female (Courtesy of Dr. Ophelia Dadzie)

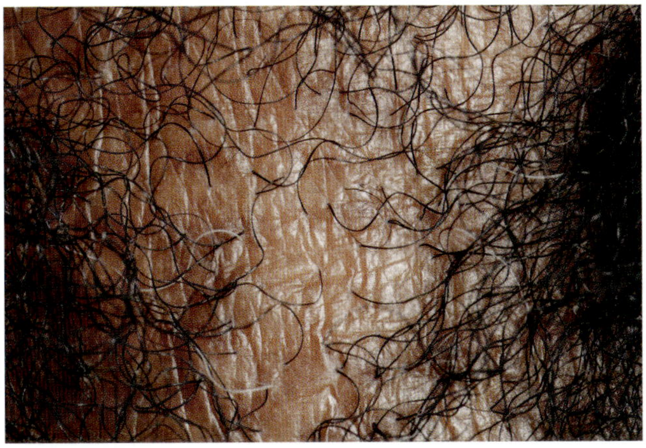

Fig. 17.3 CCCA in an African American female, close-up (Courtesy of Dr. Ophelia Dadzie)

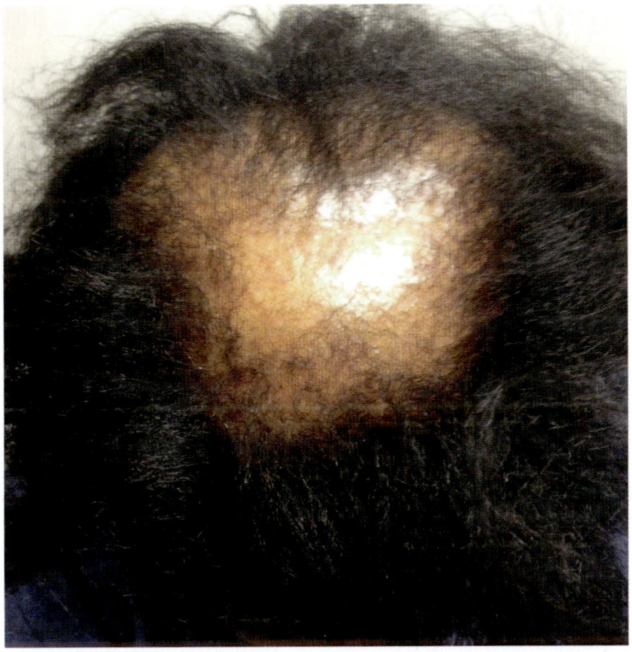

Fig. 17.4 Moderate to severe CCCA in an African American female

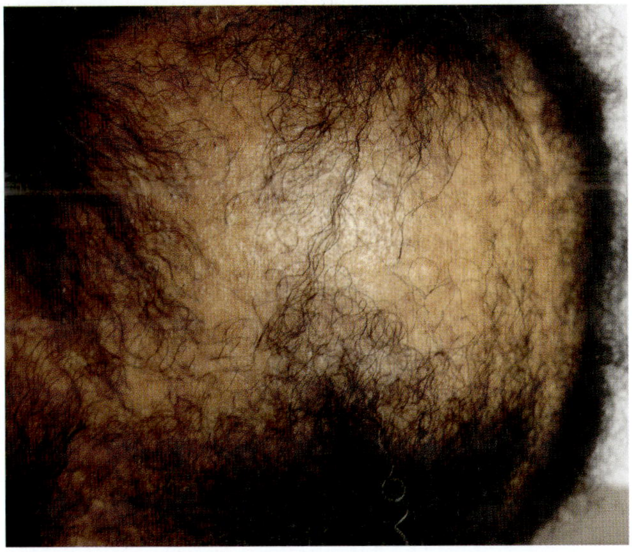

Fig. 17.5 Severe CCCA in an African American female

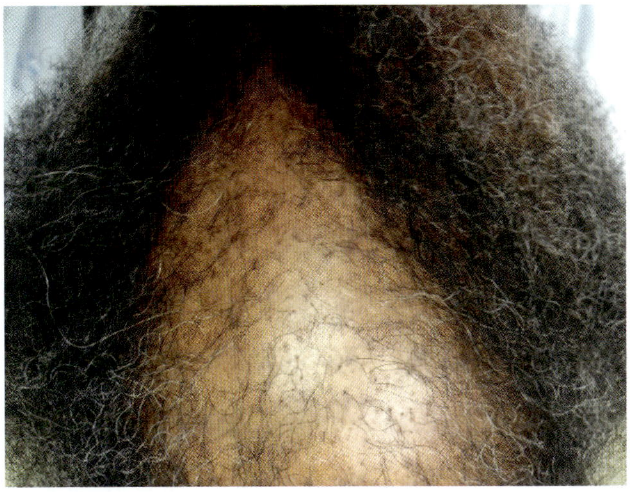

Fig. 17.6 Severe CCCA in an African American female

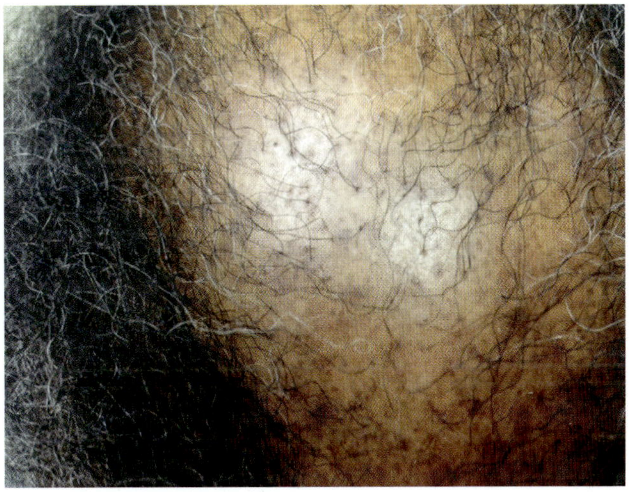

Fig. 17.7 Severe CCCA in an African American female, close-up

17.3 Histopathologic Features

Early histopathologic findings show a perifollicular lymphocytic infiltrate involving the infundibulum and isthmus. There is concentric lamellar fibrosis around the mid and upper follicle and displacement of the follicular canal to an eccentric position. Premature desquamation of the inner root sheath has been noted by Sperling; however, this finding has also been seen in other forms of scarring alopecias. Atrophy of the external root sheath leads to follicular distention and rupture. Hair fiber granulomas are seen within fibrous tracts. Sebaceous glands are lost, but this is also seen in other forms of cicatricial alopecia. In contrast to lesions of discoid lupus, there is no interface change at the dermal-epidermal junction and no follicular plugging, mucin is absent, and direct immunofluorescence testing is negative. In late-stage disease, widened fibrous tracts are marginated by thickened elastic fibers. These histopathologic changes are almost indistinguishable from pseudopelade of Brocq, however, CCCA has a much different clinical presentation, helping to make the distinction between the two disorders [4, 5].

17.4 Diagnosis and Differential Diagnosis

Diagnosis should include a careful medical and hair care history, physical exam, and scalp biopsy to rule out other possible causes of hair loss. Differential diagnosis includes pseudopelade of Brocq, lichen planopilaris, and female pattern hair loss.

17.5 Treatment

Early intervention is important, but there are no studies examining response to various therapies. Discontinuation of possible damaging hairstyling practices should be encouraged and may alleviate progression of disease. Topical corticosteroids and intralesional triamcinolone acetonide, 3–10 mg/ml injections performed monthly into affected areas for at least 6 months, may be helpful. Any coincidental seborrheic dermatitis, tinea or bacterial folliculitis should be treated. Treatment may prevent progression of disease but usually does not reverse existing hair loss; therefore, reasonable expectations must be discussed with patients.

References

1. Olsen EA, Callender V, McMichael A, Sperling L, Anstrom K, Shapiro J, Roberts J, Durden F, Whiting D, Bergfeld W. Central hair loss in African American women: incidence and potential risk factors. J Am Acad Dermatol. 2011;64(2):245–52.
2. Gathers R, Jankowski M, Eide M, Lim H. Hair grooming practices and central centrifugal cicatricial alopecia. J Am Acad Dermatol. 2009;60:574–8.
3. McMichael AJ. Hair and scalp disorders in ethnic populations. Dermatol Clin. 2003;21:629–44.
4. Whiting DA, Olsen EA. Central centrifugal cicatricial alopecia. Dermatol Ther. 2008;21(4):268–78.
5. Somani N, Bergfeld WF. Cicatricial alopecia: classification and histopathology. Dermatol Ther. 2008;21:221–37.

Folliculitis Decalvans and Dissecting Cellulitis

18

Diane Jackson-Richards

Contents

18.1 Etiology

Folliculitis decalvans (FD) is an inflammatory, cicatricial scalp disorder in which the cellular infiltrate is primarily neutrophilic [1]. The most widely accepted theory for the pathogenesis for FD postulates that *Staphylococcus aureus* secretes cytotoxins or superantigens that bind to major histocompatibility complex (MHC) class II molecules [2, 3]. This stimulates T-lymphocytes, leading to release of proinflammatory mediators (IFN-gamma and TNF-alpha) and pro-fibrotic mediators (TGF-beta and IL-4) [4]. An abnormal host immune response is thought to be responsible for allowing this cascade of events to occur. *S. aureus* is usually isolated from mostly all cases of untreated folliculitis decalvans. *S. aureus* is present in 20–30 % of the general population, but less than 0.05 % of these normal carriers suffer from infection.

Dissecting cellulitis or dissecting folliculitis is a chronic, inflammatory scalp disorder also known as perifolliculitis capitis abscedens et suffodiens or Hoffmann disease. It can occur with hidradenitis suppurativa, pilonidal cysts, and acne conglobata as part of the follicular occlusion tetrad. Coexistence with acne conglobata and hidradenitis occur in one-third of patients. These disorders are felt to share a common pathogenesis. Occlusion of the follicles with keratinous and sebaceous material occurs. The follicles then rupture and lead to a neutrophilic inflammatory reaction.

18.2 Epidemiology

Although sufficient epidemiologic studies are not available, FD accounts for approximately 10–11 % of all cases of primary cicatricial alopecias. This disorder occurs in young adults, affecting men more than women and African Americans more than Caucasians [3, 5]. There may be a genetic predisposition, as there are a number of familial cases reported. Dissecting cellulitis usually affects black males in the second to fourth decades of life; however, 10 % of cases have been in white males and more rarely females.

D. Jackson-Richards, MD
Department of Dermatology, Multicultural Dermatology Center, Henry Ford Hospital, 3031 West Grand Blvd., Detroit, MI 48202, USA
e-mail: djackso1@hfhs.org

D. Jackson-Richards, A.G. Pandya (eds.), *Dermatology Atlas for Skin of Color*, DOI 10.1007/978-3-642-54446-0_18, © Springer-Verlag Berlin Heidelberg 2014

18.3 Clinical Features

Folliculitis decalvans first involves the vertex and occipital scalp, presenting with erythematous perifollicular papules and yellow scale at follicular openings (Figs. 18.1 and 18.2). Pustules, erosions, and hemorrhagic crusts then develop and, finally, scarring alopecia. Tufted folliculitis is seen with multiple hairs emerging from a single follicular orifice (Fig. 18.3). Although tufting is commonly seen in folliculitis decalvans, it is also seen in other cicatricial alopecias. Patients often experience pruritus, pain, and disfiguring alopecia. The course of FD is chronic and treatment is difficult.

Dissecting cellulitis affects the vertex and occipital scalp beginning as perifollicular pustules. This folliculitis progresses into painful nodules and deep-seated abscesses that are interconnected by sinus tracts (Figs. 18.4, 18.5, and 18.6). The formation of sinus tracts are a hallmark finding of dissecting cellulitis and distinguishes it from folliculitis decalvans (Figs. 18.7 and 18.8). Secondary bacterial infection with *S. aureus* is common. This progressive inflammation leads to marked, scarring alopecia. Dissecting cellulitis is a painful chronically relapsing condition that's cosmetically disfiguring. When part of the follicular occlusion tetrad, there is a 30 % risk of HLA-B27 negative spondyloarthropathy associated with SAPHO (synovitis, acne, palmoplantar pustolosis, hyperostosis, osteitis) syndrome.

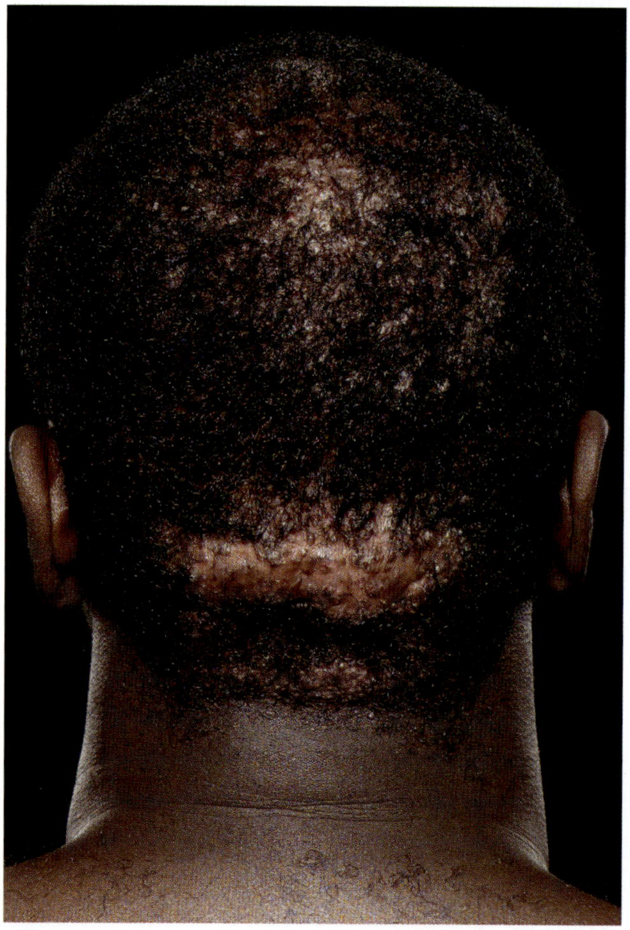

Fig. 18.1 Folliculitis decalvans of scalp along with acne keloidalis nuchae on occiput in an African American male

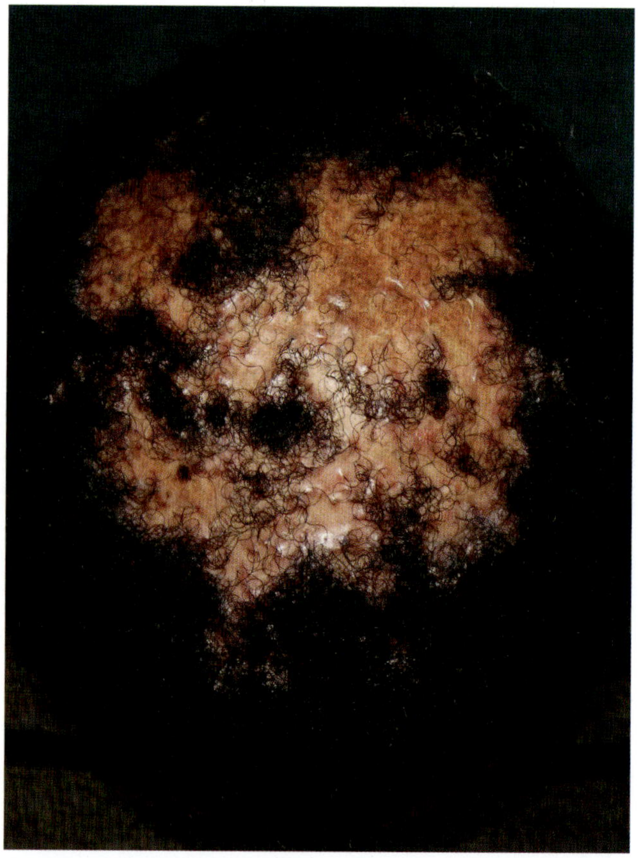

Fig. 18.2 Folliculitis decalvans in an African male (Courtesy of Service de Dermatologie, APHP Hospital Saint-Louis, Paris, France)

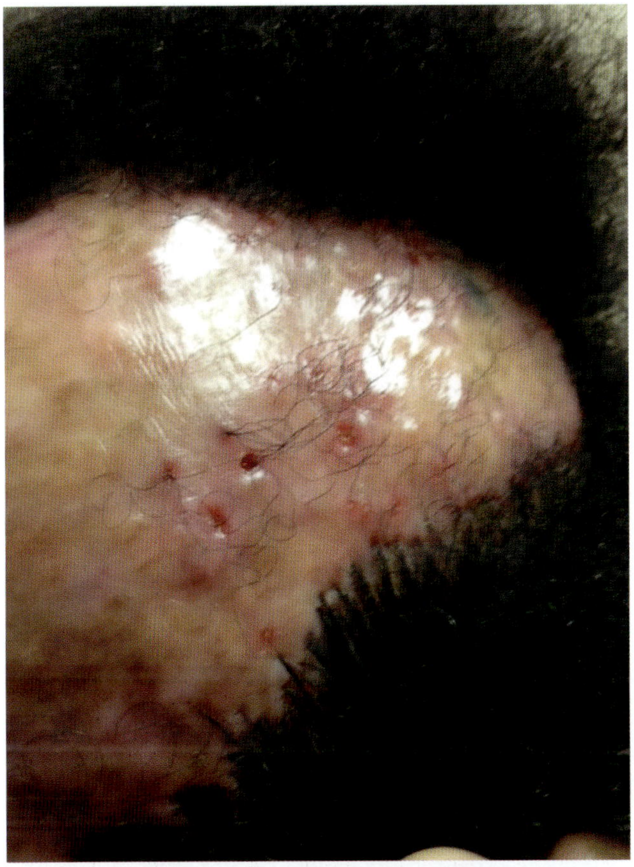

Fig. 18.3 Severe folliculitis decalvans keloidal scarring and tufted folliculitis in an African American male

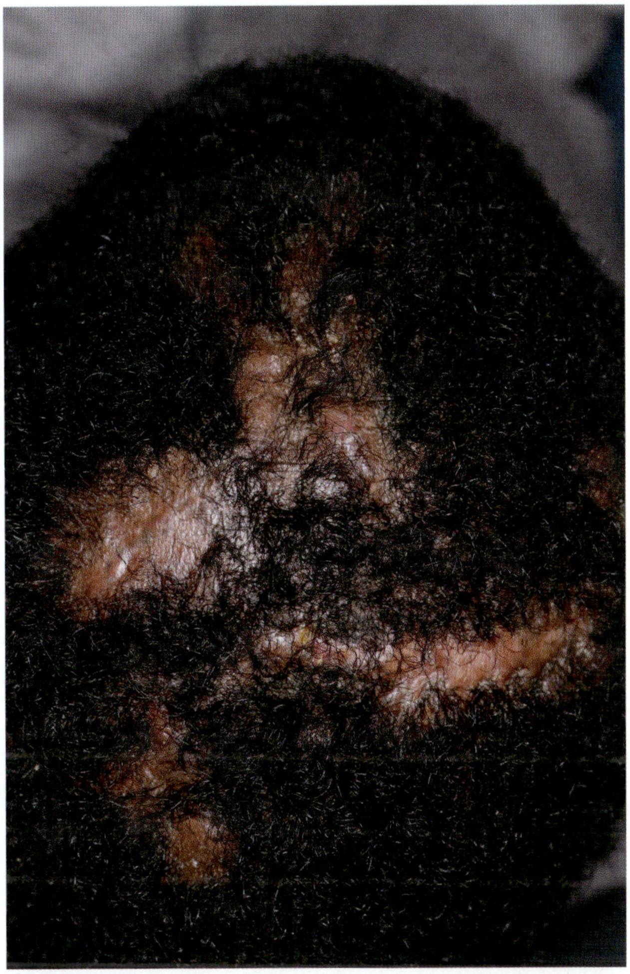

Fig. 18.4 Dissecting cellulitis in an African male (Courtesy of Service de Dermatologie, APHP Hospital Saint-Louis, Paris, France)

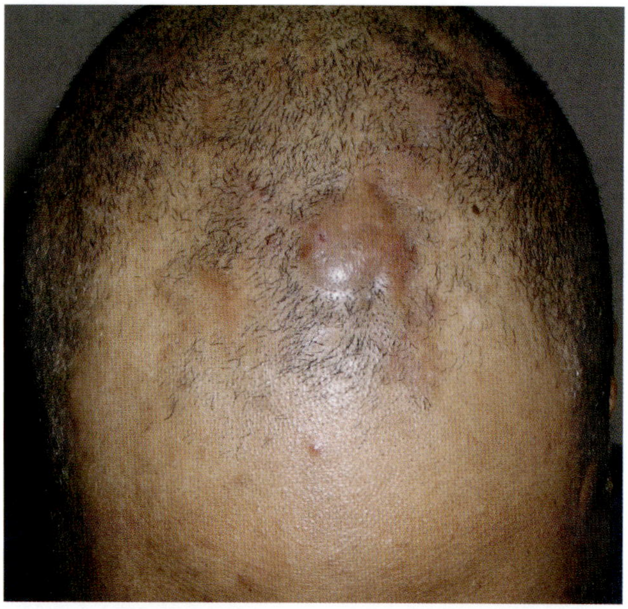

Fig. 18.5 Dissecting cellulitis in an African American male (Courtesy of Dr. Iltefat Hamzavi)

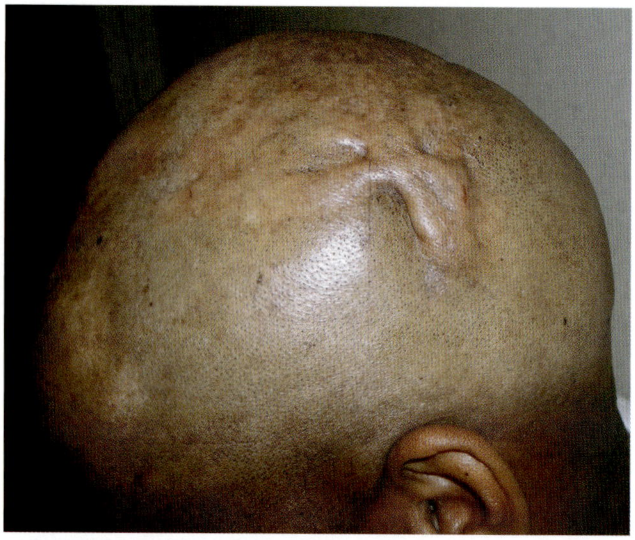

Fig. 18.7 Dissecting cellulitis with sinus tracts in an African American male (Courtesy of Dr. Iltefat Hamzavi)

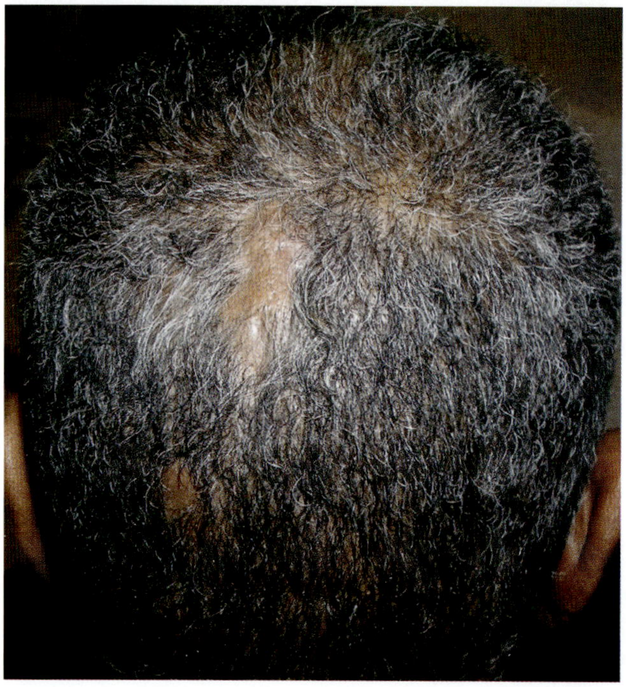

Fig. 18.6 Dissecting cellulitis in a Middle Eastern male (Courtesy of Dr. Iltefat Hamzavi)

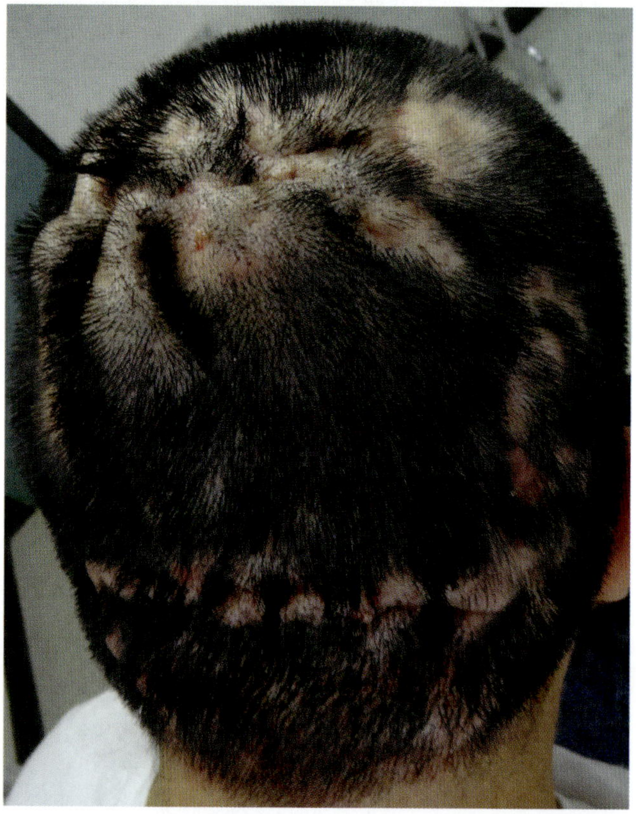

Fig. 18.8 Dissecting cellulitis with sinus tracts in a Hispanic male

18.4 Histopathologic Features

Histopathology of early lesions of FD shows keratin aggregation and a dilated infundibulum with an intrafollicular neutrophilic infiltrate [3, 5]. Even in early lesions there is a loss of sebaceous glands. More advanced lesions show a mixed infiltrate of neutrophils, lymphocytes, and plasma cells. Granulomatous inflammation with foreign body giant cells is seen around ectopic hair shafts. Follicular tufts with multiple hairs merging into one infundibulum are often seen. End-stage lesions exhibit fibrosis. Biopsies of dissecting cellulitis show distension of the follicular infundibula with a perifollicular neutrophilic infiltrate of the upper and middle portion of the hair follicle. Follicular rupture occurs and the infiltrate becomes a mixed pattern that includes lymphocytes, histiocytes, and plasma cells. Abscesses form in the adventitial dermis. Late-stage disease shows sinus tracts that are partially lined by squamous epithelium and dense fibrous scarring replacing follicular units.

18.5 Differential Diagnosis

Differential diagnosis of FD includes acne keloidalis nuchae, which affects males, especially African American males, disproportionately. Both disorders can have similar clinical and histopathologic features. Lichen planopilaris, discoid lupus, pseudopelade of Brocq, and central centrifugal cicatricial alopecia are lymphocytic primary cicatricial alopecias. Pustules are not the primary lesion in those disorders unless there is secondary bacterial infection. Tinea capitis can cause hair loss and pustules can be seen in inflammatory cases. Fungal cultures to rule out a dermatophyte infection such as kerion are recommended in all cases. Differential diagnosis of dissecting cellulitis includes folliculitis decalvans and acne keloidalis nuchae as well. These conditions may demonstrate perifollicular pustules and scarring alopecia; however, large abscesses and sinus tracts are usually not seen. Folliculotropic mycosis fungoides can sometimes resemble dissecting cellulitis and can be ruled out with a skin biopsy.

18.6 Treatment

Folliculitis decalvans often affects individuals for years and treatment is difficult. Topical treatment alone is not sufficient. Various oral antibiotics are used but relapse is common. Oral doxycycline, minocycline, clarithromycin, sulfamethoxazole-trimethoprim, and fusidic acid have been used alone and in combination. Rifampin is a very good antistaphylococcal agent, but resistance often occurs when used alone. A combination of rifampin 300 mg twice daily and clindamycin 300 mg twice daily has been used successfully and has reportedly given the best outcomes, with remission for months to years after treatment. Patients must be monitored for hepatitis, oral contraceptive failure, interaction with warfarin, hemolytic anemia, and thrombocytopenia when using rifampin. Pseudomembranous colitis is a side effect of clindamycin. Topical antibiotics such as mupirocin, clindamycin, fusidic acid, and erythromycin have also been used with oral antibiotics [2, 3, 6]. Intralesional, topical, and oral corticosteroids are used to reduce inflammation when used with oral antibiotics. Other reported treatments include dapsone, isotretinoin, topical tacrolimus [7], and ND-YAG laser [8].

Dissecting cellulitis is chronic and recalcitrant to a number of treatments and multiple modalities are usually necessary [9]. Oral antibiotics such as doxycycline and ciprofloxacin have been used, but relapse is common [10]. Concomitant use of topical antibiotics and intralesional and oral corticosteroids is useful [11]. Large abscesses should be incised and drained. Scerri et al. have reported long-standing remission with oral isotretinoin, 1 mg/kg/day for 4 months followed by a maintenance dosage of 0.75 mg/kg/day for 5–7 months [12]. Adalimumab has been used successfully to control dissecting cellulitis in a number of reported cases [13]. When medical treatment fails, follicular destruction with radiation, lasers, or surgical resection with skin grafting may be necessary.

References

1. Olsen EA, Bergfeld WF, Cotsarelis G, et al. Workshop on Cicatricial Alopecia. Summary of North American Hair Research Society (NAHRS)-sponsored Workshop on Cicatricial Alopecia. Duke University Medical Center, Feb 10 and 11, 2001. J Am Acad Dermatol. 2003;48:103–10.
2. Powell JJ, Dawber RP, Gatter K. Folliculitis decalvans including tufted folliculitis: clinical, histological and therapeutic findings. Br J Dermatol. 1999;140:328–33.
3. Whiting DA. Cicatricial alopecia: clinico-pathological findings and treatment. Clin Dermatol. 2001;19:211–5.
4. Chiarini C, Torchia D, Bianchi B, Volpi W, Caproni M, Fabbri P. Immunopathogenesis of folliculitis decalvans. Am J Clin Pathol. 2008;130:526–34.
5. Tan E, Martinka M, Ball N, Shapiro J. Primary cicatricial alopecias: clinicopathology of 112 cases. J Am Acad Dermatol. 2004;50: 25–32.
6. Otberg N, Kang H, Alzolibani A, Shapiro J. Folliculitis decalvans. Dermatol Ther. 2008;21:238–44.
7. Bastida J, Valeron-Almazon P, Santana-Molina N, Medina-Gil C, Carretero-Hernandez G. Treatment of folliculitis decalvans with tacrolimus ointment. Int J Dermatol. 2012;51:216–20.
8. Parlette E, Kroeger N, Ross V. Nd:YAG laser treatment of recalcitrant folliculitis decalvans. Dermatol Surg. 2004;30:1152–4.
9. Mundi JP, Marmon S, Fischer M, Kamino H, Patel R, Shapiro J. Dissecting cellulitis of the scalp. Dermatol Online J. 2012; 18(12):8.
10. Otberg N. Primary cicatricial alopecias. Dermatol Clin. 2013;31(1):155–66. W.B. Saunders.
11. Somani N, Bergfeld WF. Cicatricial alopecia: classification and histopathology. Dermatol Ther. 2008;18:12.
12. Scerri L, et al. Dissecting cellulitis of the scalp: response to isotretinoin. Br J Dermatol. 1996;134:1105.
13. Sukhatme SV, Lenzy YM, Gottlieb AB. Refractory dissecting cellulitis of the scalp treated with adalimumab. J Drugs Dermatol. 2008;7(10):981–3.

Traction Alopecia

19

Diane Jackson-Richards

Contents

19.1 Etiology

Traction alopecia (TA) is a common form of hair loss seen along the frontal and temporal hair line areas. Although any area of the scalp where tension is placed on the hair can be involved, it is usually seen in the frontotemporal areas. It is due to chronic use of tight hairstyles such as tight ponytails, tight braids, hair weaves, and hair rollers [1, 2]. Although not limited to one ethnic group, it is most often seen in African American women and girls, as these hairstyles are popular in this group. Traction alopecia is also commonly seen in young girls due to the custom of using tight hairstyles, which begins at a young age (Figs. 19.1 and 19.2). It is also seen in Sikh men and boys due to the cultural practice of pulling the hair back tightly [3]. The tight tension on the hair leads to loosening of the hair shaft from the follicle, after which folliculitis ensues. Traction alopecia has been classified as a "biphasic" or "transitional" alopecia as it is initially non-scarring, but later on becomes a scarring alopecia [4].

D. Jackson-Richards, MD
Department of Dermatology, Multicultural Dermatology Center,
Henry Ford Hospital, 3031 West Grand Blvd.,
Detroit, MI 48202, USA
e-mail: djackso1@hfhs.org

D. Jackson-Richards, A.G. Pandya (eds.), *Dermatology Atlas for Skin of Color*,
DOI 10.1007/978-3-642-54446-0_19,

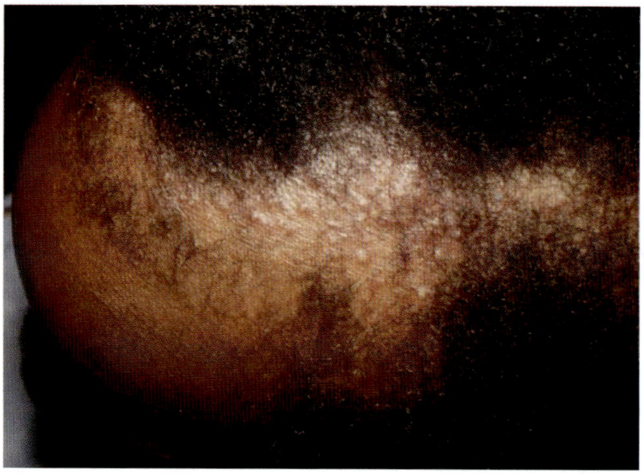

Fig. 19.1 Traction alopecia with pustules on the scalp of a young African American girl

19.2 Epidemiology

Studies on the incidence of traction alopecia have not been done; however it is usually seen in women of African descent. Hairstyles with tight cornrow braids and hair weaves are popular in this group. Although it has been observed in Sikh men and boys, it is mostly seen in African American women. Khumalo et al. studied 574 African schoolgirls and 604 women in the community in Cape Town, South Africa. Participants were evaluated for the presence of TA along with past and present hairstyling history. There were increased odds of TA appearing in adults compared to children, most likely related to a longer history of hairstyles that ultimately produces TA. The odds of TA in natural hair with traction in the form of braids, with or without added extensions, was higher than in those wearing long natural hair without extensions. In this study there seemed to be an even higher incidence of TA when extensions such as braids or weaves (Fig. 19.3) were added to chemically relaxed hair [5].

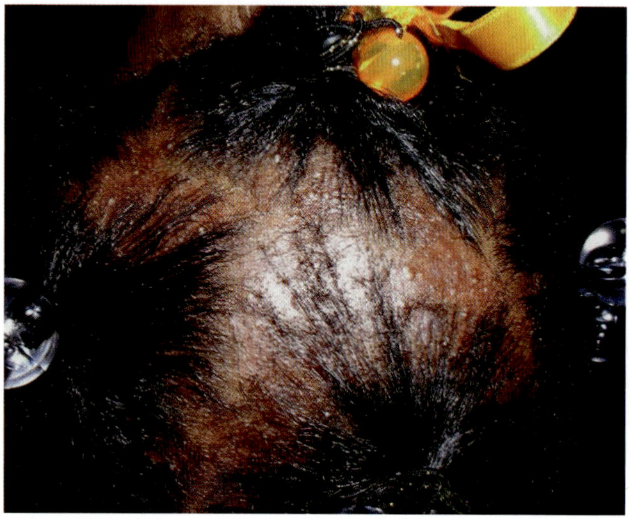

Fig. 19.2 Traction alopecia with pustules on the scalp of a young African American girl

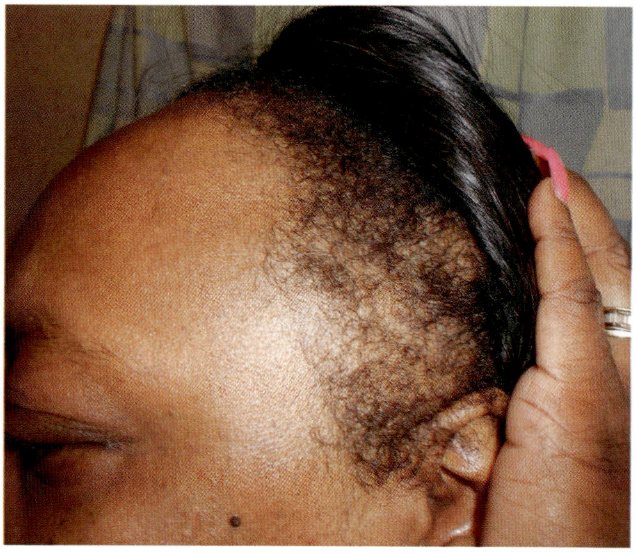

Fig. 19.3 Traction alopecia in an African American female wearing a hair weave

19.3 Clinical Features

Early on there may be mild perifollicular erythema, scaling, and pustules, usually at the frontotemporal hairline. Symptoms of pruritus or tenderness are usually mild or absent and erythema is subtle (Fig. 19.4). As the follicles atrophy, only short, thin vellus type hairs remain. Examination reveals a reduced number or absent follicular openings (Figs. 19.5 and 19.6). Eventually follicles atrophy and with chronic tension, permanent hair loss often results. A study by Samrao et al. looked at women with TA over a 3 ½ year period [3]. The groups studied included 29 % Hispanic women and 58.5 % African American women. This study described the "fringe" sign as a clinical feature of TA involving the marginal hairline. The "fringe" sign refers to those short, thin hairs that remain in TA and involve the frontotemporal hairline. This feature was felt to be a unique feature of TA not usually seen in other forms of hair loss affecting the frontotemporal areas. Although thin vellus-like hairs can be seen in alopecia areata with an ophiasis pattern, it is not usually prominent and symmetrical. The "fringe" sign is felt to be absent in frontal fibrosing alopecia.

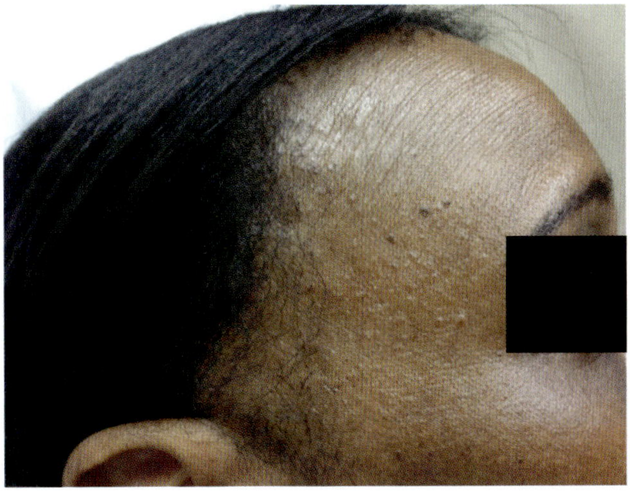

Fig. 19.5 Traction alopecia in an African American female

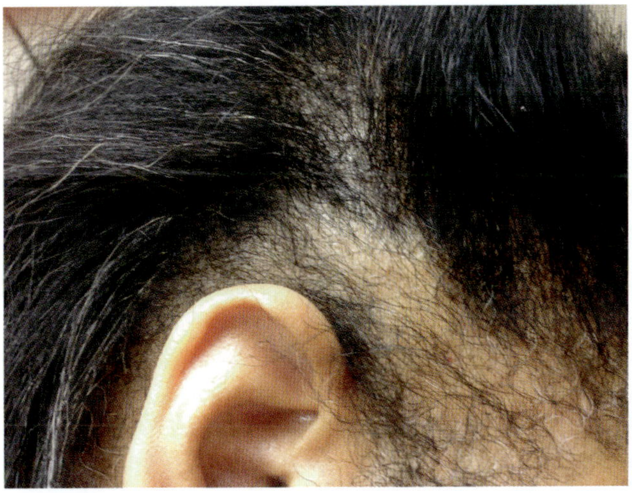

Fig. 19.4 Mild traction alopecia in an African American female

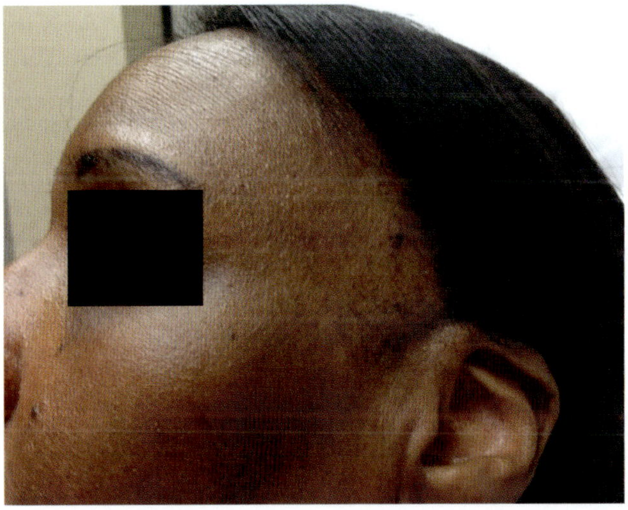

Fig. 19.6 Severe traction alopecia in an African American female

19.4 Histopathologic Features

Histopathology of early stages of traction alopecia shows trichomalacia and increased telogen and catagen hairs along with preserved sebaceous glands. With progression of TA there is follicular dropout of terminal hairs with vellus-sized hairs remaining. Inflammation in biopsies varies from mild in early disease to absent in more advanced cases. In late-stage TA, terminal follicles are replaced by fibrous tracts. In other forms of primary cicatricial alopecias, there is perifollicular inflammation and fibrosis along with loss of sebaceous glands. Histopathology of alopecia areata shows a peribulbar, lymphocytic infiltrate and lack of fibrous tracts [3].

19.5 Differential Diagnosis

Differential diagnosis for traction alopecia includes trichotillomania, ophiasis pattern alopecia areata, frontal fibrosing alopecia, and androgenetic alopecia.

19.6 Treatment

Discontinuation of the tension-producing hairstyle is the key to treatment of TA. If this is done early, permanent hair loss may be averted. Since patients may have discontinued tension-producing hairstyles for quite some time, a careful history of past hairstyling practices must be taken. If a bacterial folliculitis or secondary fungal process is present, these should be treated. Although there are no controlled studies, topical and intralesional corticosteroids may reduce inflammation and hair may regrow, providing follicles have not been permanently damaged. There have been reports of topical minoxidil being helpful in some patients [6]. Severe cases of traction alopecia can be treated with hair transplantation or rotation flap transplantation, but consideration must be given to scarring as a result of these procedures.

References

1. McMichael A. Hair and scalp disorders in ethnic populations. Dermatol Clin. 2003;21(4):629–44.
2. Callender V, McMichael A, Cohen G. Medical and surgical therapies for alopecias in black women. Dermatol Ther. 2004;17:164–76.
3. Samrao A, Price V, Zedek D, Mirmirani P. The "Fringe Sign"- a useful clinical finding in traction alopecia of the marginal hair line. Dermatol Online J. 2011;17(11):1.
4. Somani N, Bergfeld W. Cicatricial alopecia: classification and histopathology. Dermatol Ther. 2008;21:221–37.
5. Khumalo N, Jessop S, Gumedze F, Ehrlich R. Determinants of marginal traction alopecia in African girls and women. J Am Acad Dermatol. 2008;59:432–8.
6. Khumalo N, Ngwanya R. Traction alopecia: 2 % topical minoxidil shows promise. Report of two cases. J Eur Acad Dermatol Venereol. 2007;21:433–44.

Part III

Papulosquamous and Eczematous Disorders

Atopic Dermatitis

20

Diane Jackson-Richards

Contents

D. Jackson-Richards, MD
Department of Dermatology, Multicultural Dermatology Center,
Henry Ford Hospital, 3031 West Grand Blvd.,
Detroit, MI 48202, USA
e-mail: djackso1@hfhs.org

20.1 Epidemiology

Atopic dermatitis (AD) is a chronic inflammatory skin condition that affects 10–20 % of children worldwide. Although it affects infants, children, and adults, 90 % of patients with atopic dermatitis have onset of the disease before the age of 5 [1]. Because of this, much of the epidemiologic data is from studies performed in children. A 1995 study by Williams et al. found a twofold prevalence of AD in black Caribbean children compared to white children born in London, England. In 2002, Janumpally et al. looked at office visits for AD using data of the National Ambulatory Medical Care Survey (NAMCS) from 1990 to 1998. Blacks were three times and Asian/Pacific Islanders six times more likely than whites to be seen for AD [2]. Kim et al. studied 4,028 Korean children and found an AD incidence of 9.5 %. Decker et al. has found an increasing incidence of AD in Africa, East Asia, and Western and Northern Europe. A study by Shaw et al. looked at the incidence in the USA overall as well as in each specific state within the USA. This study used the 2003 data of the National Survey of Children's Health sponsored by the federal Maternal and Child Health Bureau. They found an incidence of 10.7 % of children overall in the USA and 15.9 % in black children. In general, this study showed a higher AD prevalence in urban environments, black race, and household education greater than high school [3].

20.2 Etiology

The etiology of atopic dermatitis is a complex interplay of genetic and environmental factors that is not fully understood. There is an association with asthma, allergic rhinitis, or family history of AD in 30–70 % of patients. A genetic tendency for a compromised epidermal barrier, along with environmental influences, is thought to produce the disease. Within anucleated stratum corneum cells, the plasma membrane is replaced by a layer of large protein molecules of which filaggrin (FLG) is a component. FLG plays an important role in

D. Jackson-Richards, A.G. Pandya (eds.), *Dermatology Atlas for Skin of Color*,
DOI 10.1007/978-3-642-54446-0_20, © Springer-Verlag Berlin Heidelberg 2014

the cohesion of the stratum corneum and the production of humectants or natural moisturizers of the skin [4]. Filaggrin (FLG) gene mutations were first proposed as a cause of ichthyosis vulgaris by Sybert et al. in 1985. Atopic dermatitis is divided into two subsets: extrinsic AD and intrinsic AD. FLG gene mutations along with elevated serum IgE (immunoglobulin E) levels are seen in extrinsic AD but not intrinsic AD. Intrinsic AD has relative late onset and milder severity. FLG gene mutations alone are not the sole factor in the disease. AD patients with FLG gene mutations are felt to have more severe and persistent disease [5].

Antigen-presenting cells such as Langerhans cells present antigens and stimulate the infiltration of Th lymphocytes. Differentiation of ThO lymphocytes is toward the Th2 subset. Th2 lymphocytes secrete the proinflammatory cytokines IL-3, IL-4, IL-5, and IL-13 and stimulate a humoral immune response. IL-13 has been associated with dermatitis and pruritus in experimental animals. In the chronic phase of the disease, there is a shift toward the Th1 subset, which secretes growth factor beta, interferon gamma, IL-12, IL-11, and IL-18 and activates the cellular immune response.

Patients with AD are often colonized with *Staphylococcus aureus*. The Th2 environment inhibits production of antimicrobial peptides which predisposes the skin to secondary infections. Inflamed, excoriated skin is more susceptible to *S. aureus* which produces superantigen-specific IgE. This superantigen-specific IgE degranulates mast cells and leads to further inflammation.

20.3 Clinical Features

Atopic dermatitis presents with erythematous, thin plaques with fine scaling and xerosis. Acute lesions may show serous drainage and crusting. Because of the intense pruritus of AD, excoriations are usually seen. In infants, lesions are typically seen on the face and extensor extremities. Although AD involves many areas of the skin, the posterior neck, hands, and antecubital and popliteal fossa are commonly involved (Figs. 20.1, 20.2, 20.3, and 20.4). Erythema is difficult to assess in darker skin and should not be relied upon to determine severity of disease. The presence of edema, warmth of the skin, and scale can help to make the diagnosis in this group of patients. Perifollicular accentuation or papular eczema is more commonly seen in African Americans (Figs. 20.5 and 20.6). As the condition becomes more chronic, lesions evolve into thickened, lichenified plaques (Figs. 20.7, 20.8, 20.9, and 20.10).

Chronic AD often results in postinflammatory hyper- and hypopigmentation in long-standing lesions (Fig. 20.11). Diffuse xerosis, even in uninvolved areas of the skin, is common and a result of impaired barrier function (Fig. 20.12). Patients with severe AD may become erythrodermic (Fig. 20.13). Dennie-Morgan lines or prominent skin folds of the lower eyelids are often present, as well as hyperlinearity of the palms.

Patients with AD are more prone to superimposed skin infections (Fig. 20.14). *S. aureus* is often cultured from the skin and nares of AD patients and should be considered when patients are unresponsive to treatment. Molluscum contagiosum and eczema herpeticum, a form of widespread herpes simplex infection, can be complications. A high percentage of AD patients also have asthma or allergic rhinitis. The American Academy of Dermatology Consensus Conference on Pediatric AD has established major and minor criteria for diagnosis of AD. Major criteria include pruritus, eczematous changes consistent with those described above, and a chronic, relapsing course. Minor criteria include periorbital involvement, perifollicular accentuation, palmar hyperlinearity, keratosis pilaris, and ichthyosis vulgaris. AD is a chronic, relapsing disorder and although some patients improve after childhood, 40 % may have disease into adulthood. A form of eczema on the hands, known as dyshidrotic eczema, presents as small papules and vesicles on the sides of the palms and fingers accompanied by pruritus (Fig. 20.15).

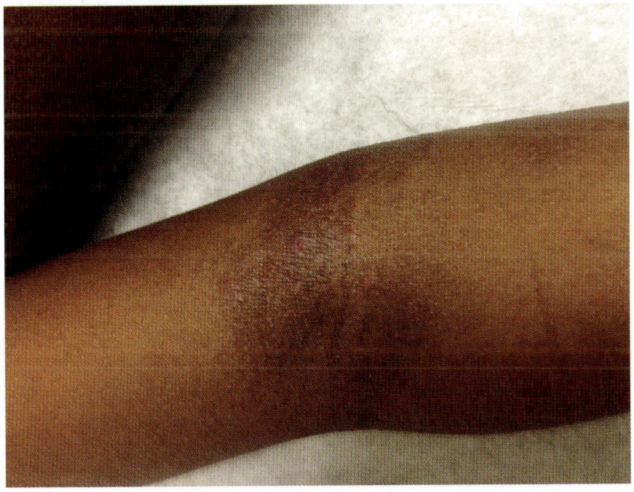

Fig. 20.1 AD involving antecubital fossa in an AA boy

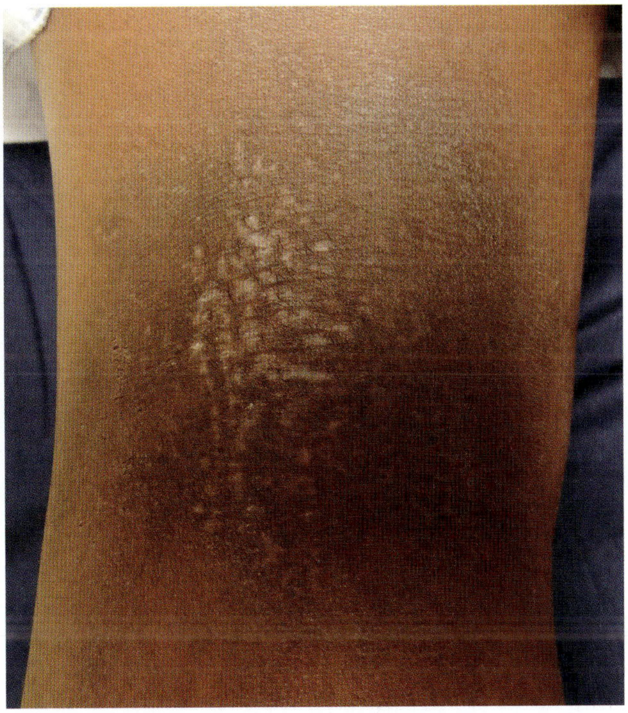

Fig. 20.2 AD on popliteal fossa in an AA girl

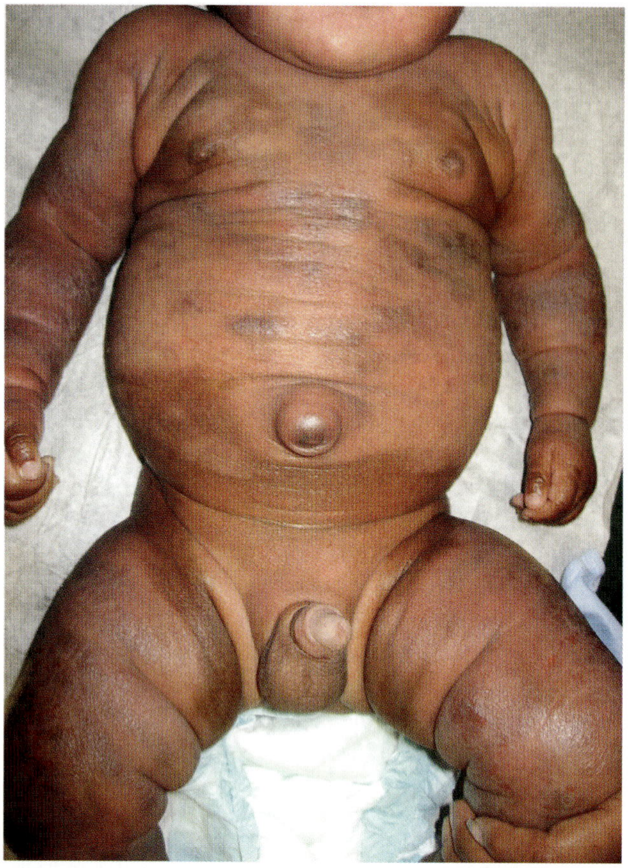

Fig. 20.3 AD in a 5-month-old AA male infant (Courtesy of Dr Tor Shwayder)

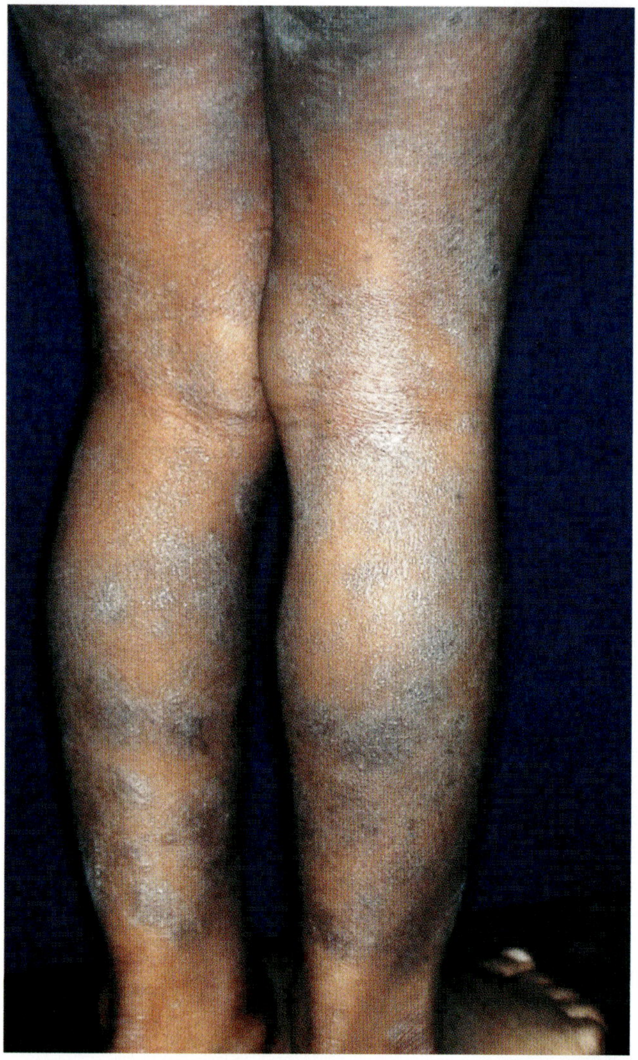

Fig. 20.4 AD on legs of a 3-year-old AA child (Courtesy of Dr Tor Shwayder)

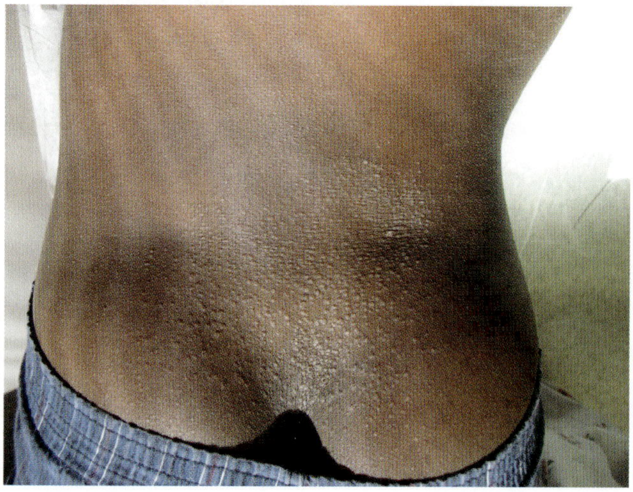

Fig. 20.5 Papular eczema on trunk of a AA male (Courtesy of Dr Tor Shwayder)

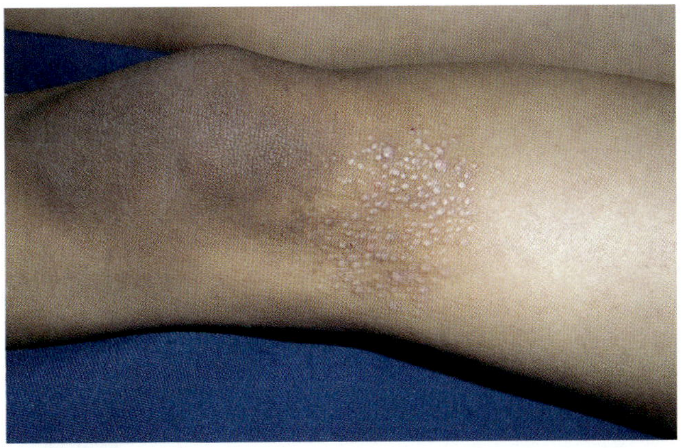

Fig. 20.6 Papular eczema on the leg of an AA girl (Courtesy of Dr Tor Shwayder)

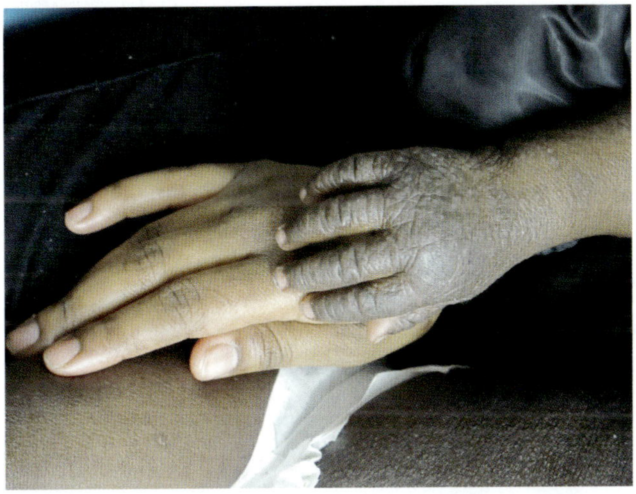

Fig. 20.7 Lichenified AD on hand of an AA infant (Courtesy of Dr Tor Shwayder)

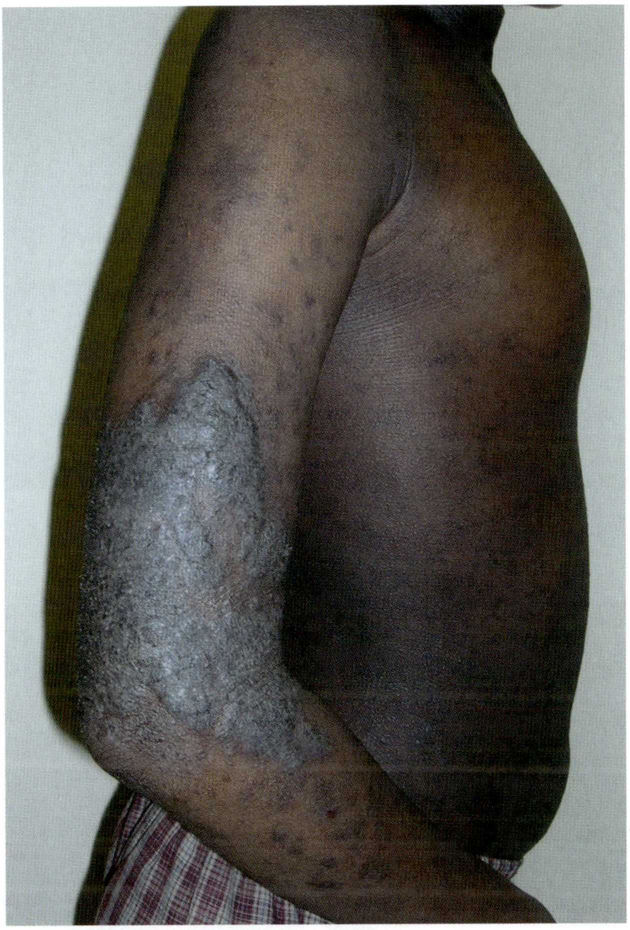

Fig. 20.8 Lichenified AD on the arm of an AA boy (Courtesy of Dr Tor Shwayder)

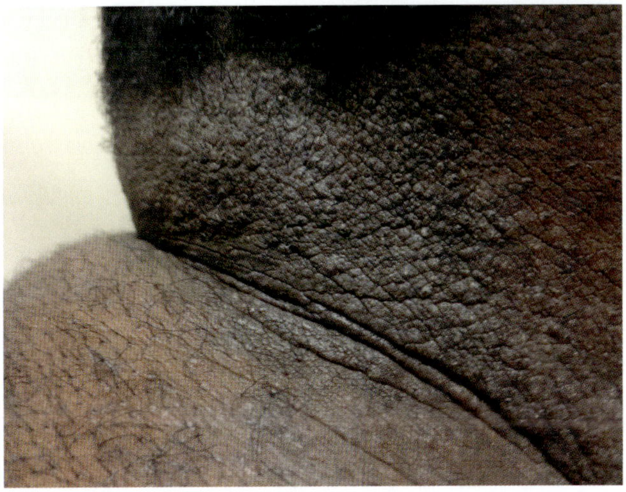

Fig. 20.9 Severe AD with lichenification in an adult AA male

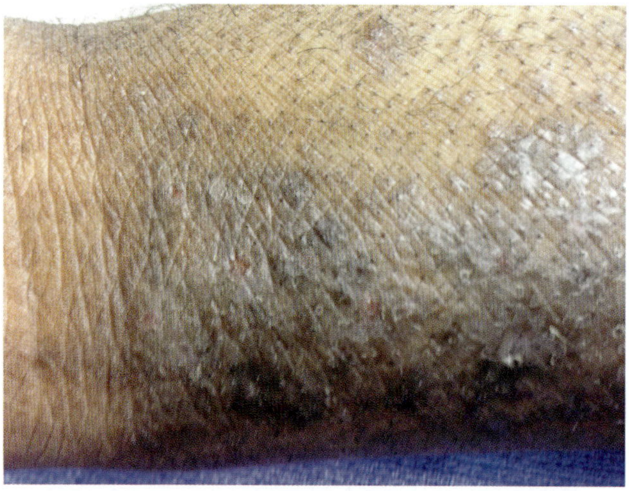

Fig. 20.10 Lichenification and excoriations in an AA male with AD

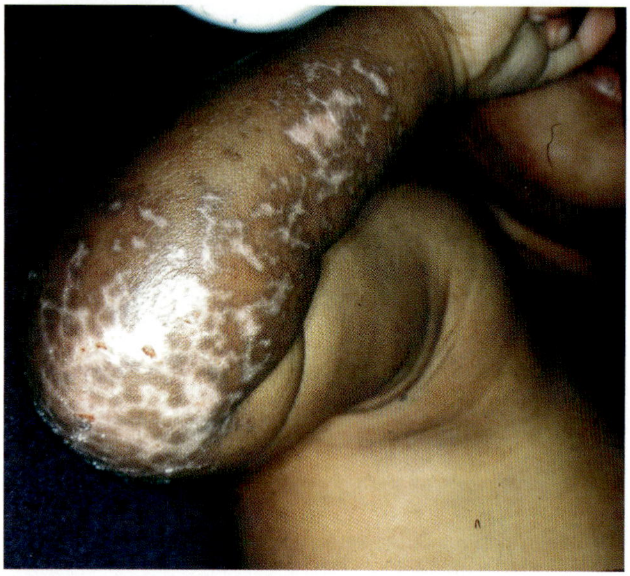

Fig. 20.11 Severe AD with dyschromia in an AA child (Courtesy of Dr Tor Shwayder)

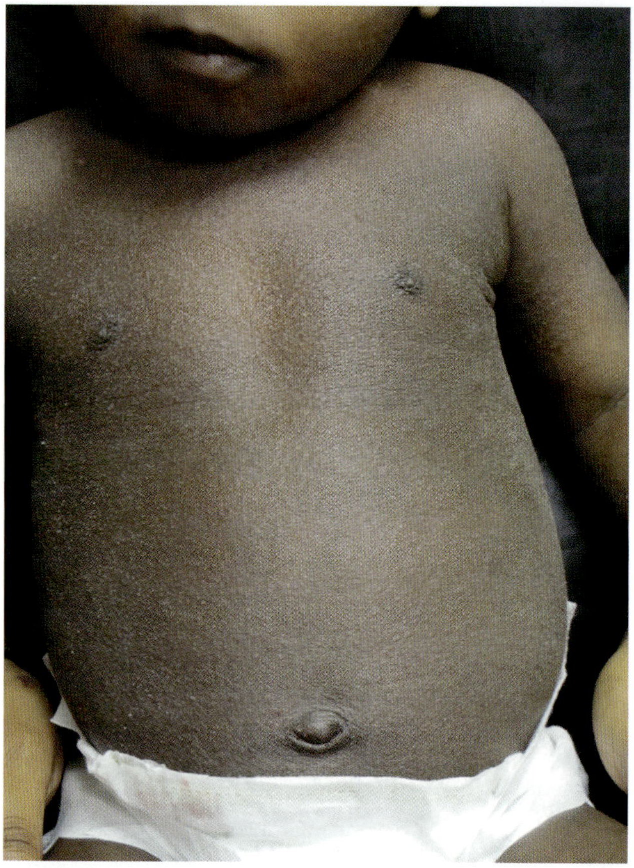

Fig. 20.12 Diffuse xerosis and extensive AD in an AA infant (Courtesy of Dr Tor Shwayder)

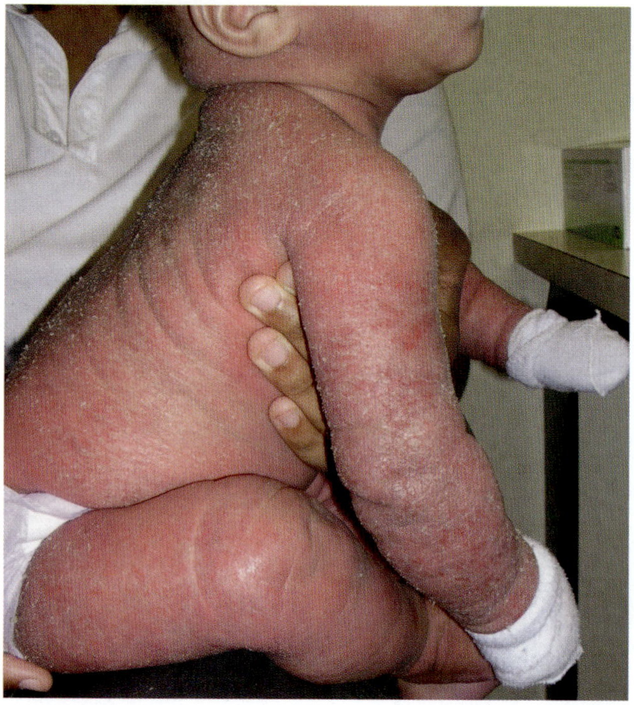

Fig. 20.13 Severe erythrodermic AD in an African American infant (Courtesy of Dr Tor Shwayder)

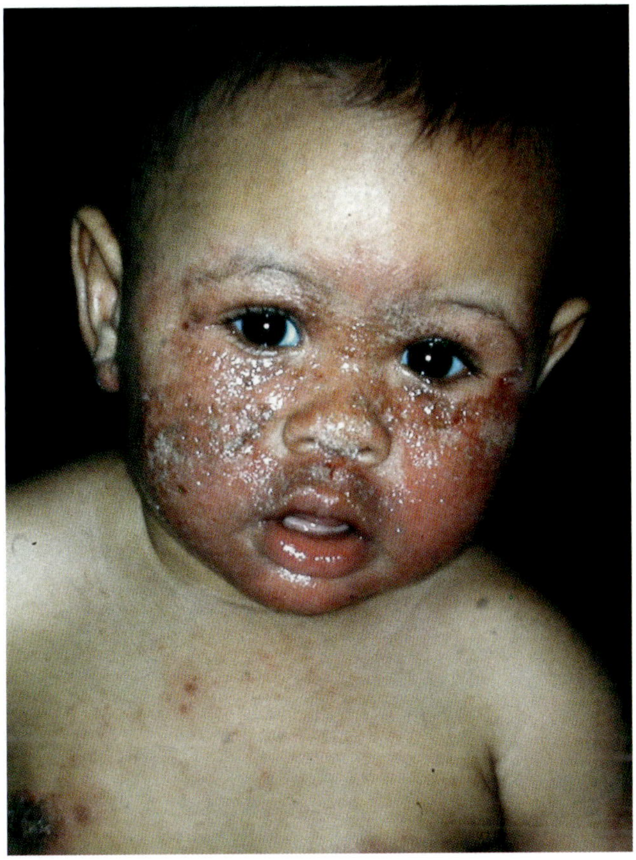

Fig. 20.14 AD with *S. aureus* infection in a Filipino infant (Courtesy of Dr Tor Shwayder)

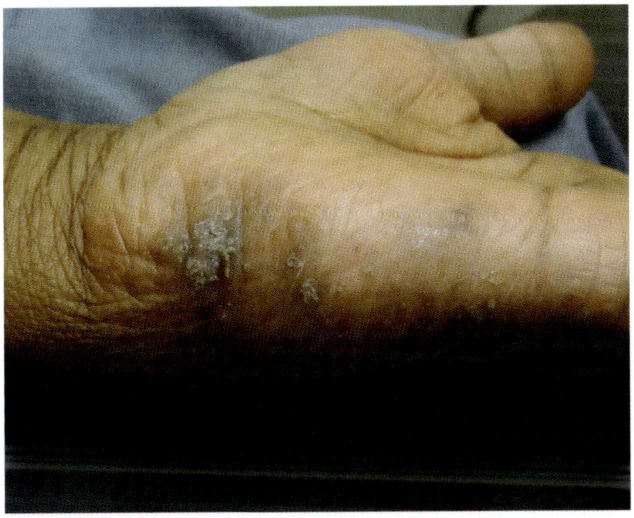

Fig. 20.15 Dyshidrotic eczema of the hand in an AA female

20.4 Histopathologic Features

The histopathology of AD shows epidermal edema or spongiosis. Lymphocytes are seen in the epidermis and in the upper dermis in a perivascular pattern. As lesions become more chronic, the epidermis may become thickened in a psoriasiform pattern and the spongiosis and lymphocytes diminish. Total serum IgE levels may be elevated but are not specific to AD.

20.5 Differential Diagnosis

Atopic dermatitis is diagnosed by the history and classic skin features described above. The pathology does not have a unique, distinguishing feature. Although rare, Wiskott-Aldrich syndrome or hyperimmunoglobulin E syndrome can present with eczematous skin changes. Adults with dermatitis that is unresponsive to corticosteroids should have a biopsy to rule out cutaneous T-cell lymphoma (CTCL). Multiple biopsies or biopsy of an untreated lesion may be necessary to rule out CTCL.

20.6 Treatment

Although topical corticosteroids and emollients are the mainstay of therapy for AD, avoiding known triggers of the disease is important. Harsh detergents, fragrances, and wool clothing should be avoided. Only mild, non-alkali soaps should be used for skin cleansing. Moisturizers that contain ceramides, petroleum, or urea are important for improving the barrier function of the skin. Sodium hypochlorite or "bleach baths" (1/4–1/2 cup of bleach in a half or full bathtub of water) two to three times a week along with intranasal mupirocin ointment [6] reduces *S. aureus* colonization of the skin. A topical corticosteroid, appropriate for the age of the patient and extent of disease, should be used twice a day along with emollients. Once the acute flare has been controlled, long-term maintenance with a mid-potency topical corticosteroid is typical, but caution must be taken to avoid skin atrophy or HPA (hypothalamus pituitary axis) suppression. Topical calcineurin inhibitors (TCIs) are macrolactams that inhibit activation of T-lymphocytes and thereby decrease the release of cytokines. Long-term maintenance with TCIs can reduce the side effects of atrophy and HPA suppression. In 2006, the FDA imposed black box warning on TCIs citing rare cases of malignancy although noting that a causal relationship was not established. The studies in animal models were based on systemic administration rather than topical and at doses that were 26–340 times greater than those given to humans. In 2012 the American Academy of Dermatology endorsed that TCIs are safe with proper use and reduce the debilitating effects of AD [7]. Antihistamines are also helpful for associated pruritus.

For more recalcitrant cases, narrowband UVB light treatments starting at 50–70 % of the minimal erythema dose (MED) and increasing by 10–20 % per treatment three times weekly may significantly improve or clear patients. On average 24–30 treatments were required and remission duration of 3–6 months or longer has been achieved. Short courses of oral corticosteroids can be used for an acute flare but should not be relied upon for frequent or long-term therapy. Cyclosporine and mycophenolate mofetil with appropriate monitoring have also been used successfully for severe cases [8].

References

1. Williams HC, Grindlay DJ. What's new in atopic eczema? An analysis of the clinical significance of systematic reviews on atopic eczema published in 2006 and 2007. Clin Exp Dermatol. 2008;33(6):685–8.
2. Janumpally SR, Feldman SR, Gupta AK, Fleischer Jr AB. In the United States, blacks and Asian/Pacific Islanders are more likely than whites to seek medical care for atopic dermatitis. Arch Dermatol. 2002;138(5):634–7.
3. Shaw T, Currie GP, Koudelka CW, Simpson EL. Eczema prevalence in the United States: data from the 2003 National Survey of Children's Health. J Invest Dermatol. 2011;131:67–73.
4. Eichenfield LF, Ellis CN, Mancini AJ, Paller AS, Simpson EL. Atopic dermatitis: epidemiology and pathogenesis update. Semin Cutan Med Surg. 2012;31:S3–5. Elsevier, Inc.
5. Kabashima K. New concept of the pathogenesis of atopic dermatitis: interplay among the barrier, allergy and pruritus as a trinity. J Dermatol Sci. 2013;70:3–11.
6. Huahg J, Abrams M, et al. Treatment of Staphylococcus aureus colonization in atopic dermatitis decreases disease severity. Pediatrics. 2009;123(5):e808–14.
7. Carr WW. Topical calcineurin inhibitors for atopic dermatitis: review and treatment recommendations. Paediatr Drugs. 2013;15(4):303–10.
8. Tan A, Gonzalez M. Management of severe atopic dermatitis in children. J Drugs Dermatol. 2012;11(10):1158–65.

Seborrheic Dermatitis

21

Diane Jackson-Richards

Contents

21.1 Etiology

Seborrheic dermatitis (SD) is a very common, chronic inflammatory skin disorder that affects areas of the skin with high sebum production. Unna first described the condition in 1887, but it was Malassez who first observed a fungal organism in flakes of skin taken from the scalp of patients with SD. Malassezia is a lipophilic fungus found in normal flora of the skin. The exact pathophysiology of SD has not been established, but Malassezia yeast on the skin is felt to play a role [1]. In 1989, Bergbrant and Faergman failed to find a difference in the amount of Malassezia on the skin of individuals with SD versus control subjects or between lesional and nonlesional skin. Bergbrant proposes that it is not the quantity of Malassezia on the skin but the quantity of lipids and an individual's immune response to the fungus that determines if SD will develop [2]. Patients with SD have normal sebum production, but the skin surface lipids show an increase in triglycerides and cholesterol along with a decrease in squalene and free fatty acids. When lymphocytes of SD patients were exposed to Malassezia extracts, there was a reduction in IL-2 and IFN-gamma but an increase in IL-10. These mechanisms may play a role in pathogenesis. Other investigators have found a normal level of circulating antibodies to Malassezia, suggesting that humoral immunity to Malassezia does not play a major role in etiology. It has also been suggested that an irritant, nonallergic response to Malassezia may be the cause of SD.

D. Jackson-Richards, MD
Department of Dermatology, Multicultural Dermatology Center, Henry Ford Hospital, 3031 West Grand Blvd., Detroit, MI 48202, USA
e-mail: djackso1@hfhs.org

D. Jackson-Richards, A.G. Pandya (eds.), *Dermatology Atlas for Skin of Color*,
DOI 10.1007/978-3-642-54446-0_21,

21.2 Epidemiology

There are two forms of seborrheic dermatitis, an infantile form and an adult form. Infantile SD occurs from birth to 3 months of age, while the adult form peaks at ages 30–60. Seborrheic dermatitis affects all races. The prevalence of adult SD in the United States is 3–5 %. The incidence may be much higher, considering that dandruff, which is a mild form of SD, is quite common and underreported. There is a higher incidence of SD in HIV-positive individuals, ranging from 31 to 85 %. A higher prevalence of SD is also seen in patients with Parkinson's disease or those with other neurological disorders such as traumatic brain or spinal cord injury and cerebrovascular accidents [1].

21.3 Clinical Findings

Infantile SD usually occurs shortly after birth with yellowish, greasy scale on the scalp that is often referred to as "cradle cap." There may be progression to erythematous, scaly lesions on the face, retroauricular area, axillae, and inguinal folds (Fig. 21.1). Infants with SD are usually not irritable and the condition resolves around 3 months of age. For adults, SD is a chronic, relapsing disorder. Typically the scalp exhibits diffuse fine, white, or greasy scale (Figs. 21.2, 21.3, and 21.4). More significant disease manifests as erythema and pruritus associated with the scale. Often, thin erythematous, scaly plaques may extend beyond the frontal scalp onto the forehead. On the face, lesions are often symmetrical with erythema and scaling of the nasolabial folds, malar areas, glabella, and eyebrows (Fig. 21.5). Other commonly involved areas are the external ear, retroauricular area, and presternal or intertriginous skin. In men, the beard and mustache areas are commonly involved. Hypopigmentation is often seen on the facial lesions of darker- skinned individuals (Figs. 21.6, 21.7, and 21.8). This postinflammatory hypopigmentation usually improves with treatment. Pruritus may be mild to moderate. Patients with HIV infection may have extensive SD on the face, neck, scalp, and upper trunk (Fig. 21.9).

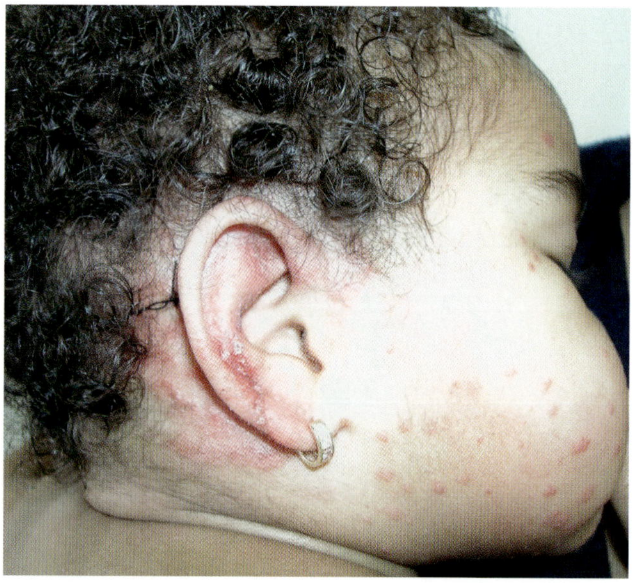

Fig. 21.1 SD in an AA infant (Courtesy of Dr Tor Shwayder)

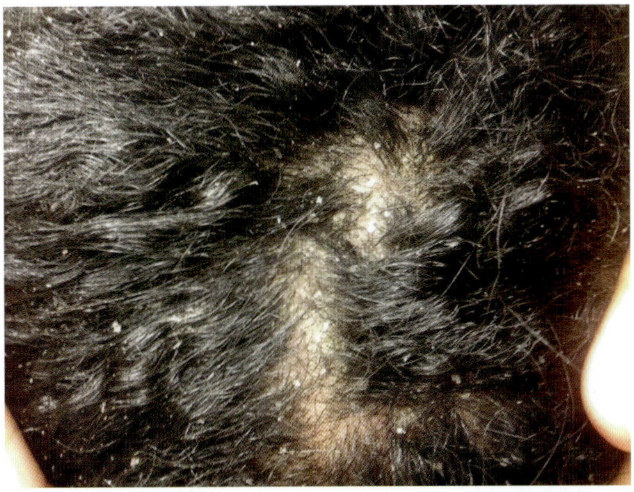

Fig. 21.2 SD of the scalp in an AA female

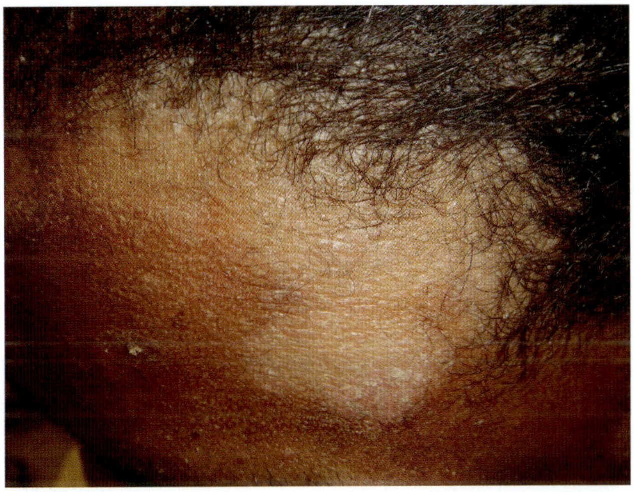

Fig. 21.3 SD of frontal scalp in an AA female (Courtesy of Dr Henry Lim)

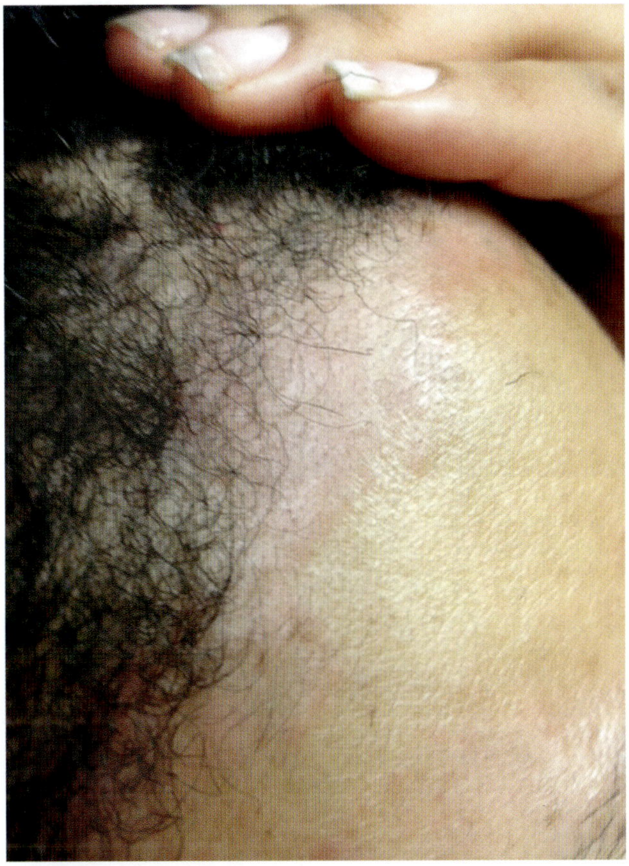

Fig. 21.4 SD along frontal hairline in an AA female

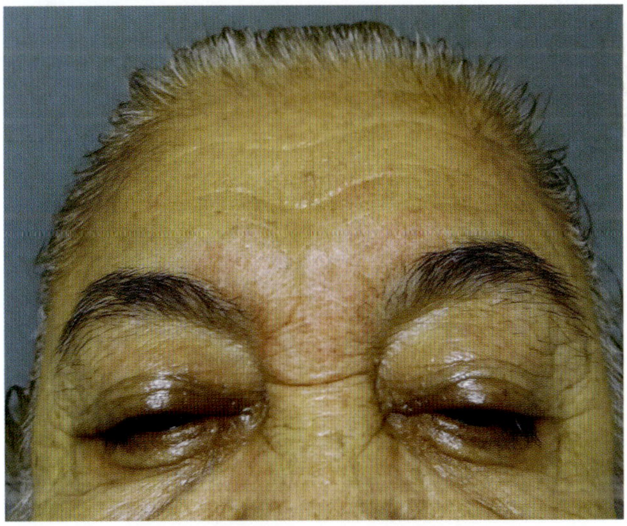

Fig. 21.5 SD of forehead in a Hispanic female

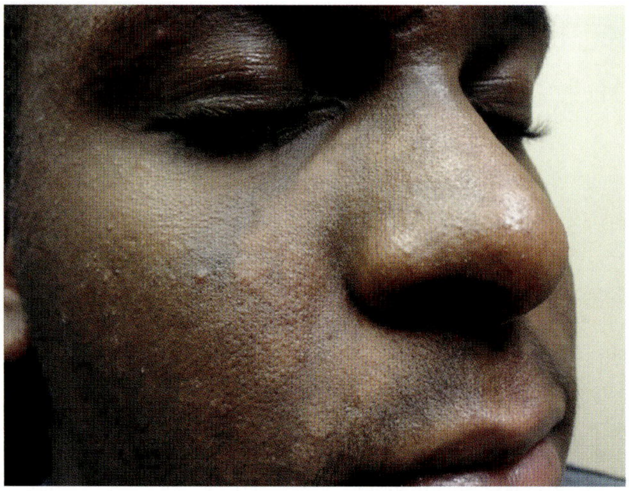

Fig. 21.6 SD of the face in an AA male with postinflammatory hypopigmentation

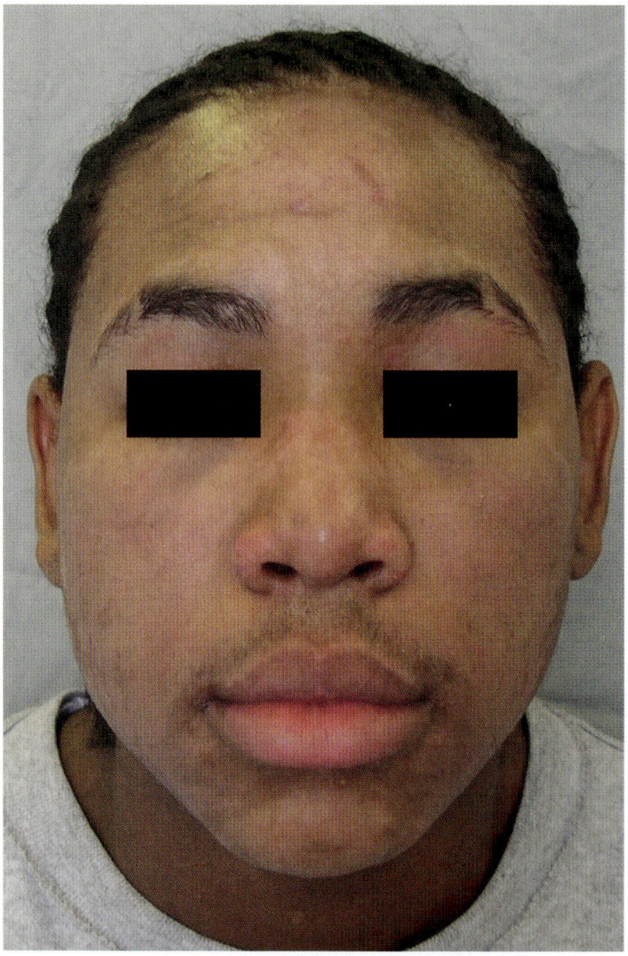

Fig. 21.7 Extensive SD of the face in an AA male with postinflammatory hypopigmentation (Courtesy of Dr. Tor Shwayder)

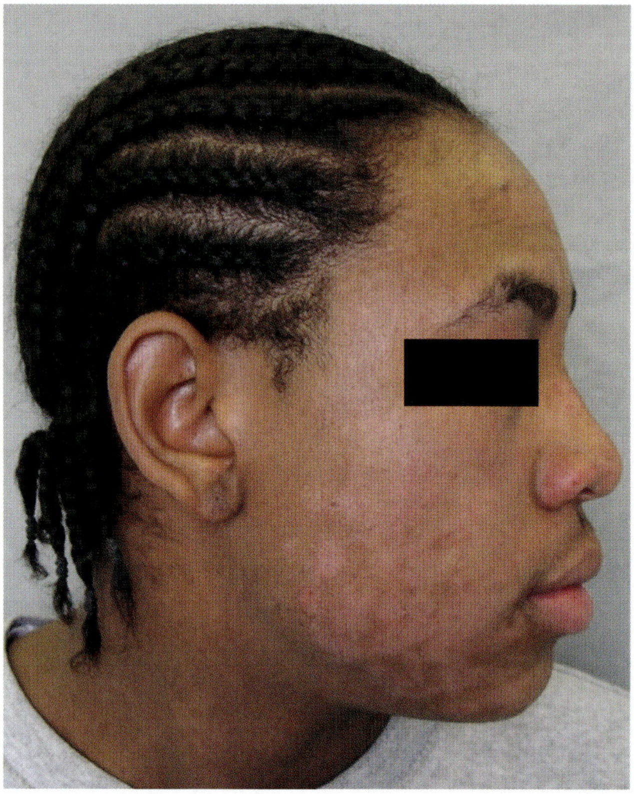

Fig. 21.8 Extensive SD of the face in an AA male with postinflammatory hypopigmentation (Courtesy of Dr. Tor Shwayder)

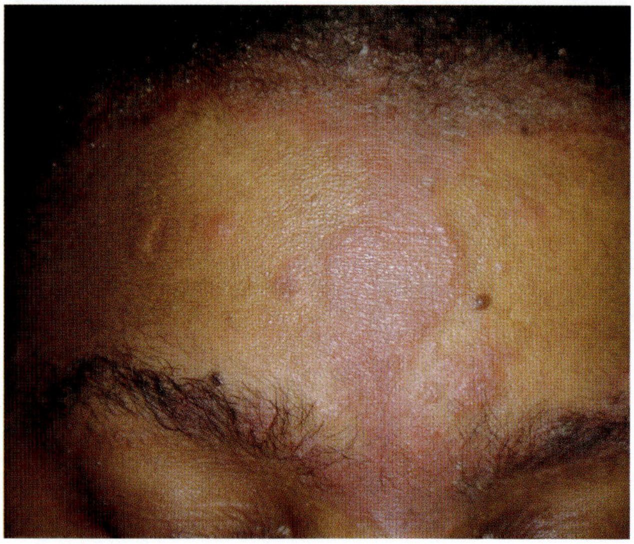

Fig. 21.9 SD of forehead in an AA female with HIV infection (Courtesy of Dr. Henry Lim)

21.4 Histopathology

The histopathology of SD shows a superficial lymphocytic infiltrate with mild to moderate spongiosis. With more chronic lesions there is psoriasiform hyperplasia with dilatation of superficial capillaries [2]. The histologic features may be difficult to distinguish from psoriasis; however, psoriasis tends not to show spongiosis, while SD tends not to have Munro's microabscesses in the epidermis.

21.5 Differential Diagnosis

In cases of extensive infantile SD, atopic dermatitis, tinea capitis, and Langerhans cell histiocytosis should be ruled out. In adults, facial lesions of acute cutaneous lupus, rosacea, and psoriasis can be confused with SD. SD in body folds can resemble inverse psoriasis, erythrasma, or irritant dermatitis. If an adult presents with marked SD for the first time or there is sudden worsening of SD, testing for HIV should be considered.

21.6 Treatment

The first reported use of ketoconazole to treat SD was in 1984. Various topical antifungals, particularly the azoles, continue to be the basis of treatment for SD. Topical azoles as well as ciclopirox are used in the form of creams, lotions, or shampoos. Ciclopirox has both anti-inflammatory and antifungal properties. Another azole, miconazole, has also been used successfully in the treatment of SD [3]. Zinc pyrithione and selenium sulfide shampoos are usually very helpful in SD treatment [4]. Topical corticosteroids are commonly used in combination with topical antifungals; however, with long-term use there is concern over tachyphylaxis, atrophy, and perioral dermatitis. Care must be given to the choice of treatment, as African American patients may find some shampoos and solution-based topicals very drying to hair that is inherently dry and brittle. Shampooing more frequently than once a week is not reasonable in this racial group, particularly for African American women. Choosing a topical corticosteroid with an emollient base is also more cosmetically acceptable for this group. Topical calcineurin inhibitors such as tacrolimus and pimecrolimus are quite helpful in the treatment of SD. These agents are particularly helpful for resistant cases and provide prolonged remission without the side effects of topical corticosteroids. A study by High and Pandya treated African American adults for facial SD with 1 % pimecrolimus cream twice daily for 16 weeks. Not only was there improvement in the erythema and scaling but significant improvement in the associated hypopigmentation seen in the affected patients [5]. Although most cases of SD can be managed with topical treatment, oral antifungals can be used in severe cases. Terbinafine 250 mg daily for 4 weeks, ketoconazole 200 mg daily for 14 days, and itraconazole 200 mg daily for 1 week followed by 200 mg once every 2 weeks have been used, but the risk of these systemic treatments should be given consideration.

References

1. Hay RJ. Malassezia, dandruff and seborrheic dermatitis: an overview. Br J Dermatol. 2011;65(2):2–8.
2. Sampaio AL, Vargas TJ, Nunes AP, Mameri AC, Ramos-e-Silva CM, Carneiro SC. Seborrheic dermatitis. An Bras Dermatol. 2011;86(6):1061–74.
3. Buechner S. Multicenter, double-blind, parallel group study investigating the non-inferiority of efficacy and safety of a 2 % miconazole nitrate shampoo in comparison with a 2 % ketoconazole shampoo in the treatment of seborrheic dermatitis of the scalp. J Dermatol Treat. 2014;25(3):226–31.
4. Stefanaki I, Katsambas A. Therapeutic update on seborrheic dermatitis. Skin Therapy Lett. 2010;15(5):1–4.
5. High WA, Pandya AG. Pilot trial of 1 % pimecrolimus cream in the treatment of seborrheic dermatitis in African American adults with associated hypopigmentation. J Am Acad Dermatol. 2006;54:1083–8.

Lichen Planus, Nitidus, and Striatus

22

Daniel Condie and Amit G. Pandya

Contents

22.1 Lichen Planus

22.1.1 Epidemiology

Lichen planus (LP) is an inflammatory disease of unknown cause affecting the skin, scalp, nails, and mucous membranes. LP primarily affects middle-aged adults (ages 30–60) and is estimated to affect 0.5–1.0 % of the population worldwide [1]. Childhood LP typically accounts for 5 % or less of cases, and some studies report a higher incidence in patients with skin of color, particularly South Asians and African-Americans [2, 3].

22.1.2 Etiology

LP is characterized by a T-cell-mediated immunological reaction affecting the dermis and epidermis, leading to keratinocyte apoptosis [4]. While the role of specific trigger factors is controversial, LP has been linked to hepatitis C infection [5].

D. Condie, BS • A.G. Pandya, MD (✉)
Department of Dermatology, University of Texas Southwestern Medical Center, 5323 Harry Hines Blvd., Dallas, TX 75235, USA
e-mail: daniel.condie@utsouthwestern.edu; amit.pandya@utsouthwestern.edu

D. Jackson-Richards, A.G. Pandya (eds.), *Dermatology Atlas for Skin of Color*,
DOI 10.1007/978-3-642-54446-0_22, © Springer-Verlag Berlin Heidelberg 2014

22.2 Clinical Features

22.2.1 Distribution and Arrangement

The lesions of LP have a predilection for the flexor wrists, trunk, medial thighs, shins, scalp, oral mucosa, and genital mucosa (Figs. 22.1, 22.2, 22.3, 22.4, 22.5, 22.6, 22.7, and 22.8). LP may also affect the palms and soles. Involvement of the face is rare. The Koebner phenomenon is a common occurrence in patients with LP (Fig. 22.9). Many clinical variants of LP have been reported, including actinic (Fig. 22.10), linear, annular (Fig. 22.11), hypertrophic, and ulcerative LP. Some variants are reported to occur more often in certain patient populations. Actinic LP is characterized by lesions in the sun-exposed areas of the face, arms, hands, and neck. It primarily affects the Middle Eastern population with usual onset in the spring and summer [6]. Linear LP, in which lesions are limited to one band or streak, has been reported in up to 10 % of cases of LP in Japan compared to less than 1 % of patients elsewhere [7]. Lichen planopilaris is a disease of the scalp which is characterized by scaly papules at the base of affected hairs leading to permanent alopecia (Figs. 22.12 and 22.13).

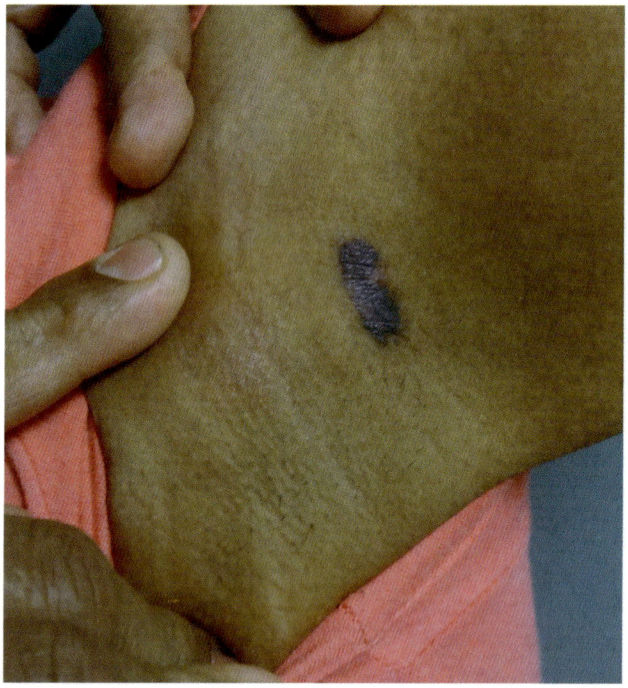

Fig. 22.1 Lichen planus of axilla in a Hispanic female

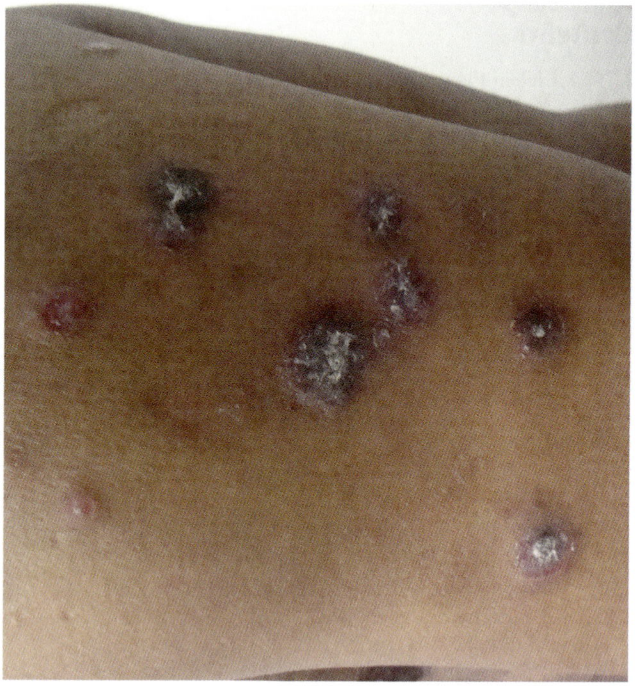

Fig. 22.3 Lichen planus of upper arm in an AA male

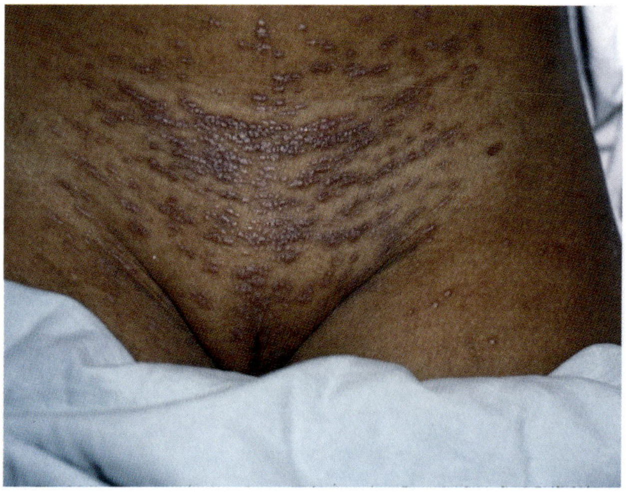

Fig. 22.2 Lichen planus of lower trunk and genital region in an AA female (Courtesy of Dr. Chauncey McHargue)

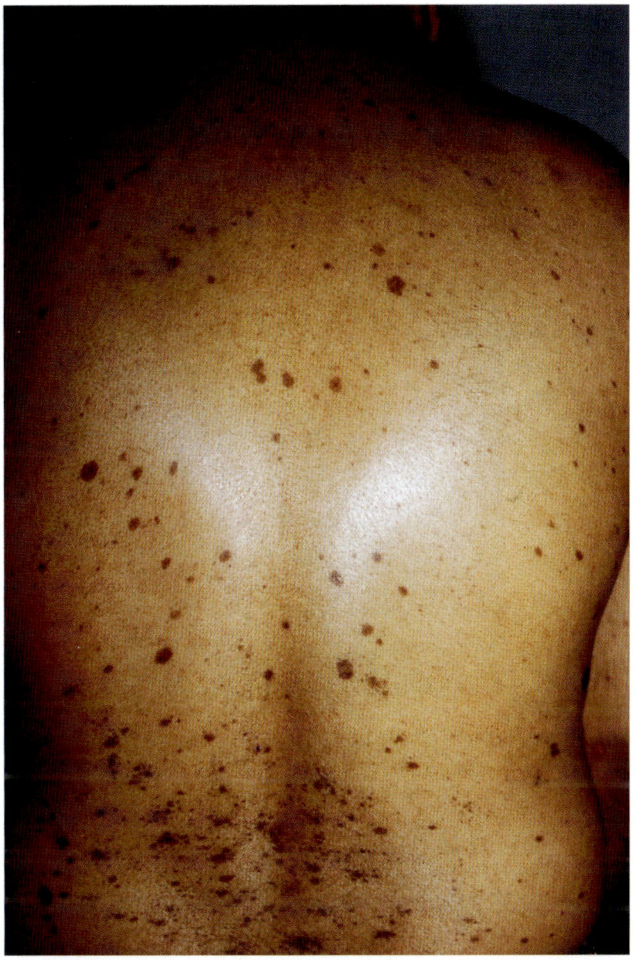

Fig. 22.4 Lichen planus of the back in a Hispanic male

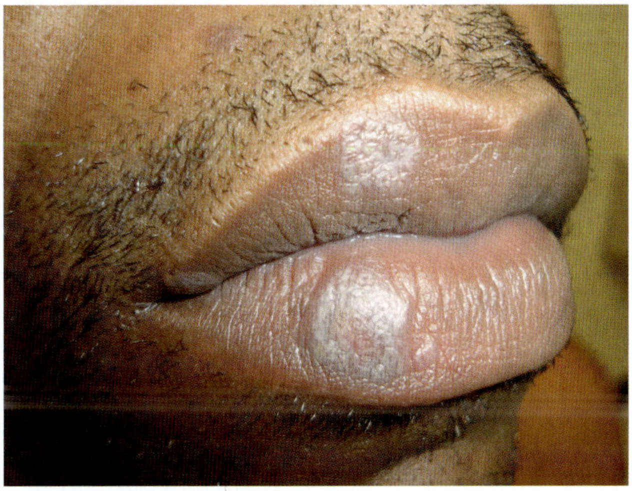

Fig. 22.5 Lichen planus of lips in an AA male

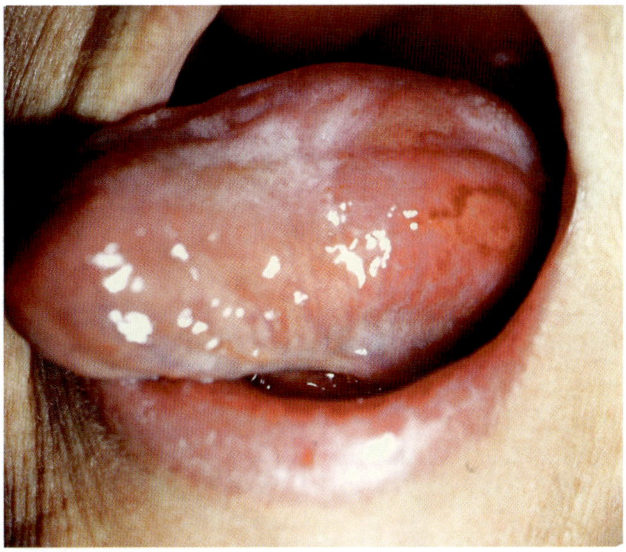

Fig. 22.6 Lichen planus of the tongue in a Hispanic female

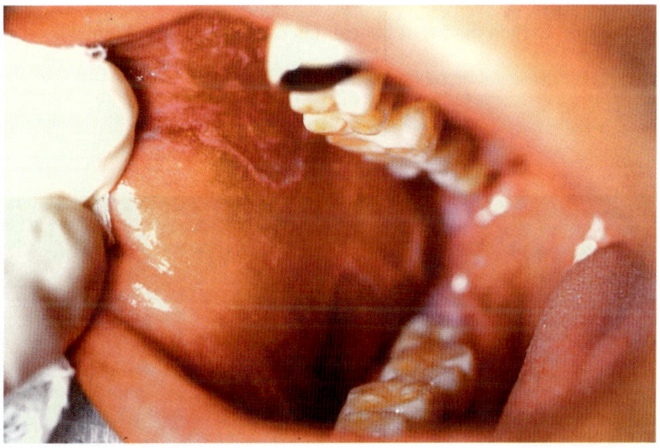

Fig. 22.7 Lichen planus of buccal mucosa in a Hispanic male

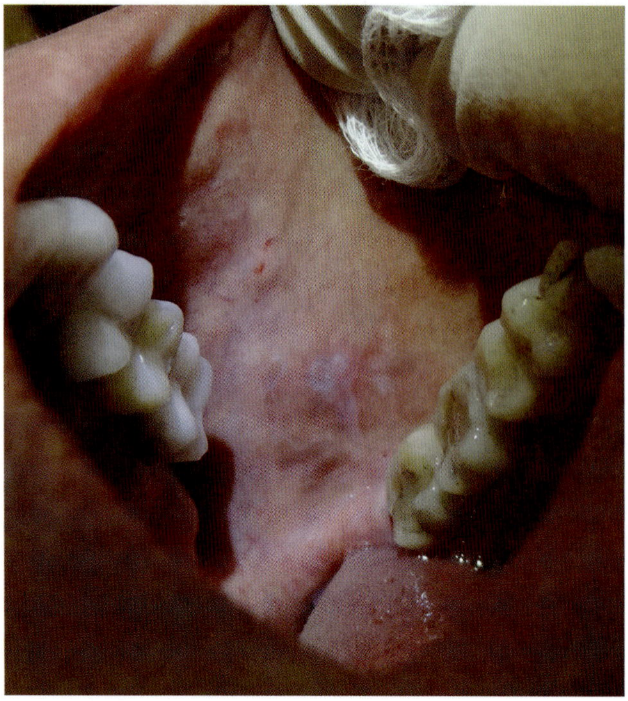

Fig. 22.8 Lichen planus of buccal mucosa in a Hispanic female

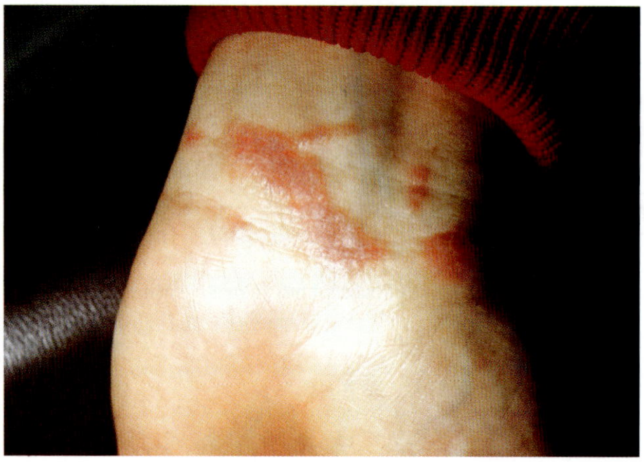

Fig. 22.9 Lichen planus of wrist in a Hispanic female

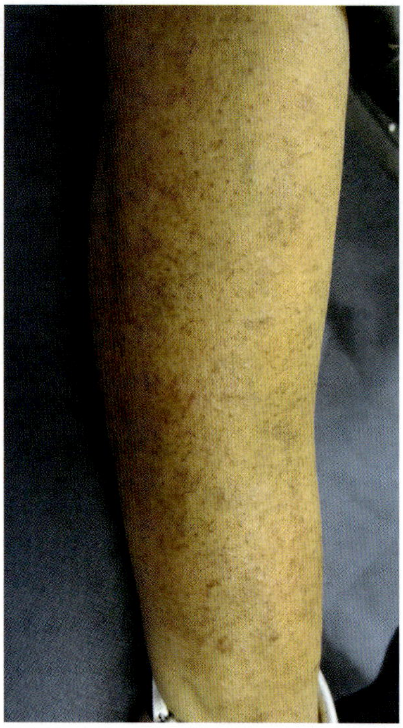

Fig. 22.10 Actinic lichen planus of the forearm in a South Asian female

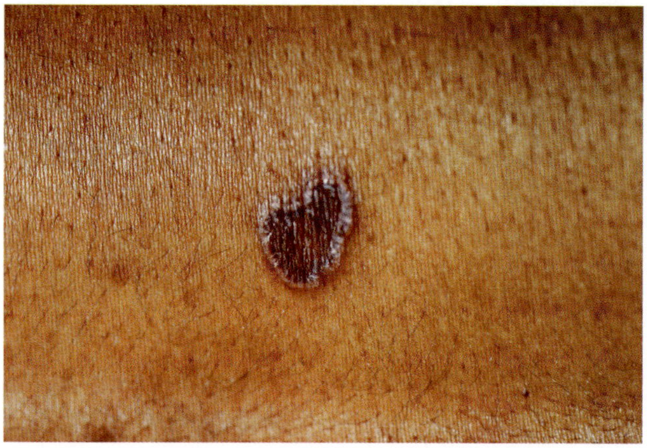

Fig. 22.11 Annular lichen planus of the arm in an AA male

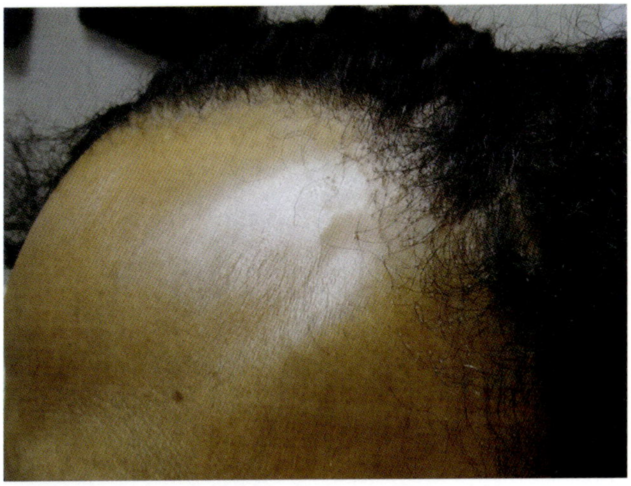

Fig. 22.12 Lichen planopilaris of scalp in an AA female

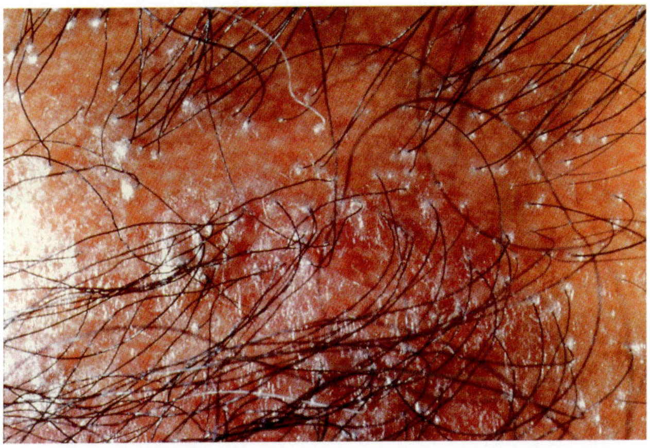

Fig. 22.13 Lichen planopilaris of scalp in a Hispanic female

22.2.2 Morphology

The primary lesions of LP are polygonal, violaceous, flat-topped papules that may coalesce into plaques. Pruritus is a prominent feature of the disease. The lesions are often covered by scant, adherent scales or a reticular network of fine white lines (Wickham striae). Postinflammatory hyperpigmentation is a common finding as the lesions clear, particularly in people with skin of color [6]. Oral lesions may be reticulate, annular, erythematous, or ulcerative and are often painful. Genital lesions are more common in men, often presenting on the glans penis, sometimes with an annular pattern. Women may have linear, white striae on the vulva and vagina. LP often affects the nails, typically with simultaneous involvement of several nails. Longitudinal ridging and splitting are common findings. Other observed changes include thinning of the nail plate, pterygium, trachyonychia, onycholysis, and subungual hyperkeratosis [1].

22.3 Natural History and Prognosis

The natural history of LP is highly variable. The majority of LP cases with skin lesions will resolve within 1–2 years. Oral disease is often chronic and resistant to treatment [4]. Recurrences of LP are common [6].

22.4 Histopathologic Features

LP is characterized by a dense, band-like lymphocytic infiltrate in the superficial dermis. Degenerative keratinocytes (Civatte or colloid bodies) are also present in the superficial dermis [4]. A "sawtooth" pattern of epidermal hyperplasia may also be seen.

22.5 Diagnosis and Differential Diagnosis

Diagnosis is often made clinically by the classic morphologic characteristics of the lesions, but a punch biopsy may be helpful to confirm the diagnosis in atypical cases. The differential diagnosis of LP includes lichenoid drug reaction, pityriasis rosea, guttate psoriasis, lichen nitidus, and lichenoid syphilid [1, 6]. The differential diagnosis of oral lesions includes leukoplakia, lupus erythematosus, candidiasis, squamous cell carcinoma, and autoimmune bullous diseases.

22.6 Treatment

For limited skin or oral lesions, high-potency topical steroids are appropriate first-line therapies. Widespread lesions may respond to oral corticosteroids. Other therapies to consider include retinoids (topical or systemic), phototherapy (UVB, UVA1, PUVA), topical calcineurin inhibitors, antifungal agents (for oral LP), and low molecular weight heparin [8, 9].

22.7 Lichen Nitidus

22.7.1 Introduction

Lichen nitidus (LN) is a chronic inflammatory condition of the skin that primarily affects children and young adults. The cause of LN is unknown although some have reported cases of LN concurrent with Crohn's disease. Others have reported an association between LN and atopic dermatitis. Familial cases of LN are rare [3].

22.7.2 Clinical Features

Lesions of LN are often localized to a few areas, including the penis, lower abdomen, upper extremities, and chest (Figs. 22.14, 22.15, and 22.16). In some cases LN assumes a widespread distribution and the lesions may coalesce into plaques with fine scale. The Koebner phenomenon is common (Figs. 22.17 and 22.18) [6].

The lesions are discrete, flat-topped, uniform papules, no larger than 1–2 mm. The color varies from yellow/brown to dark red in contrast to the violaceous lesions of LP. Unlike LP, LN is usually asymptomatic. LN occasionally affects the palms and soles with multiple hyperkeratotic papules that may coalesce into plaques.

Variants of LN have been reported in African-Americans and dark-skinned patients from the Middle East and Indian subcontinent. This disease is called summertime LN actinicus, actinic LN, or actinic lichenoid eruption. LN actinicus affects both children and adults. Lesions are identical in appearance and histology to LN but with a distribution in sun-exposed areas of the dorsal hands, forearm, and posterior neck [3]. Facial presentation of LN actinicus in three African-American girls has also been reported [10].

22.7.3 Histologic Features

LN is characterized by a focal, circumscribed infiltrate of lymphocytes and histiocytes. The epidermis often grows around this infiltrate, giving a "ball and claw" appearance. The inflammation is often granulomatous with multinucleate giant cells and epithelioid histiocytes [3].

22.7.4 Natural History and Treatment

The course of LN is slowly progressive with spontaneous remission after several years. Treatment is unnecessary in most cases. Patients who desired treatment can be treated with topical corticosteroids, dinitrochlorobenzene, PUVA, astemizole, or acitretin [3].

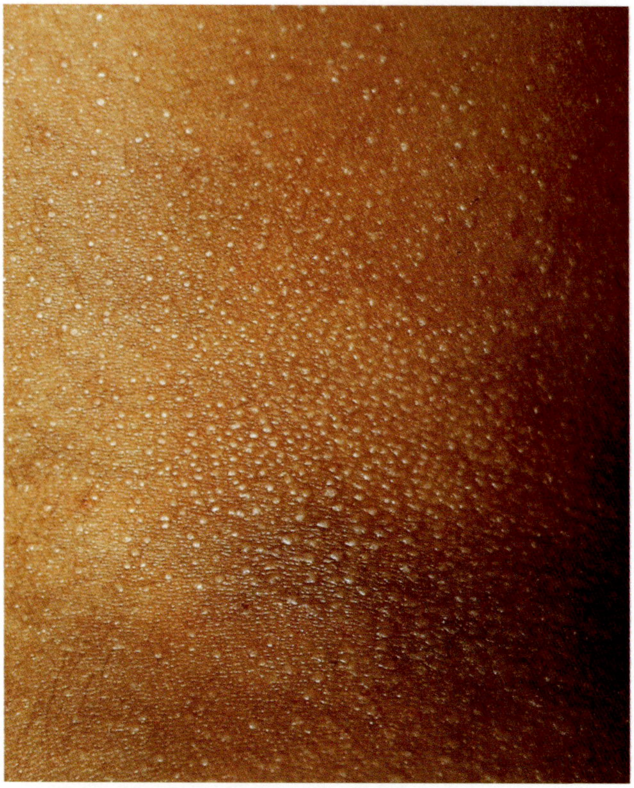

Fig. 22.14 Lichen nitidus of trunk in a Hispanic girl

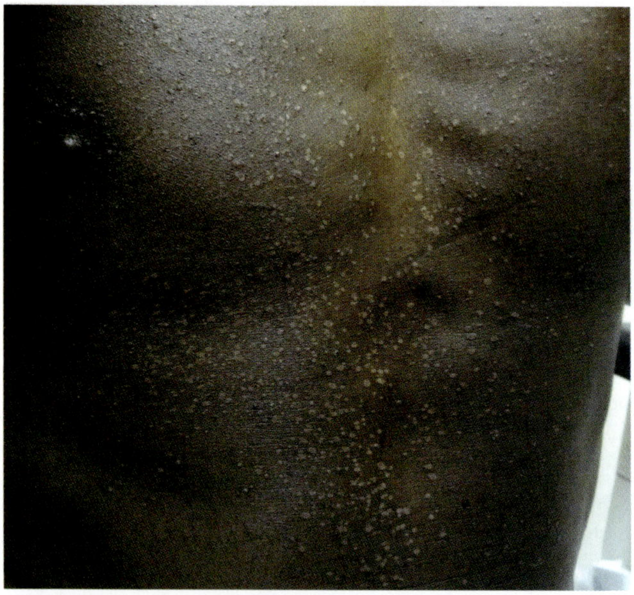

Fig. 22.15 Lichen nitidus of trunk in an African male

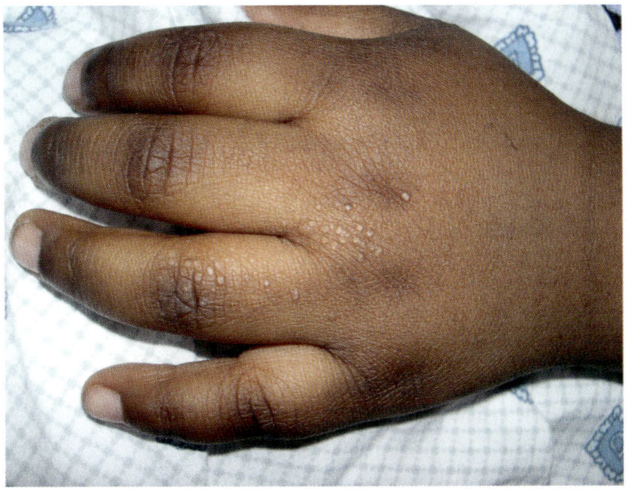

Fig. 22.16 Lichen nitidus of hand in an AA male (Courtesy of Dr Tor Shwayder)

Fig. 22.17 Lichen nitidus in an AA male with Koebner phenomenon (Courtesy of Dr Tor Shwayder)

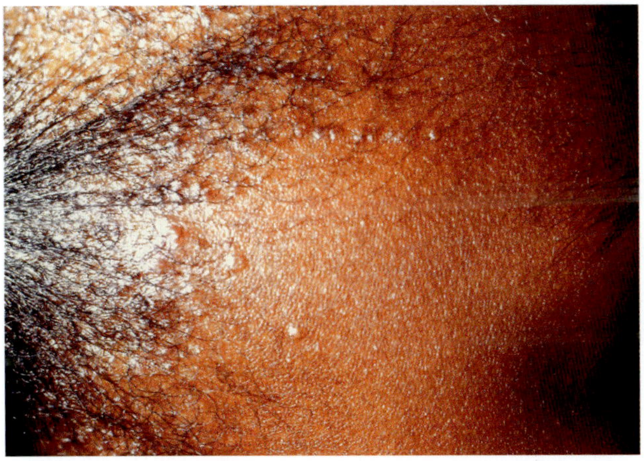

Fig. 22.18 Lichen nitidus of the temple in an African-American girl

22.8 Lichen Striatus

22.8.1 Introduction

Lichen striatus is an asymptomatic, self-limited eruption of small, scaly, erythematous papules seen primarily in children. The cause of lichen striatus is unknown [3].

22.8.2 Clinical Features

The 1–3 mm papules characteristic of lichen striatus coalesce to form a band which progresses down the extremity (more common) or around the trunk (less common) and characteristically follows the lines of Blaschko (Fig. 22.19). Hypopigmentation is prominent in persons with skin of color. Nail lesions are rare and typically restricted to a single nail [3].

22.8.3 Brief Description of Histopathologic Features

The histologic appearance of lichen striatus is variable. There is a dense lymphocytic infiltrate of the dermis which may be perivascular or band-like. Often there is a dense infiltrate around the eccrine sweat glands and ducts as well, which may help distinguish lichen striatus from LP [3].

22.8.4 Natural History and Treatment

On average lichen striatus spontaneously resolves within 1 year, but it may persist for up to 4 years. Postinflammatory hypopigmentation may last for months or several years as

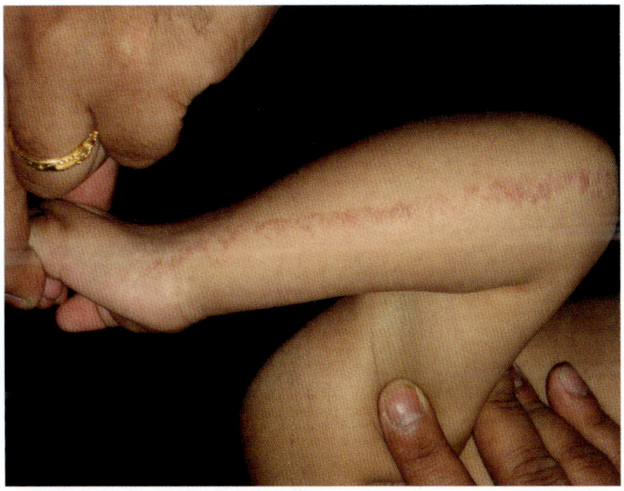

Fig. 22.19 Lichen striatus in a South Asian girl (Courtesy of Dr Tor Shwayder)

well. Recurrences are uncommon. The diagnosis is usually straightforward, but the differential diagnoses may include linear lichen planus, linear psoriasis, and inflammatory linear verrucous epidermal nevus. Treatment is usually not necessary although corticosteroids may be used to help the appearance of the lesions [3].

References

1. Wagner G, Rose C, Sachse MM. Clinical variants of lichen planus. J Dtsch Dermatol Ges. 2013;11:309–19.
2. Walton KE, Bowers EV, Drolet BA, Holland KE. Childhood lichen planus: demographics of a U.S. population. Pediatr Dermatol. 2010;27:34–8.
3. Tilly JJ, Drolet BA, et al. Lichenoid eruptions in children. J Am Acad Dermatol. 2004;51(4):606–24.
4. Sugerman PB, Savage NW, Walsh LJ, et al. The pathogenesis of oral lichen planus. Crit Rev Oral Biol Med. 2002;13:350–65.
5. Lodi G, Pellicano R, Carrozzo M. Hepatitis C virus infection and lichen planus: a systematic review with meta-analysis. Oral Dis. 2010;16:601–12.
6. Boyd AS, Neldner KH. Lichen planus. J Am Acad Dermatol. 1991;25:593–619.
7. Handa S, Sahoo B. Childhood lichen planus: a study of 87 cases. Int J Dermatol. 2002;41:423–7.
8. Lodi G, Scully C, et al. Current controversies in oral lichen planus: report of an international consensus meeting. Part 2. Clinical management and malignant transformation. Oral Surg Oral Med Oral Pathol Oral Radiol Endod. 2005;100(2):164–78.
9. Stefanidou MP, Ioannidou DJ, Panayiotides JG, Tosca AD. Low molecular weight heparin; a novel alternative therapeutic approach for lichen planus. Br J Dermatol. 1999;141:1040–5.
10. Modi S, Harting M, et al. Lichen nitidus actinicus: a distinct facial presentation in 3 pre-pubertal African-American girls. Dermatol Online J. 2008;14(4):10.

Pityriasis Rosea

23

Diane Jackson-Richards

Contents

23.1 Etiology

Pityriasis rosea (PR) is a self-limited harmless, skin eruption first described by Robert William in 1798 and later termed pityriasis rosea by Camille Melchior Gibert in 1860 (Bolognia). Although the etiology is unknown, it is postulated to be caused by a virus, specifically human herpes viruses 6 and 7 (HHV-6 and HHV-7). Drago et al. detected herpes virus via electron microscopy around collagen fibers and blood vessels of the mid and upper dermis in 70 % of PR patients [1]. Another study by Watanabe et al. found HHV-7 in the plasma of 50 % of patients with acute PR and none in healthy controls. In 2002 Watanabe et al. found HHV-6 and HHV-7 in the skin and serum of patients with PR. PR is not caused by a direct herpes viral infection of the skin but possibly by cutaneous infiltration of latently infected lymphocytes during systemic viral replication. Although these studies are compelling, they have not been reproduced and thus the exact etiology has yet to be definitively proven.

23.2 Epidemiology

Pityriasis rosea occurs worldwide and some reports attribute 2 % of outpatient dermatology visits to this condition. It affects both sexes equally as well as all ages and races. Seventy-five percent of PR cases occur within the range of 10–35 years. There have been reports of an increased incidence during the spring and fall.

D. Jackson-Richards, MD
Department of Dermatology, Multicultural Dermatology Center,
Henry Ford Hospital, 3031 West Grand Blvd.,
Detroit, MI 48202, USA
e-mail: djackso1@hfhs.org

D. Jackson-Richards, A.G. Pandya (eds.), *Dermatology Atlas for Skin of Color*,
DOI 10.1007/978-3-642-54446-0_23, © Springer-Verlag Berlin Heidelberg 2014

23.3 Clinical Features

Classic cases present with the acute onset of a "herald patch" which is a solitary 1–4 cm pink or hyperpigmented patch or plaque. Lesions typically have a fine collarette of scale at their periphery. The herald patch or initial lesion occurs in 80 % of cases (Fig. 23.1). Within a few days of the initial lesion, there is an outbreak of papules and plaques on the trunk and upper extremities that are similar to the herald patch but smaller in size (Figs. 23.2, 23.3, and 23.4). In darker pigmented individuals, lesions may be hyperpigmented rather than pink. Lesions may follow Langer's lines and often are referred to as resembling a "Christmas tree" pattern. Facial lesions may be seen in up to 30 % of cases in African Americans (Fig. 23.5). Amer et al. studied the clinical presentation of PR in black children presenting to a pediatric clinic in Detroit, Michigan. They found facial lesions in 30 % and scalp involvement in 8 % of cases [2]. In addition, lesions may consist of small papules as opposed to plaques, especially in darker-skinned patients. Oral lesions are rare and consist of punctate hemorrhages, erythematous macules, or plaques. Oral lesions tend to be more common in children, black patients, and those with more widespread PR [3]. An atypical presentation referred to as inverse pityriasis (Fig. 23.6) presents with lesions in the inguinal and perineal region and axillae as opposed to the trunk. Associated pruritus may vary from nonexistent to moderately severe. PR usually spontaneously resolves in 8 weeks and rarely lasts as long as 5 months. As with many inflammatory disorders, residual hyper- or hypopigmentation is more common in darker skin.

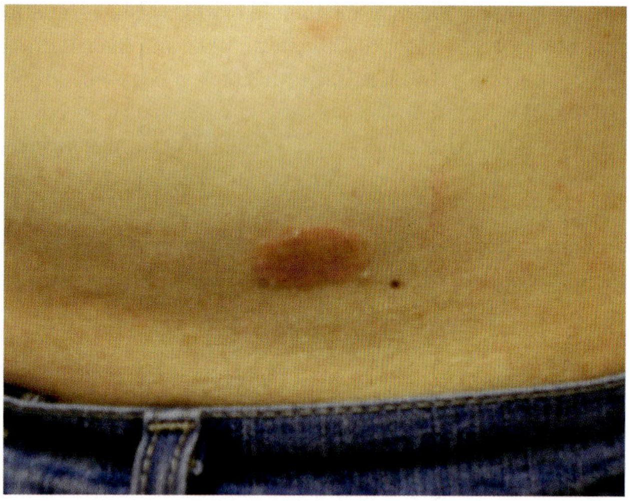

Fig. 23.1 Herald patch of PR in a Hispanic male

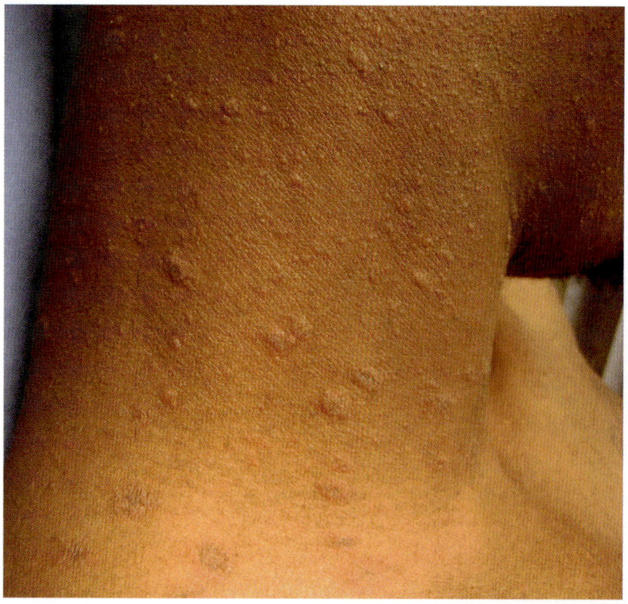

Fig. 23.2 PR on the neck of an African American male

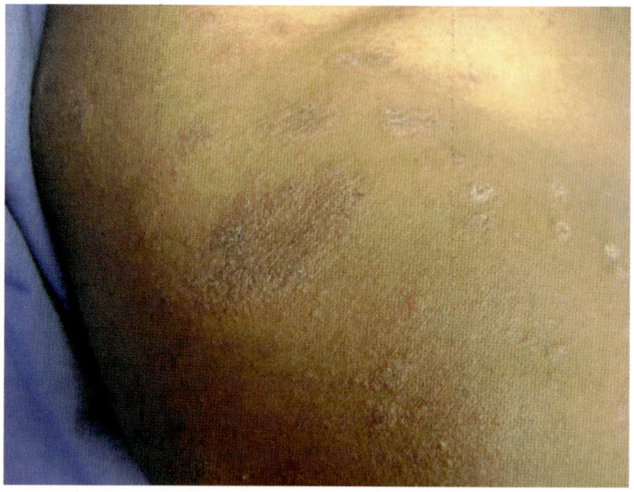

Fig. 23.3 PR on the shoulder of an African American male

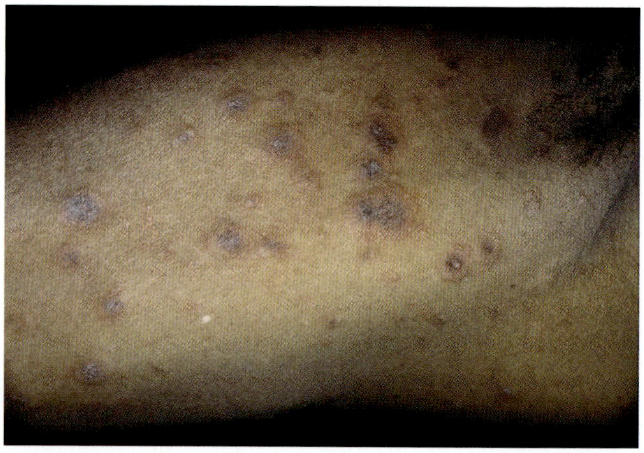

Fig. 23.4 PR on the proximal arm of an African American male

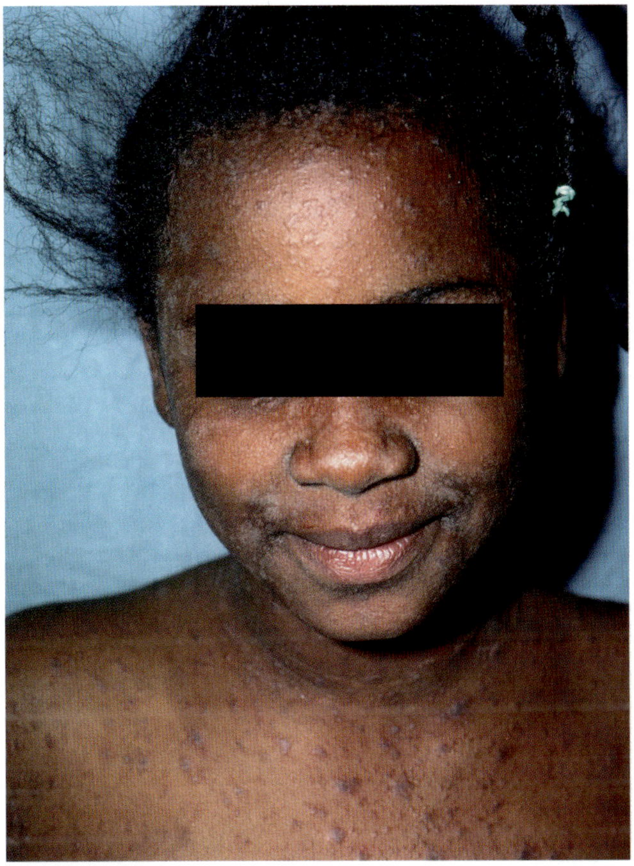

Fig. 23.5 PR lesions on the face of a young African American girl

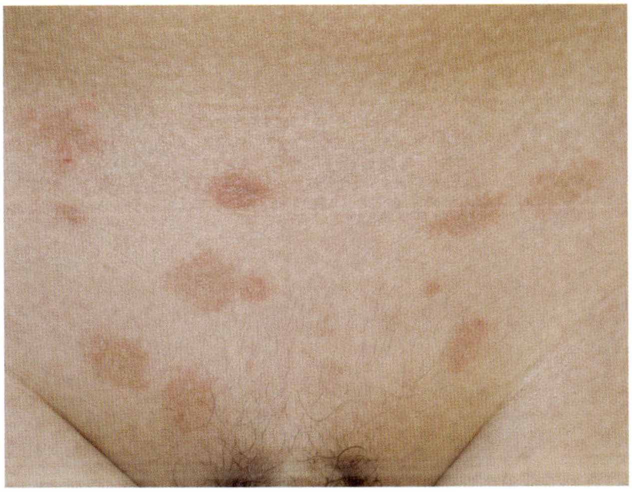

Fig. 23.6 Inverse PR in an AA boy (Courtesy of Dr. Tor Shwayder)

23.4 Histopathologic Features

Histopathology shows spongiosis with a mild lymphohistiocytic, perivascular infiltrate. Small areas of parakeratosis can be seen. In general the pathology is rather nonspecific. When in doubt VDRL and FTA-ABS are recommended to rule out syphilis.

23.5 Differential Diagnosis

The herald patch is often mistaken for tinea corporis or nummular dermatitis. Most importantly secondary syphilis can resemble pityriasis rosea. Secondary syphilis may have palm and sole involvement and can be ruled out with serologic tests. Other disorders to include in the differential diagnosis are a viral exanthem, nummular dermatitis, drug eruption, and guttate psoriasis.

23.6 Treatment

Since PR is self-limited, reassurance is often all that is needed. Some patients may have more intense pruritus and topical corticosteroids, emollients, and antihistamines are helpful. UVB phototherapy has been shown to lessen the severity of extensive pityriasis rosea and hasten clearing of the condition. Oral erythromycin, 250 mg four times daily, resulted in resolution of PR within 2 weeks in 73 % of cases [4].

References

1. Drago F, Broccolo F, Rebora A. Pityriasis rosea: an update with a critical appraisal of its possible herpesviral etiology. J Am Acad Dermatol. 2009;61:303–18.
2. Amer A, Fischer H, Li X. The natural history of pityriasis rosea in black American children. Arch Pediatr Adolesc Med. 2007;161:503–6.
3. Gonzalez LM, Allen R, Janniger CK, Schwartz RA. Pityriasis rosea: an important papulosquamous disorder. Int J Dermatol. 2005;44:757–64.
4. Sharma PK, Yadav TP, Gautam RK. Erythromycin in pityriasis rosea: a double-blind, placebo-controlled clinical trial. J Am Acad Dermatol. 2000;42:241–4.

Pityriasis Lichenoides Chronica

24

Alfred Wang and Amit G. Pandya

Contents

A. Wang, BS • A.G. Pandya, MD (✉)
Department of Dermatology,
University of Texas Southwestern Medical Center,
5323 Harry Hines Boulevard, Dallas, TX 75390, USA
e-mail: alfred.wang@utsouthwestern.edu;
amit.pandya@utsouthwestern.edu

24.1 Introduction

First reported in 1894 by Neisser and Jadassohn, pityriasis lichenoides chronica (PLC) is one of three variants of pityriasis lichenoides—the other two being pityriasis lichenoides et varioliformis acuta (PLEVA) and febrile ulceronecrotic Mucha-Habermann disease (FUMHD) [1].

24.1.1 Epidemiology

PLC may present in any geographic area and in individuals of any age or race, but the exact prevalence and incidence is unknown. PLC has been reported to occur more often in males and often presents in late childhood/early adulthood with an average age of presentation of 29 years. PLC has rarely been reported to occur in infants [1–3].

24.1.2 Etiology

Although the pathogenesis of PLC is still unknown, there are three current hypotheses regarding possible etiologies. First, PLC has been theorized to be an atypical immune response triggered by a foreign/infectious agent, including HIV, EBV, VZV, Parvovirus B19, HHV8, *Toxoplasma gondii*, *Staphylococcus aureus*, and group A beta-hemolytic streptococci. However, this theory is more often associated with PLEVA, the acute form of pityriasis lichenoides [1, 2, 4]. A second hypothesis is that PLC is a monoclonal T-cell disorder that precedes mycosis fungoides. PCR amplification in some cases of PLC has shown dominant T-cell clonality, with the atypical T cells showing predominant CD7 deletions. The third pathogenic theory, and the least substantiated, postulates that PLC is caused by an immune-complex-mediated vasculitis [1].

D. Jackson-Richards, A.G. Pandya (eds.), *Dermatology Atlas for Skin of Color*,
DOI 10.1007/978-3-642-54446-0_24, © Springer-Verlag Berlin Heidelberg 2014

24.2 Clinical Features

24.2.1 Distribution and Arrangement

PLC is a benign chronic papulosquamous skin disorder that presents initially as an erythematous papule with central micaceous scale. Over time, PLC evolves into multiple benign-appearing papules scattered across the trunk and proximal extremities (Figs. 24.1, 24.2, 24.3, 24.4, 24.5, and 24.6). Although acral and segmental distributions have also been described, PLC usually spares the face, palms and soles, and mucous membranes [1, 2].

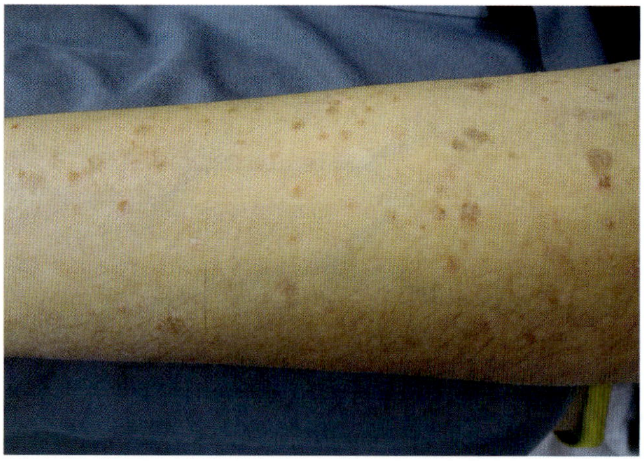

Fig. 24.1 PLC of the forearm in a South Asian female

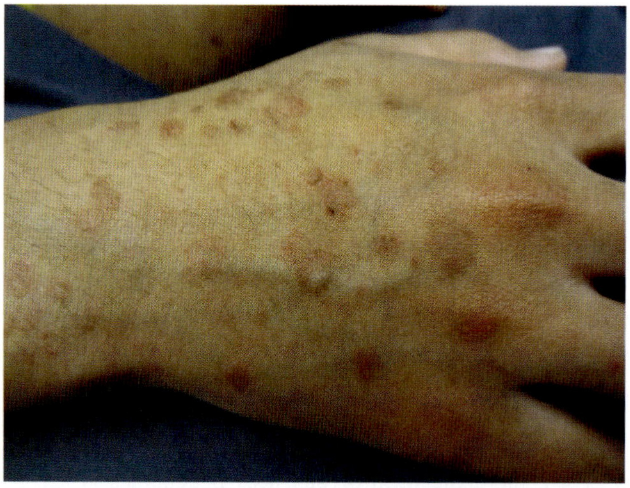

Fig. 24.2 PLC of the dorsal hand in a South Asian female

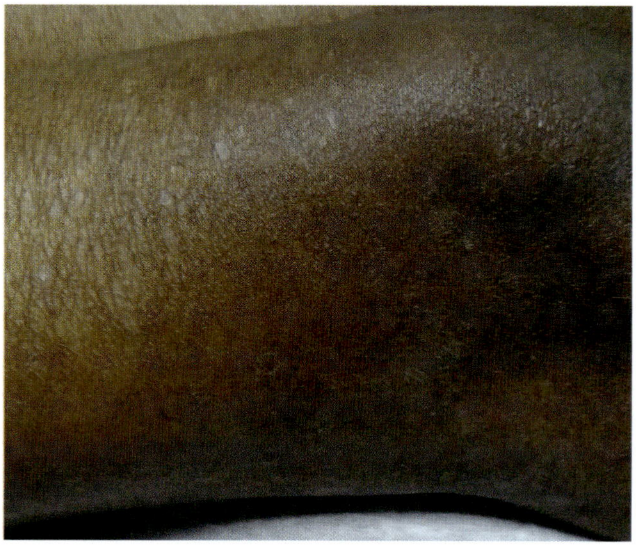

Fig. 24.3 PLC of the knee in an AA female

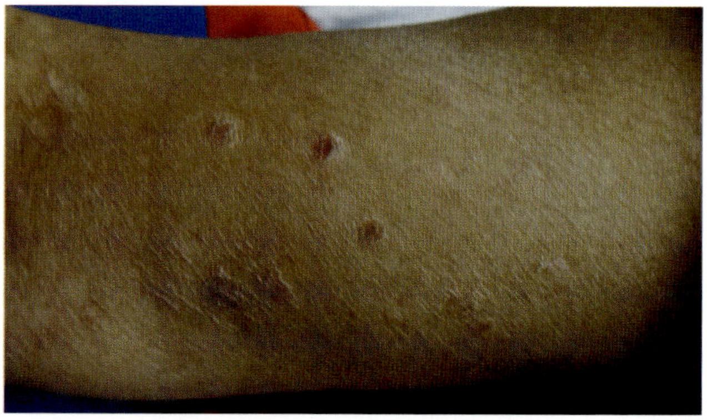

Fig. 24.4 PLC of the upper arm in a Hispanic female

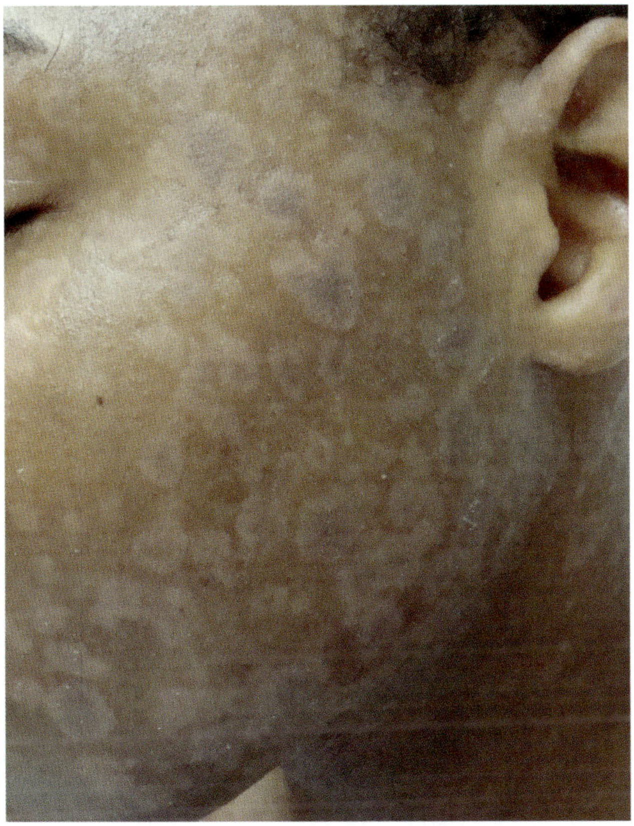

Fig. 24.5 Severe PLC of the face in an AA male

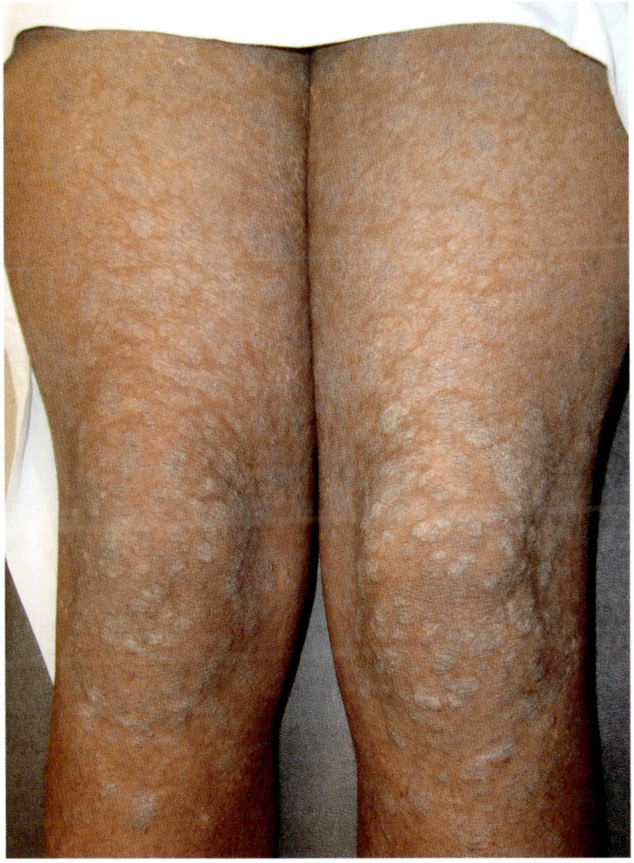

Fig. 24.6 Severe PLC of the legs in an AA male

24.2.2 Morphology of Lesions

PLC presents as gradually developing small maculopapules that are reddish-brown with fine centrally attached fine epidermal, mica-like scale. Over the span of weeks or months, these lesions may spontaneously regress and flatten, leaving a hyper- or hypopigmented macule. In dark-skinned individuals, PLC may present as generalized hypopigmented macules without scale [1, 2].

24.3 Natural History and Prognosis

PLC has an indolent course, with the generalized eruption lasting months to years before resolving. However, PLC often presents with exacerbations and long periods of remissions over time; therefore, lesions can present at all stages of development. Patients with PLC have a good prognosis in terms of overall general health, but have rarely been reported to progress to PLEVA and mycosis fungoides [1, 5]. Because of the possibility of progressing to other disorders, frequent visits and skin biopsy of suspicious lesions are suggested as patients are followed. Clonality, which can be present in lesions of PLC, does not seem to be associated with progression or adverse clinical outcome [6].

24.4 Histopathology

PLC is typified by epidermal parakeratosis, mild acanthosis, and spongiosis with mild basal cell vacuolation; band-like dermal CD4+ T-dominant lymphocytic infiltrates, dermal edema with occasional extravasated erythrocytes and neutrophils; and sparse perivascular infiltrate with dilation of superficial vessels. Over time, these interface changes become less prominent and may be undetectable in regressing lesions [1, 7, 8].

24.5 Diagnosis and Differential Diagnosis

PLC is often clinically confused with various other papulosquamous skin disorders and requires a thorough history combined with histopathologic examinations in order to distinguish PLC from other disorders. The differential diagnosis includes guttate psoriasis, papular eczematous dermatitis, tinea versicolor, mycosis fungoides, Gianotti-Crosti syndrome, pityriasis rosea, arthropod bite reaction, secondary syphilis, papulonecrotic tuberculid, polymorphous light reaction, and toxic epidermal necrolysis. The most common dermatosis confused with PLC is lymphomatoid papulosis. Lymphomatoid papulosis can be differentiated from PLC as the former is a cutaneous lymphoproliferative disorder with papules that often crust over and can develop into nodules and plaques. Lymphomatoid papulosis has distinct histologic findings and CD 30+lymphocytes in the inflammatory infiltrate, unlike PLC. In addition, patients with PLC may have hundreds of lesions, whereas patients with lymphomatoid papulosis usually have less than 50 lesions on exam [1, 2, 4].

24.6 Treatment

Currently, there is no standard of treatment for PLC; instead, there are various treatment options. These options include phototherapy, oral antimicrobials, antivirals, topical corticosteroids, antihistamines, methotrexate, acitretin, cyclosporine, and calciferol/ergocalciferol. Phototherapy is currently the first-line treatment, including the pediatric population, and includes UVB, narrow-band UVB, psoralen plus UVA, and UVA-1. To help prevent relapses of PLC, light therapy is usually slowly tapered during the course of treatment [2].

If PLC was triggered by a foreign antigen such as a bacterial or viral source, treating with antibiotics or antivirals is recommended. Topical corticosteroids and antihistamines are used as symptomatic treatment options to help relieve any inflammation and pruritus. For more severe PLC in the adult population, cyclosporine, retinoids, calciferol, and methotrexate have proven to be effective. Because PLC is resistant to many of the available treatments, combination therapy is often superior to monotherapy [1].

References

1. Bowers S, Warshaw EM. Pityriasis lichenoides and its subtypes. J Am Acad Dermatol. 2006;55:557–72.
2. Khachemoune A, Blyumin ML. Pityriasis lichenoides: pathophysiology, classification, and treatment. Am J Clin Dermatol. 2007;8(1): 29–36.
3. Chand S, Srivastava N, Khopkar U, Singh S. Pityriasis lichenoides chronica: onset at birth. Pediatr Dermatol. 2008;25(1):135–6.
4. Kim JE, Yun WJ, Mun SK, Yoon GS, Huh J, Choi JH, Chang S. Pityriasis lichenoides et varioliformis acuta and pityriasis lichenoides chronica: comparison of lesional T-cell subsets and investigation of viral associations. J Cutan Pathol. 2011;38:649–56.
5. Magro CM, Crowson AN, Morrison C, Li J. Pityriasis lichenoides chronica: stratification by molecular and phenotypic profile. Hum Pathol. 2007;38:479–90.
6. Shieh S, Mikkola DL, Wood GS. Differentiation and clonality of lesional lymphocytes in PLC. Arch Dermatol. 2001;137:305–8.
7. Joshi R. Stratum corneum findings as clues to histological diagnosis of pityriasis lichenoides chronica. Indian J Dermatol Venereol Leprol. 2008;74(2):156–7.
8. Nair PS. A clinical and histopathological study of pityriasis lichenoides. Indian J Dermatol Venereol Leprol. 2007;73(2):100–2.

Psoriasis

25

Ryan Thorpe and Amit G. Pandya

Contents

R. Thorpe, BS • A.G. Pandya, MD (✉)
Department of Dermatology,
University of Texas Southwestern Medical Center,
5323 Harry Hines Boulevard, Dallas, TX 75390, USA
e-mail: ryan.thorpe@utsouthwestern.edu;
amit.pandya@utsouthwestern.edu

25.1 Introduction

Psoriasis is a chronic immune-mediated, hyperproliferative disease of the skin. Though rarely life threatening, psoriasis is associated with high morbidity and poor quality of life [1]. The disease has several presentations, which are similar across races and ethnicities. There is relatively little data on psoriasis in non-Caucasian populations [2].

25.1.1 Epidemiology

The prevalence of psoriasis worldwide is approximately 2 % [3]. Prevalence is generally lower in populations with skin of color. In one population-based study, the prevalence of psoriasis was 1.3 % in African Americans compared with 2.5 % for Caucasians [4]. Prevalence is highest among Northern Europeans (5 %) [5]. Many countries and regions have reported psoriasis prevalence rates, including Mexico (3 %), Western Africa (0.3–0.8 %), Kenya (3.5 %), Uganda (2.8 %), Tanzania (3 %), India (0.5–2.3 %), China (0.05–1.23 %), Japan (0.29–1.18 %), Italy (2.9 %), France (2.58 %), Spain (1.43 %), and Taiwan (0.2 %) [1].

25.1.2 Etiology

Evidence supports strong roles for both genetic and environmental factors in the etiopathogenesis of psoriasis.

Environmental factors include psychological stress, smoking, trauma, obesity, weather, HIV, streptococcal pharyngitis, other infections, and drugs, especially β-blockers, lithium, antimalarial medications, and interferon [1, 3].

The genetic influence on developing psoriasis is supported by an increased incidence of psoriasis in first- and second-degree relatives of psoriatic patients [6]. A two- to threefold increase in risk of developing psoriasis is found in monozygotic twins compared with dizygotic twins, and

D. Jackson-Richards, A.G. Pandya (eds.), *Dermatology Atlas for Skin of Color*,
DOI 10.1007/978-3-642-54446-0_25, © Springer-Verlag Berlin Heidelberg 2014

monozygotic twins are more likely to share distribution, severity, and age of onset [3].

Much of the genetic predisposition for psoriasis can be traced to the major histocompatibility complex on chromosome 6 and the associated human leukocyte antigens (HLAs) found on human cells. For example, the HLA-Cw6 allele is the principal allele associated with psoriasis in Caucasians, Northern Indians, and the Japanese (relative risk = 25). Only 17 % of Chinese psoriasis patients carry the HLA-Cw6 allele compared with 50–80 % of Caucasian patients [5]. Aside from HLA-Cw6, substantial evidence has accumulated associating psoriasis with HLA-A1, HLA-A2, HLA-B17, HLA-B13, HLA-B37, HLA-B39, HLA-Bw57, HLA-Cw6, HLA-Cw7, HLA-Cw11, and HLA-DR7 [5].

Psoriasis was once considered an epidermal disease with defects confined to keratinocytes. In the late 1970s and early 1980s, however, it was discovered that T-cell immunosuppressive agents such as cyclosporine were efficacious as treatments for psoriasis. This paradigm shift led to further research resulting in the current view that psoriasis is a product of a dysregulated immune system and is actually a T-cell-mediated disease [3, 6]. This new avenue of investigation has led to the development of several novel therapeutic approaches.

25.2 Clinical Features

Psoriasis presents in several different forms, and at any one time, more than one variant may coexist in the same patient. Most lesions share features of erythema, thickening, and scale [3]. In one survey of dermatologists, 66 % reported more dyspigmentation, thicker plaques, and less erythema in African Americans [7].

25.2.1 Distribution, Arrangement, and Morphology

The distribution and arrangement of psoriasis variants present similarly across skin types [5]:

1. Chronic plaque psoriasis
   (a) This is the most common form of psoriasis, in which relatively symmetric, sharply defined plaques are found on the scalp, elbows, knees, trunk, and presacral area (Figs. 25.1, 25.2, 25.3, 25.4, and 25.5). Plaques may also be found on the hands, feet, and genitalia in 45 % of affected patients. The characteristic lesion is a sharply demarcated erythematous plaque with adherent micaceous scale [3]. The silvery scale results from premature maturation of keratinocytes and incomplete cornification with parakeratosis or retention of nuclei in the stratum corneum [6]. In skin of color, lesions are typified by more violaceous and gray colors [3, 5, 6].
2. Guttate psoriasis
   (a) This category often presents explosively in adolescents and children with small, red-salmon-colored papules and plaques with or without silvery scale (Figs. 25.6 and 25.7). It is frequently preceded by an upper respiratory infection and over half have elevated antistreptolysin O, anti-DNase B, or streptozyme titers [3, 5].
3. Erythrodermic psoriasis
   (a) This variant is more unusual, can occur at any time in any psoriasis patient, and can be acute or gradual. It consists of diffuse, generalized redness of the skin and extensive scaling (Fig. 25.8). Clues that erythroderma is due to psoriasis include lesions in classic locations, nail changes, and facial sparing. This form can also be induced by withdrawal of systemic corticosteroid therapy [3, 5].
4. Pustular psoriasis
   (a) This is often seen in pregnancy or after rapid corticosteroid taper. Neutrophils dominate the picture histologically, and groups of macroscopic sterile pustules are observed with or without plaques [3, 5].
5. Palmoplantar psoriasis or pustulosis of palms and soles
   (a) Sterile pustules are characteristically involved on the palmoplantar surfaces. It can be regularly mistaken for dyshidrotic eczema [3, 5].
6. Scalp psoriasis
   (a) Scalp psoriasis can be difficult to distinguish from seborrheic dermatitis, and the two may even coexist. Psoriasis, however, frequently will advance onto the periphery of the face, retroauricular areas, and the upper neck (Fig. 25.9).
7. Inverse psoriasis or flexural psoriasis
   (a) Inverse psoriasis is distinguished for characteristic lesions found in the axillae, inframammary region, retroauricular folds, and intergluteal cleft. Localized dermatophyte, candidal, or bacterial infections can incite flexural psoriasis [3].
8. Nail psoriasis
   (a) Patients with psoriasis may develop oil spots onycholysis and pitting of the nails (Figs. 25.10 and 25.11).
9. Koebner phenomenon
   (a) Patients with psoriasis exhibit the Koebner phenomenon, in which psoriasis develops in areas of trauma (Fig. 25.12)

In a review of 1,220 Asian Indian patients, 93 % had chronic plaque psoriasis, followed by pustular, guttate, and erythrodermic types. In a survey of 28,628 Japanese patients, 86 % had plaque-type psoriasis, followed by guttate (2.8 %), generalized pustular (0.9 %), erythrodermic (0.8 %), and localized pustular forms (0.5 %). One percent had psoriatic arthritis. Studies on African Americans and Native Americans found similar results [5].

25.2.2 Associated Symptoms

Although itching is not usually a common feature, severe pruritus, edema, and pain are seen in some patients, particularly with certain variants, such as erythrodermic psoriasis. Bacteria infrequently secondarily infect psoriatic lesions, but concomitant candidal infections are more common [3]. Interestingly, less atopic dermatitis, less asthma, less urticaria, and less allergic contact dermatitis are reported in psoriasis patients [3].

25.2.3 Systemic Findings

Metabolic syndrome, depression, and even cancer, including lymphoma, are more prevalent in psoriatic patients [6]. Myocardial infarction, pulmonary embolism, peripheral arterial disease, and cerebrovascular accidents are also all more common. It remains unclear if these precede or result from psoriasis. For example, depression may be related to the psychological distress and cancer is potentially related to treatment [3]. Psoriatic arthritis occurs in 5–30 % of patients. In a minority (10–15 %), arthritis actually appears prior to skin lesions [5].

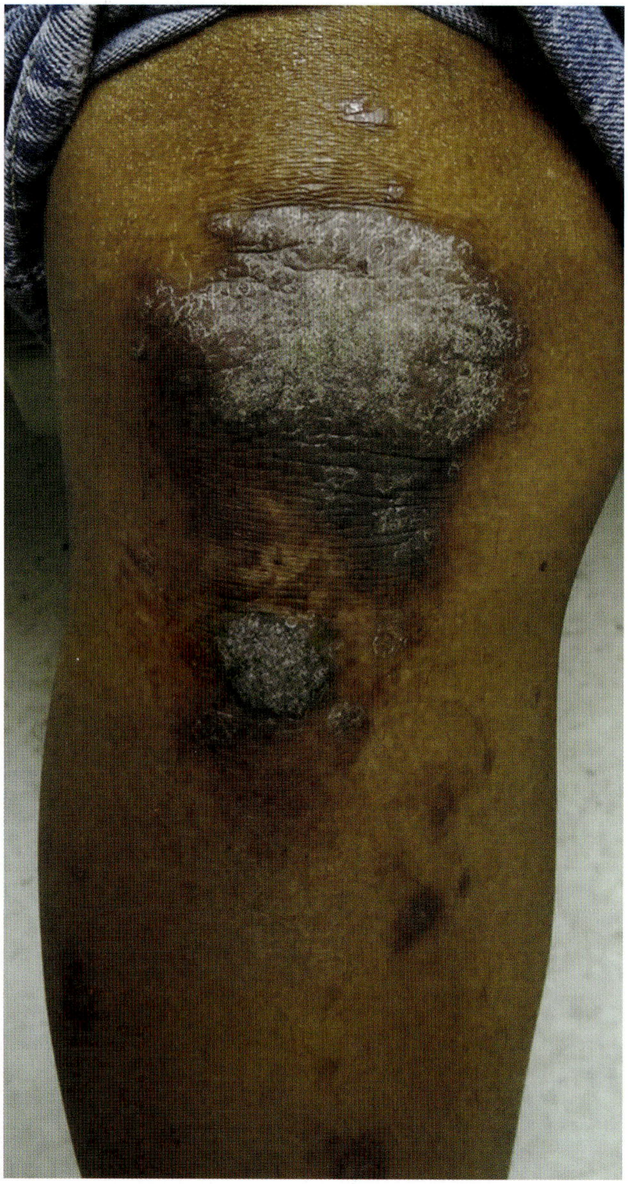

Fig. 25.1 Chronic plaques of psoriasis on the knee of an AA male

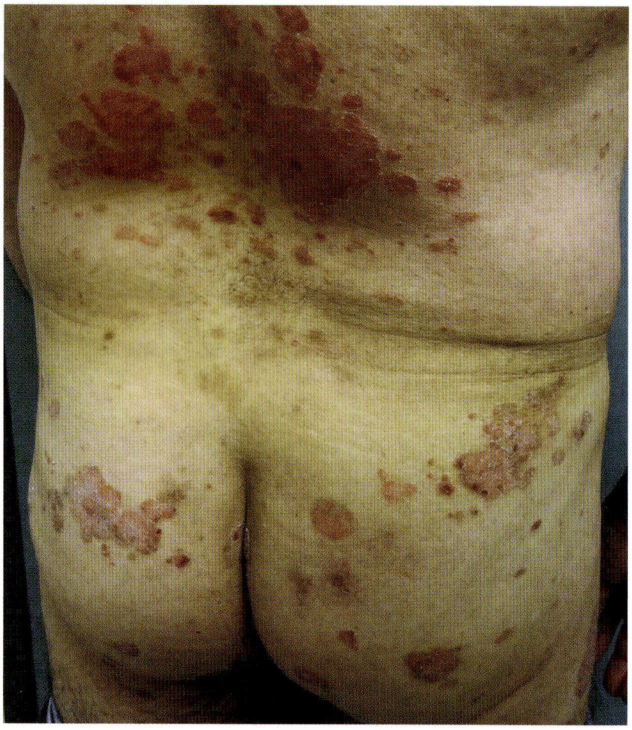

Fig. 25.2 Chronic plaques of psoriasis on the back and buttocks of a Hispanic male

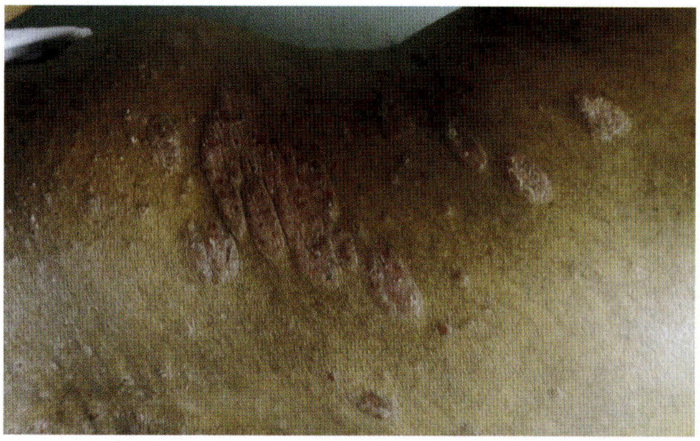

Fig. 25.3 Chronic plaques of psoriasis on the back of a South Asian male

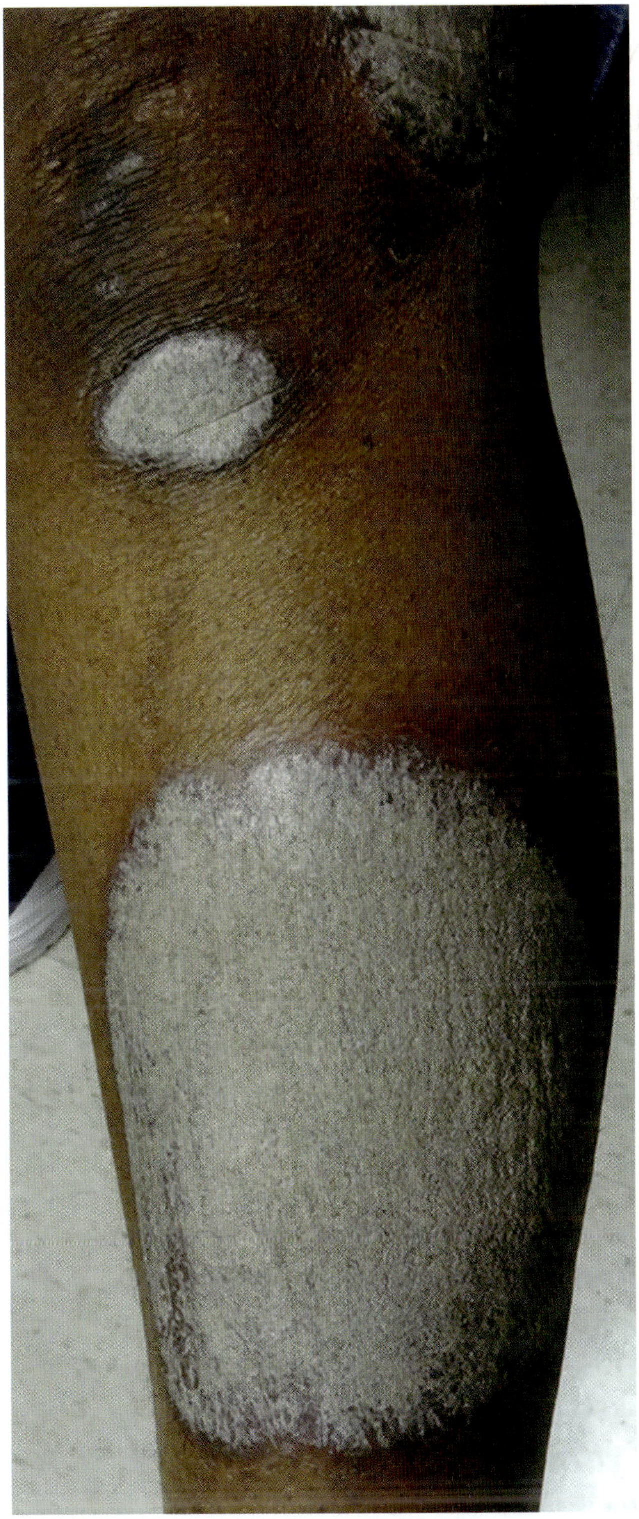

Fig. 25.4 Chronic plaques of psoriasis on the knee and shin of an AA female

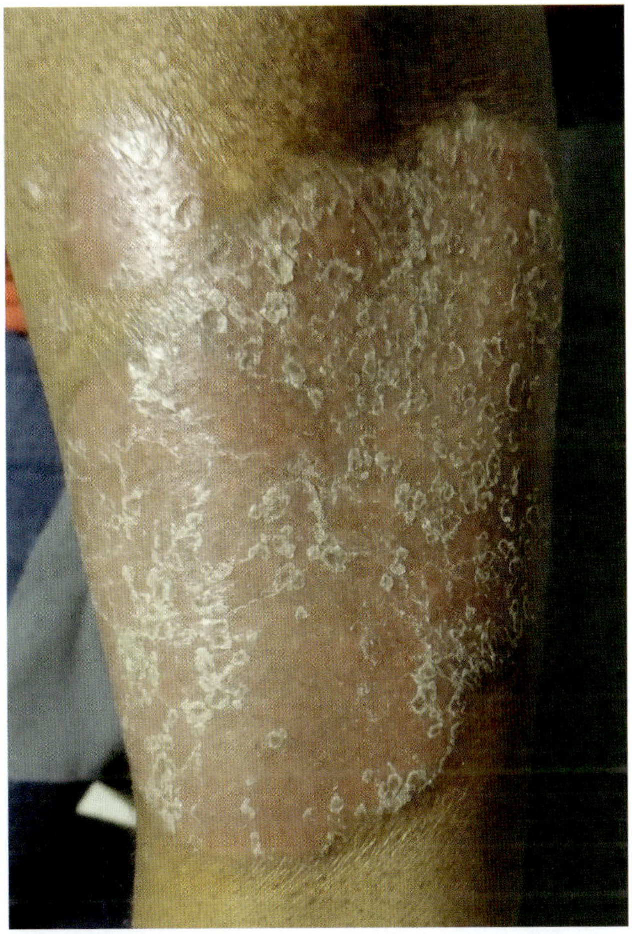

Fig. 25.5 Chronic plaque of psoriasis on the extensor arm of an AA female

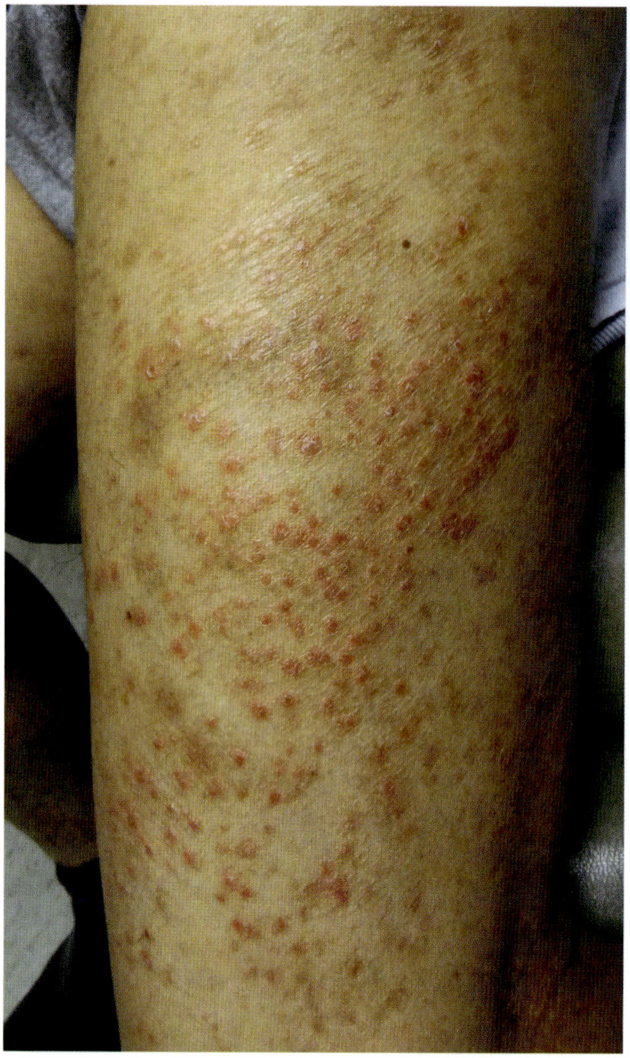

Fig. 25.6 Guttate psoriasis on the leg of a South Asian male

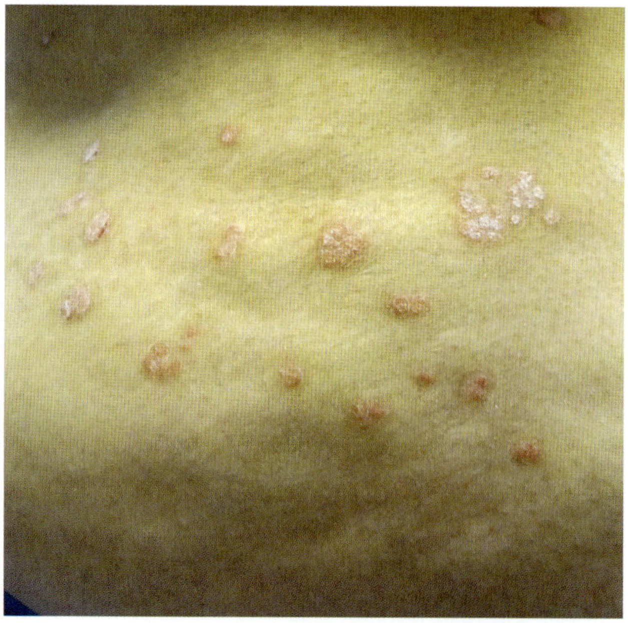

Fig. 25.7 Guttate psoriasis on the abdomen of a Hispanic female

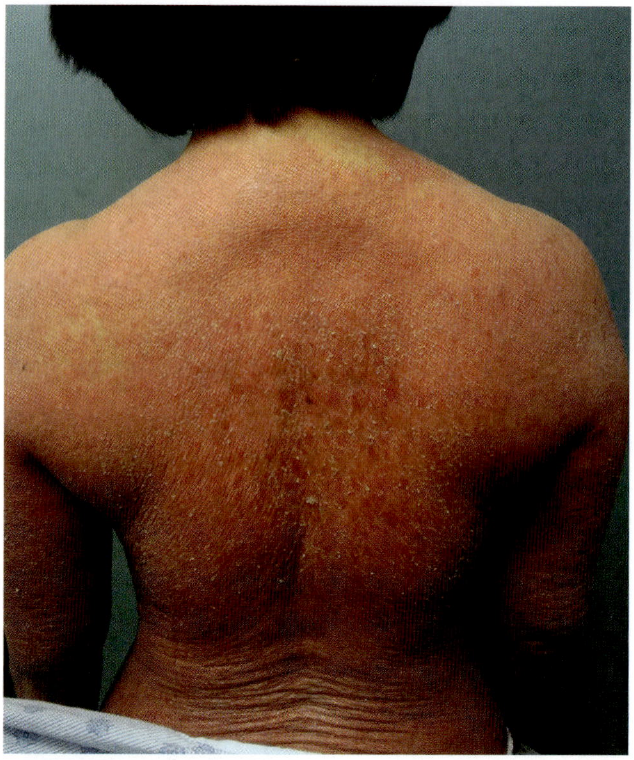

Fig. 25.8 Erythrodermic psoriasis in an Asian female

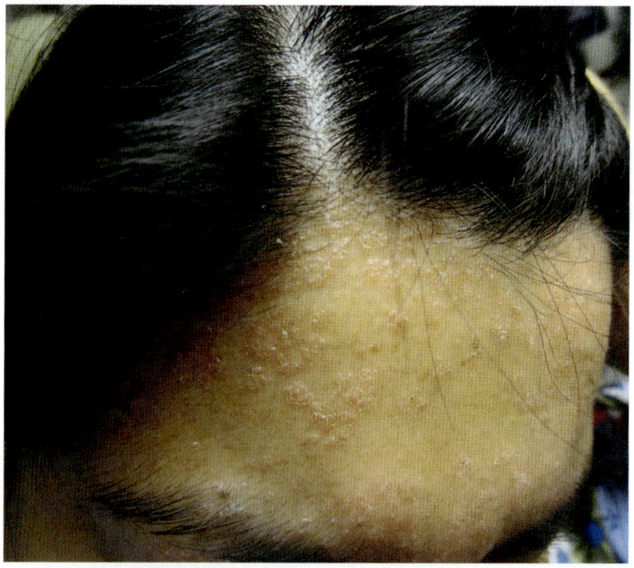

Fig. 25.9 Scalp and forehead psoriasis in a Hispanic female

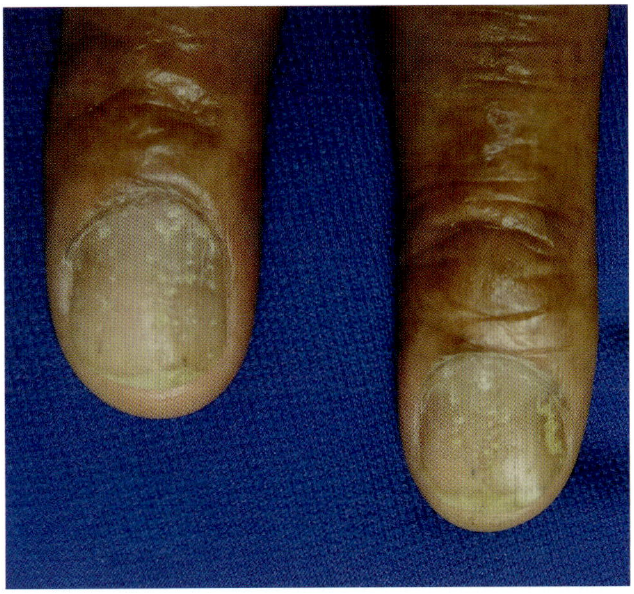

Fig. 25.10 Oil spots and pitting of the nail in a Hispanic male with psoriasis

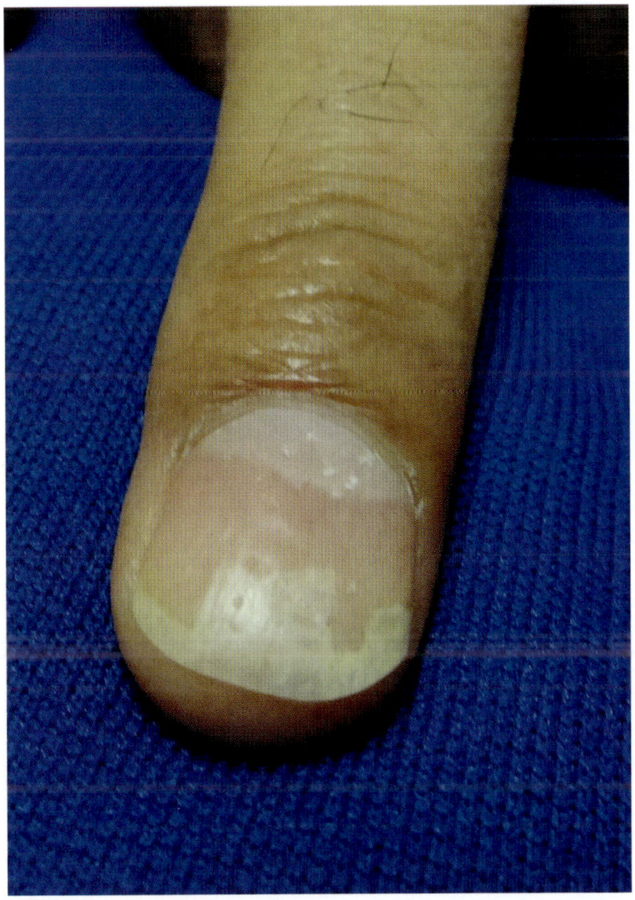

Fig. 25.11 Onycholysis and pitting of the nail in a Hispanic male with psoriasis

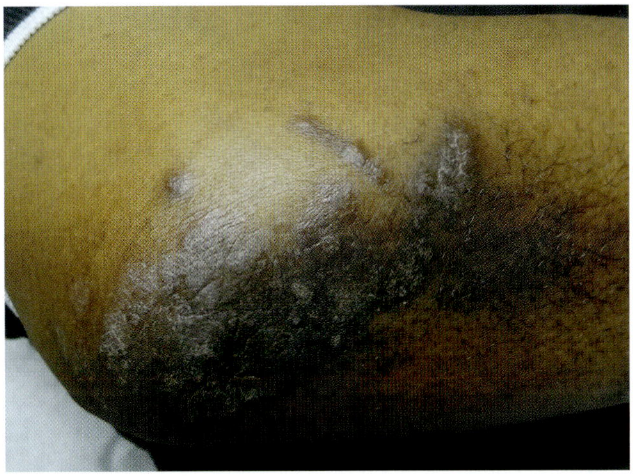

Fig. 25.12 Chronic plaque psoriasis of the elbow in an AA male showing the Koebner phenomenon

25.3 Natural History and Prognosis

Psoriasis is a chronic disease that can manifest at any age with two peaks of presentation, one at 20–30 years of age and the other at 50–60 years. Because of increased comorbidities, physicians should consider screening for atherosclerotic disease, metabolic syndrome, diabetes, hypertension, nonalcoholic steatohepatitis, and alcoholic fatty liver disease. Overall, life expectancy is reduced by 3.5–4.4 years [3, 5, 6].

25.4 Histopathological Features

Histopathological features are consistent across different races and ethnicities. Hyperkeratosis, parakeratosis, and acanthosis are hallmarks of psoriasis. Tortuous and dilated blood vessels are seen with a predominantly lymphocytic infiltrate [3]. The thickened epidermis is secondary to an increased mitotic rate and reduced cell transit time [3, 5, 6].

25.5 Diagnosis and Differential Diagnosis

Psoriasis may appear atypical in patients with skin of color because the key features are masked by pigmentation [7]. Lichen simplex chronicus and seborrheic dermatitis can both mimic and coexist with psoriasis. If there are only one or a few plaques, particularly those resistant to treatment, squamous cell carcinoma in situ should be ruled out with a biopsy. Occasionally, the mycosis fungoides variant of cutaneous T-cell lymphoma or even dermatomyositis may be mistaken for psoriasis. Palmoplantar psoriasis is sometimes diagnosed as keratotic eczema. Erythrodermic psoriasis can be confused with any condition causing generalized erythema, such as Sézary syndrome or drug reactions. Guttate psoriasis can be mistaken for secondary syphilis or pityriasis rosea. Many conditions including cutaneous candidiasis, extramammary Paget's disease, and contact dermatitis can imitate inverse psoriasis [3]. Any diagnostic confusion is usually resolved over time as characteristic lesions become manifested or with a skin biopsy.

25.6 Treatment

Treatment is similar across ethnic populations. Typically, combination therapy yields the best results. Management options include topical and systemic glucocorticoids, topical and oral retinoids, anthralins, calcipotriene, immunosuppressants, phototherapy, biologics that target either T cells or cytokines, and various other herbal remedies [3, 5, 6].

Coal tar, calcipotriol, anthralin, and topical steroids have proven efficacy in Indian patients. The newer "biologics" have been found effective in several populations, including infliximab in China, etanercept in African Americans and Hispanics, and ustekinumab in Taiwan and Korea, to name a few [2, 8, 9]. Other therapies used around the world include neem oil, turmeric (found in curry powder), acupuncture, indirubin, and many others [3, 5].

Phototherapy, a leading treatment for patients with lesions covering greater than 10 % of body surface area, poses a risk of hyperpigmentation because patients with skin of color have a more active melanogenic response to UV light. To protect from this outcome, changing from two treatments of PUVA (psoralens plus UVA) per week to three per week lowered the total dose without changing efficacy in one study. Further, some physicians push for higher doses to achieve erythrogenic levels, but a recent study showed that suberythrogenic doses of narrowband UVB are just as effective in skin of color [10]. These strategies reduce melanogenesis by reducing the dose of UV radiation.

Modified endpoints may be needed when treating patients with darker skin to account for the propensity for skin of color for hypo- or hyperpigmentation. For example, the resolution of dyschromia would likely be an equal or greater endpoint than improvement in scale or thickness in affected patients [2].

References

1. Chandran V, Raychaudhuri SP. Geoepidemiology and environmental factors of psoriasis and psoriatic arthritis. J Autoimmun. 2010;34(3):J314–21.
2. Shah SK, Arthur A, Yang YC, Steven S, Alexis AF. A retrospective study to investigate racial and ethnic variations in the treatment of psoriasis with etanercept. J Drugs Dermatol. 2011;10(8): 866–72.
3. Bolognia JL, Jorizzo JL, Schaffer JV. Dermatology, vol. 1. 3rd ed. China: Elsevier; 2012. p. 135–55.
4. Gelfand JM, Stern RS, Nijsten T, Feldman SR, Thomas J, Kist J, Rolstad T, Margolis DJ. The prevalence of psoriasis in African Americans: results from a population-based study. J Am Acad Dermatol. 2005;52(1):23–6.
5. Kelly AP, Taylor SC, editors. Dermatology for skin of color. New York: McGraw Hill; 2009. p. 139–45.
6. Nestle FO, Kaplan DH, Barker J. Psoriasis. N Engl J Med. 2009;361(5):496–509.
7. McMichael AJ, Vachiramon V, Guzman-Sanchez DA, Camacho F. Psoriasis in African-Americans: a Caregivers' survey. J Drugs Dermatol. 2012;11(4):478–82.
8. Yang HZ, Wang K, Jin HZ, Gao TW, Xiao SX, Xu IH, Wang BX, Zhang FR, Li CY, Liu XM, Tu CX, Ji SZ, Zhu XJ. Infliximab monotherapy for Chinese patients with moderate to severe plaque psoriasis: a randomized, double-blind, placebo-controlled multicenter trial. Chin Med J. 2012;125(11):1845–51.
9. Tsai TF, Ho JC, Song M, Szapary P, Guzzo C, Shen YK, Li S, Kim KJ, Kim TY, Choi JH, Youn JI. Efficacy and safety of ustekinumab for the treatment of moderate-to-severe psoriasis: a phase III, randomized, placebo-controlled trial in Taiwanese and Korean patients (PEARL). J Dermatol Sci. 2011;63(3):154–63.
10. Syed ZU, Hamzavi IH. Role of phototherapy in patients with skin of color. Semin Cutan Med Surg. 2011;30(4):184–9.

Part IV

Granulomatous Diseases

Sarcoidosis

26

Diane Jackson-Richards

Contents

D. Jackson-Richards, MD
Department of Dermatology, Multicultural Dermatology Center,
Henry Ford Hospital, 3031 W. Grand Blvd.,
Detroit, MI 48202, USA
e-mail: djackso1@hfhs.org

26.1 Epidemiology

Sarcoidosis has a worldwide distribution affecting all races and both sexes. Annual incidence has been reported as high as 64/100,000 in Sweden and lowest in Spain and Japan, with a reported rate of 1.4/100,000 [1]. There is significant racial variation of sarcoidosis in the United States with 10–14/100,000 in whites and 36–64/100,000 in African Americans. Rybicki et al. studied the incidence of sarcoidosis in the Detroit, MI, metropolitan area and findings were the following: African American females, 39/100,000; African American males, 30/100,000; white females, 12/100,000; and white males, 9/100,000. African American women, aged 30–39, had the highest incidence, at 107/100,000 [2].

26.2 Etiology

The etiology of sarcoidosis is unknown; however, hypotheses include infectious, genetic, and immunologic etiologies. Several studies have implicated mycobacteria as causative agents; however, detection of mycobacteria DNA in sarcoidal tissue has been inconclusive, and it has never been cultured from sarcoidal tissue [3]. Martinetti et al. [4] found a positive association of HLA-1, HLA-B8, and HLA-DR3 with sarcoidosis in a study of European patients. Rybicki et al. [5] found that familial clusters occurred more commonly in African Americans. The immunologic theory is that an unknown antigen is presented to CD4+, Th1 subtype T-helper cells by macrophages, bearing MHC class II molecules. Cytokines from CD4+ T-cells, IL-2, and interferon gamma stimulate lymphocytes and induce granuloma formation in the target organ. The recruitment of CD4+ T-cells from the circulation leads to a decreased delayed-type hypersensitivity reaction. Anergy is often seen in patients in the early stages of the disease. Cytokines also stimulate B-cells, leading to hypergammaglobulinemia [6].

D. Jackson-Richards, A.G. Pandya (eds.), *Dermatology Atlas for Skin of Color*,
DOI 10.1007/978-3-642-54446-0_26, © Springer-Verlag Berlin Heidelberg 2014

26.3 Clinical Findings

Sarcoidosis involves the skin in 25 % of cases [7], and dermatologists are often involved in confirming the diagnosis. Cutaneous lesions are divided into specific (those containing granulomas) and nonspecific or reactive (those without granulomas). Classic specific skin lesions are asymptomatic red-brown papules, nodules, and plaques. These lesions are commonly found on the face, lips, neck, upper back, and extremities (Figs. 26.1, 26.2, 26.3, 26.4, 26.5, and 26.6). Lupus pernio is the most common cutaneous presentation, consisting of red-brown to violaceous papules and nodules on the nose, lips, cheeks, and ears which can lead to scarring (Figs. 26.7 and 26.8). Lupus pernio is most common in African Americans and is usually associated with chronic, fibrotic sarcoidosis of the upper respiratory tract, nasopharynx, and lungs (Figs. 26.9 and 26.10). Sarcoidosis is often called the "great imitator" because of its wide variety of presentations. Other less common cutaneous lesions include subcutaneous nodules, ichthyosiform dermatitis, psoriasiform plaques, hypopigmented macules and plaques (Fig. 26.11), cicatricial alopecia, lichenoid papules and plaques, erythroderma, and ulcers.

Erythema nodosum is a nonspecific presentation of sarcoidosis. Sarcoidosis is referred to as Lofgren's syndrome when presenting as erythema nodosum and accompanied by hilar adenopathy, fever, iritis, and migratory arthritis. Erythema nodosum associated with sarcoidosis spontaneously resolves in 83 % of patients within 2 years. Other nonspecific cutaneous lesions include onychodystrophy and clubbing of the fingers, with or without bone cysts.

Pulmonary involvement occurs in 90 % of sarcoid cases and may be asymptomatic or present with cough, dyspnea, or chest pain. Chest x-ray most commonly shows hilar and paratracheal adenopathy, but pulmonary infiltrates may also be seen, with pulmonary fibrosis in end-stage disease. Ocular involvement presenting as acute anterior uveitis, lacrimal gland enlargement, and iritis is seen in 30–50 % of cases. Granulomas occur in the liver and spleen in 50–80 % of patients. Although hepatic granulomas may be asymptomatic, splenomegaly is usually associated with extensive fibrosis of other organs and poor prognosis. Musculoskeletal changes present as bone cysts, arthralgias, and myalgias. Central and peripheral nervous systems as well as the cardiac and endocrine systems may also be involved. Hypercalcemia caused by alveolar macrophage secretion of 1,25-dihydroxyvitamin D3 is seen in 17 % of cases. Cardiac involvement occurs in only 5 % of cases, presenting as an infiltrative myopathy, pericarditis, and even sudden death. Iwai et al. examined racial differences in cardiac sarcoidosis seen at autopsy. Cardiac granulomas were seen in 10–20 % of cases in the United States compared to 67 % in Japan [8].

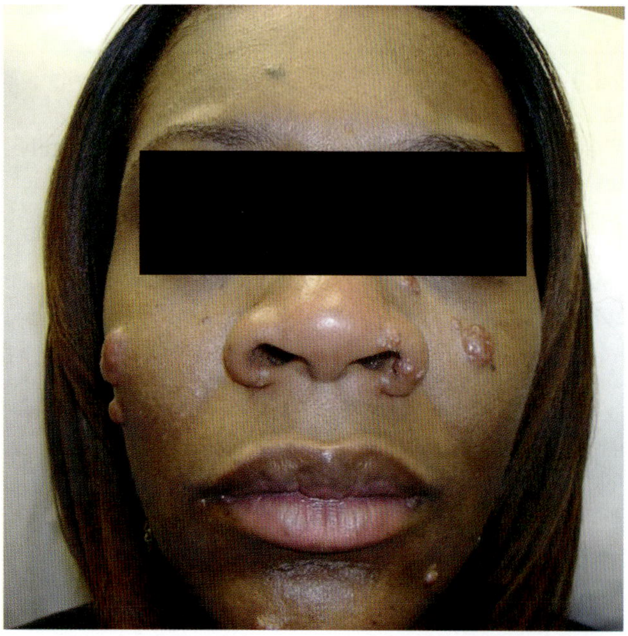

Fig. 26.1 African American female with sarcoidosis on the face

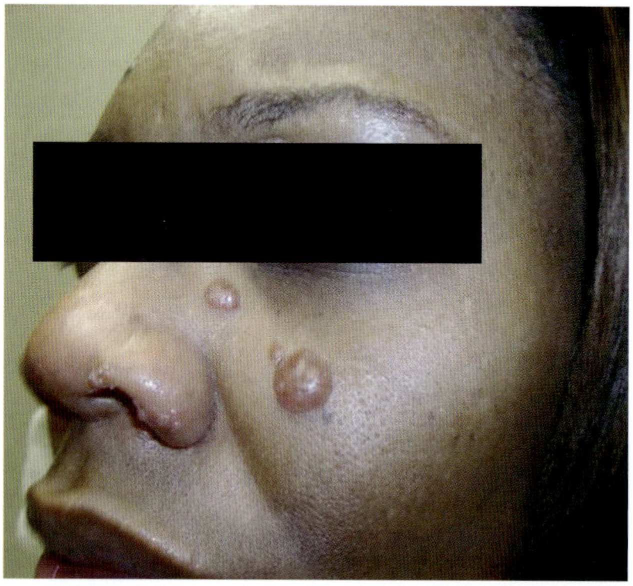

Fig. 26.2 African American female with sarcoidosis on the left cheek

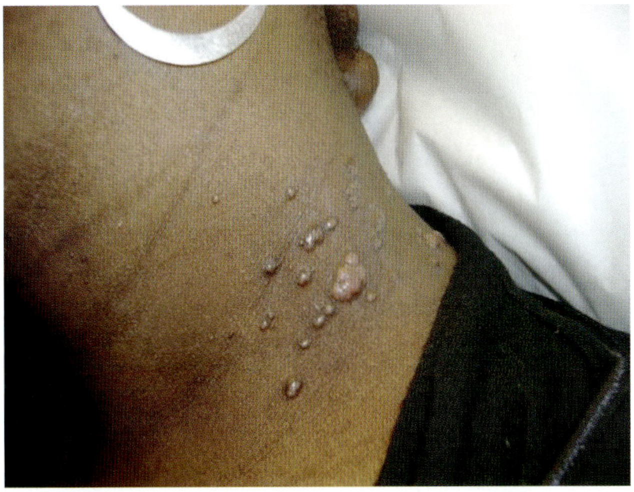

Fig. 26.3 African American female with sarcoidosis on the left neck

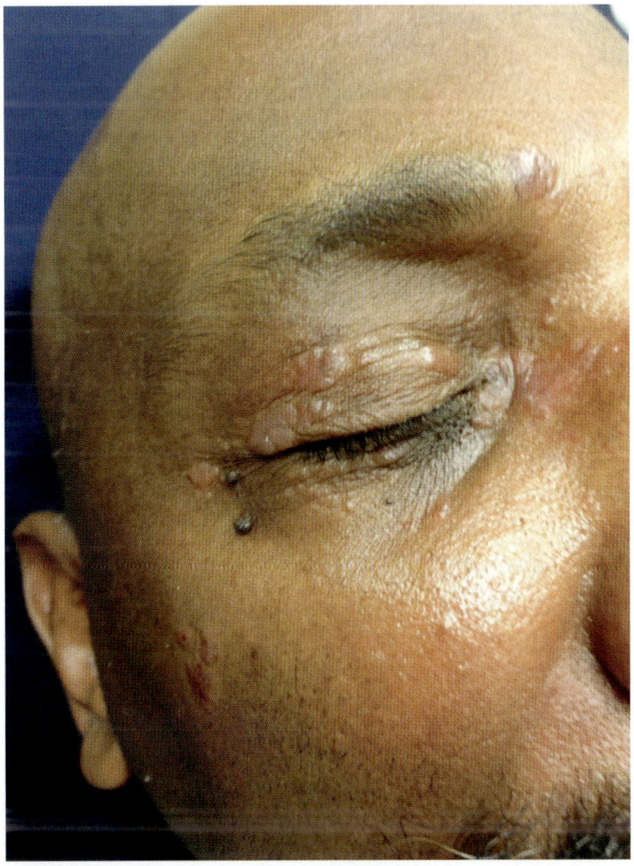

Fig. 26.4 Sarcoidosis in an African American male, right face

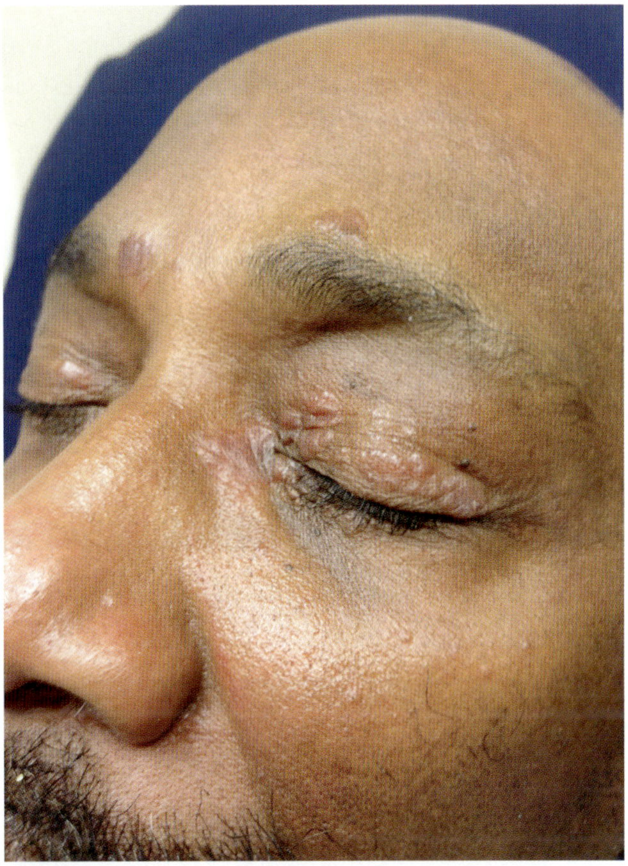

Fig. 26.5 Sarcoidosis in an African American male, left face

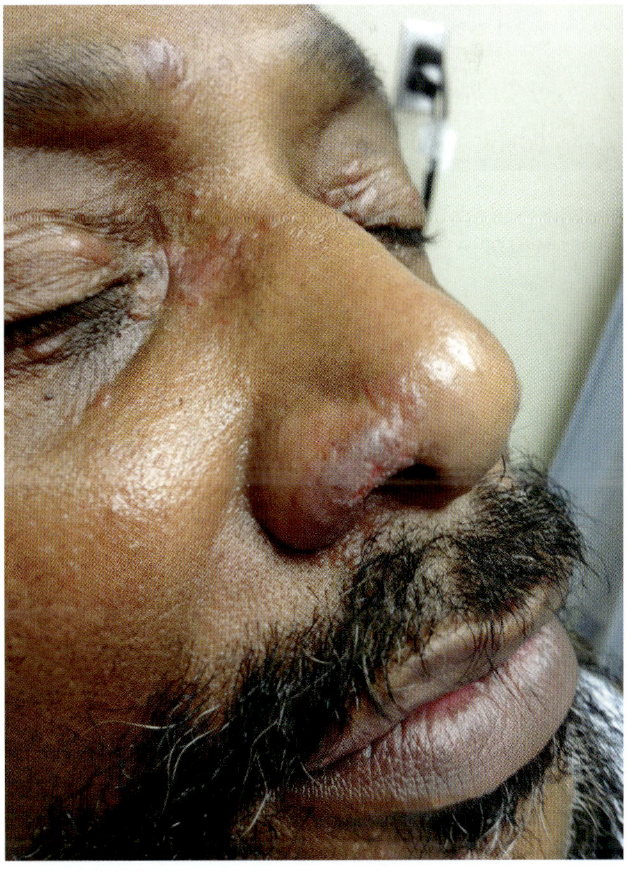

Fig. 26.6 Sarcoidosis in an African American male, right nasal ala

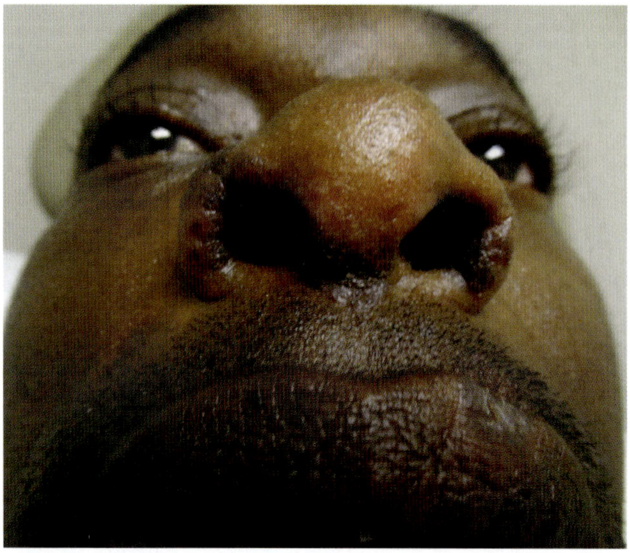

Fig. 26.7 Sarcoidosis in an African American male, nose

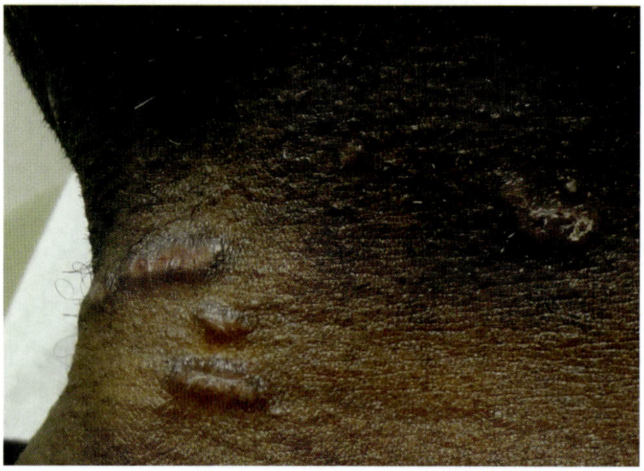

Fig. 26.8 Sarcoidosis in areas of trauma of an African American male, lower beard region of the neck

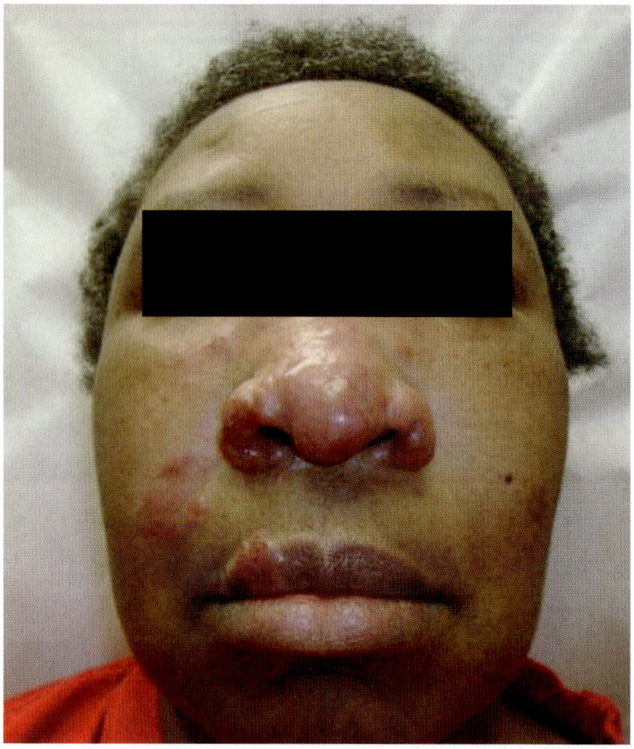

Fig. 26.9 Lupus pernio in an African American female

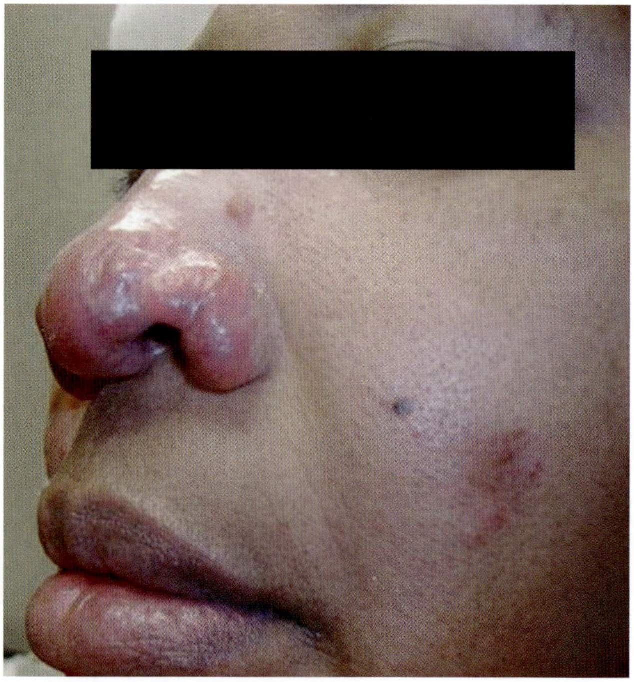

Fig. 26.10 Lupus pernio in an African American female, left face

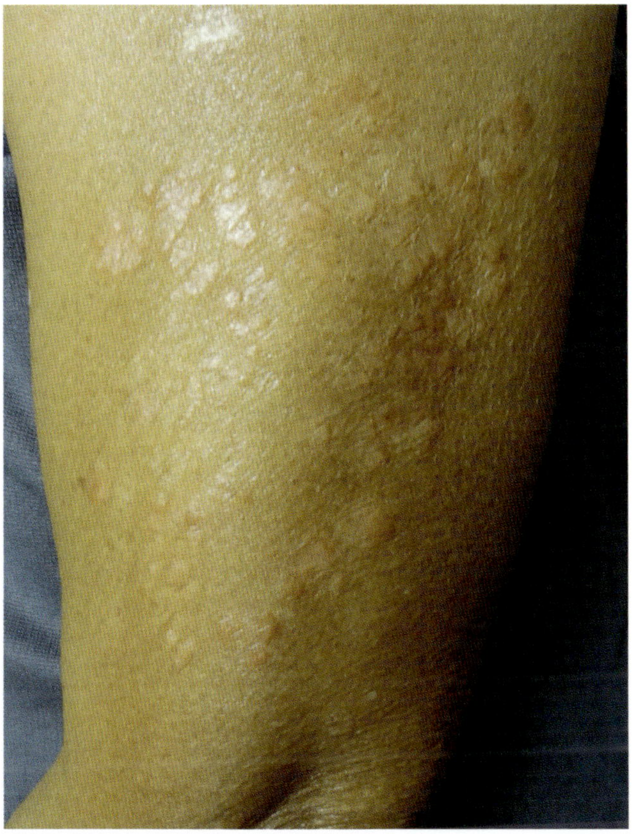

Fig. 26.11 Sarcoidosis of the left upper arm in a Hispanic female

26.4 Diagnosis

Diagnosis of sarcoidosis is one of the exclusions and should include a supportive history and histological evidence of noncaseating granulomas in the tissue, typically in the skin or paratracheal nodes. Histology shows noncaseating epithelioid granulomas with a sparse lymphocytic infiltrate at the periphery of the granulomas and occasional giant cells. Biopsies should be polarized to rule out foreign body reactions and tissue cultures done to rule out an infectious etiology. Workup should include chest x-ray, pulmonary function tests, CBC, ESR, creatinine, hepatic tests, calcium, ACE, and G6PD if antimalarials are considered. ACE levels may be elevated but are not diagnostic of sarcoidosis and have a false-negative rate of 40 %.

26.5 Treatment

Treatment of sarcoidosis is dependent on the severity of the patient's symptoms and the extent of organ involvement. Localized cutaneous lesions are often treated with topical corticosteroids or intralesional triamcinolone 5–10 mg/ml injections performed monthly. Systemic corticosteroids are used for more extensive cutaneous lesions or systemic sarcoidosis [7]. Other therapies include hydroxychloroquine, chloroquine, methotrexate, allopurinol, isotretinoin, infliximab, adalimumab, and thalidomide [9]. Patients with sarcoidosis may have spontaneous resolution of disease in 50–60 % of cases and even as high as 86 %, when presenting with erythema nodosum. The disease is chronic and progressive in 20 % of affected patients. African Americans generally have more prolonged disease, requiring more aggressive therapy, compared to Caucasians. Because of a higher incidence of G6PD deficiency in the skin of color patients, G6PD should be checked prior to initiating antimalarials. Caution should be used in vitamin D supplementation in sarcoidosis patients due to risk of hypercalcemia.

References

1. Hosoda Y, Yamaguchi M, Hirag Y. Global epidemiology of sarcoidosis: what story do prevalence and incidence tell us? Clin Chest Med. 1997;18:681–94.
2. Rybicki BA, Major M, Popovich Jr J, Maliarik MJ, Ianuzzii MC. Racial differences in sarcoidosis incidence: a 5-year study in a health maintenance organization. Am J Epidemiol. 1997;145:234–41.
3. Richter E, Greinert U, Kirsten D, Rusch-Gerdes S, Schluter C, Duchrow M, et al. Assessment of mycobacterial DNA in cells and tissues of mycobacterial and sarcoid lesions. Am J Respir Crit Care Med. 1996;153:375–80.
4. Martinetti M, Tinelli C, Kolek V, Cuccia M, Salvaneschi L, Pasturenzi L, et al. The sarcoidosis map: a joint survey of clinical and immunogenetic findings in two European countries. Am J Respir Crit Care Med. 1995;152:557–64.
5. Rybicki BA, Maliarek MJ, Major M, Popovich Jr J, Ianuzzii MC. Epidemiology demographics and genetics of sarcoidosis. Semin Respir Infect. 1998;13:166–73.
6. Kataria YP, Hotter JF. Immunology of sarcoidosis. Clin Chest Med. 1997;18:719–39.
7. English J, Patel BA, Greer K. Sarcoidosis. J Am Acad Dermatol. 2001;44:725–43.
8. Iwai K, Sekiguti M, Hosoda Y, et al. Racial difference in cardiac sarcoidosis incidence observed at autopsy. Sarcoidosis. 1994;11:26–31.
9. Baughman RP, Lower EE. Steroid-sparing alternative treatments for sarcoidosis. Clin Chest Med. 1997;18:853–64.

27 Granuloma Annulare

Bassel Mahmoud and Diane Jackson-Richards

Contents

B. Mahmoud, MD • D. Jackson-Richards, MD (✉)
Department of Dermatology, Multicultural Dermatology Center, Henry Ford Hospital, 3031 W. Grand Blvd., Detroit, MI 48202, USA
e-mail: djackso1@hfhs.org

27.1 Introduction

Granuloma annulare (GA) is a benign, commonly self-limiting dermatosis, which presents as flesh-colored or erythematous papules, frequently arranged in an annular configuration on the distal extremities. The descriptive term of granuloma annulare comes from the combination of the granulomatous appearance histopathologically and the annular configuration clinically.

27.2 Epidemiology

GA is more common in young adults; two-thirds of patients are less than 30 years of age. The female-to-male ratio is approximately 2:1. GA does not favor a specific race or ethnic group [1].

27.3 Etiology

Familial cases of GA have been reported, including cases in identical twins, and an association may exist between generalized GA and HLA-Bw35 [2]. The etiology of GA is unknown; however, multiple inciting factors have been proposed, such as trauma and vaccination for tetanus and diphtheria, hepatitis B, and tuberculosis (BCG). GA-like reaction patterns have been reported in association with localized lesions, such as tuberculosis skin tests, viral infections such as Epstein-Barr virus [3], and systemic illnesses such as sarcoidosis. A possible association with diabetes mellitus is controversial.

Other associations with GA include solid organ tumors of the breast, ovary, cervix, prostate, testicle, lung, stomach, and colon and myeloproliferative disorders and myelodysplasia [4–6].

D. Jackson-Richards, A.G. Pandya (eds.), *Dermatology Atlas for Skin of Color*,
DOI 10.1007/978-3-642-54446-0_27,

27.4 Clinical Features

GA classically presents as annular to semi-annular asymptomatic skin-colored to erythematous papules and plaques located on the extremities of young people (Figs. 27.1, 27.2, 27.3, and 27.4). In darker-skinned individuals, skin lesions may not appear erythematous and in contrast may appear brown or gray in color. The distribution of GA is primarily on the upper and lower extremities and to less extend on the trunk, while facial lesions are rare. Clinical variants include localized (most common), generalized (15 % of patients), micropapular, nodular, perforating, patchy, and subcutaneous forms. Generalized or disseminated GA has a symmetric distribution on the trunk and extremities with a later age of onset and poorer response to therapy. Perforating GA may show focal ulceration and is located on the dorsal hands. Deep dermal or subcutaneous GA presents as large nodules.

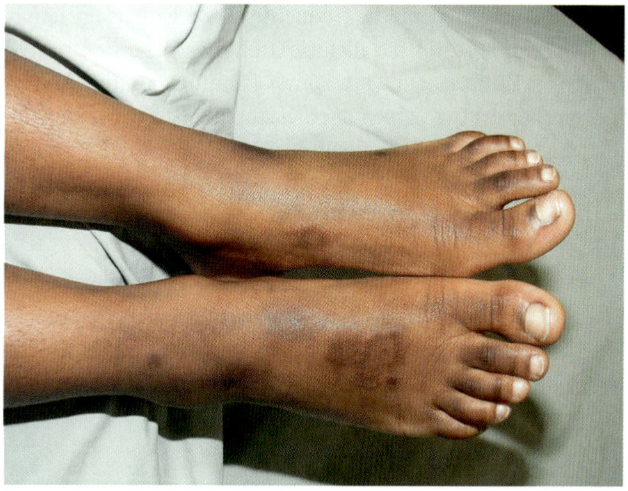

Fig. 27.1 GA in a young African American female (Courtesy of Dr. Tor Shwayder)

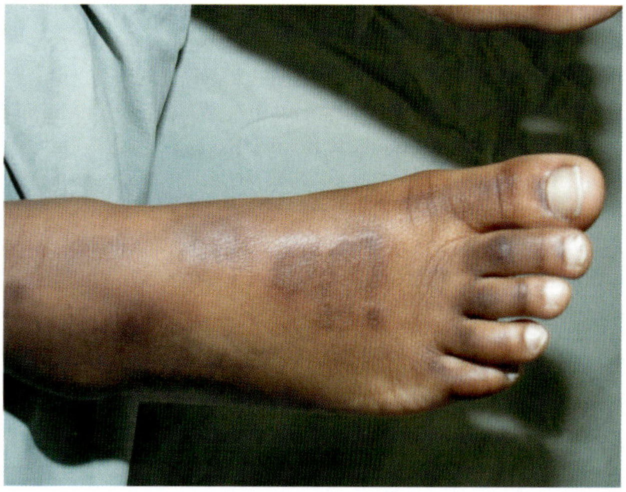

Fig. 27.2 GA in a young African American female (Courtesy of Dr. Tor Shwayder)

Clinical presentation may be atypical, with some lesions being painful, pustular, or follicular. It can also appear in patches or unusual locations, particularly in paraneoplastic GA when it is associated with a malignant neoplasm. Studies showed that the onset of GA ranges from 5 years before to 27 years after the diagnosis of a lymphoma. GA-like eruption can be a clinical indicator of neoplasm progression in patients, and although primarily a reactive pattern, it can rarely harbor malignant neoplastic cells [3–6].

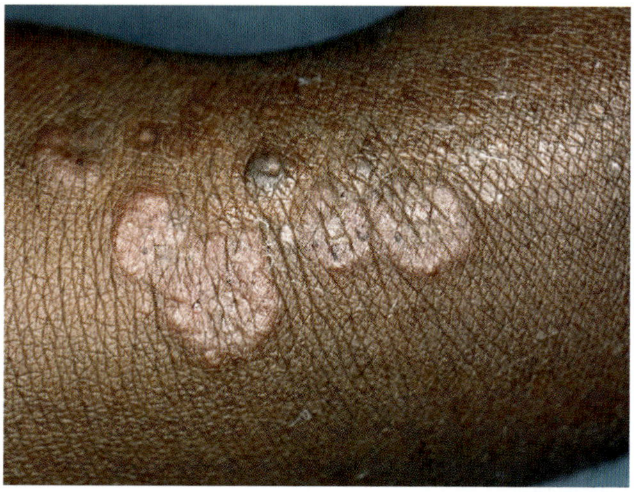

Fig. 27.3 GA in an adult African American female

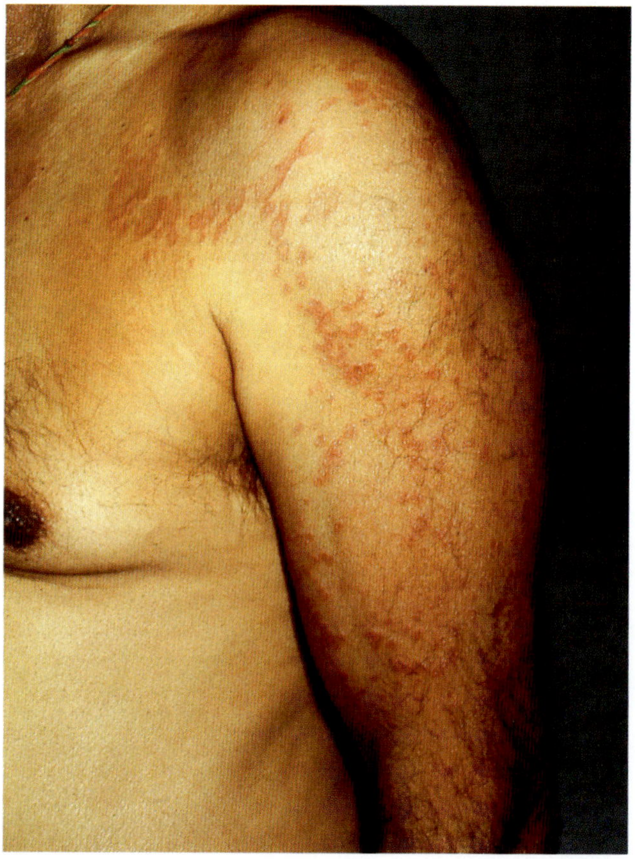

Fig. 27.4 GA on the arm and shoulder of a South Asian male

27.5 Histopathologic Features

The most prominent histologic feature of GA is the palisading granuloma, which consists of a central core of necrobiotic collagen, surrounded by a radially arranged infiltrate of lymphocytes, histiocytes, and fibroblasts. There is also mucin deposition, identified with Alcian blue and colloidal iron stains. Histiocytes exist in three different patterns: the interstitial pattern in which scattered histiocytes are distributed between collagen fibers. The second pattern is palisading granulomas with central connective tissue degeneration surrounded by histiocytes and lymphocytes. The third pattern consists of epithelioid histiocytic nodules. In deep GA, the palisaded granulomas extend into the deep dermis or subcutaneous fat. In perforating GA, there is transepidermal elimination of necrobiotic collagen.

27.6 Differential Diagnosis

GA is diagnosed mainly on its clinical and histopathologic features. The clinical differential diagnosis of GA includes annular sarcoidosis, warts, and eruptive xanthomas. It also includes annular plaques of mycosis fungoides and leprosy. Subcutaneous GA can resemble rheumatoid nodules and deep granulomatous infections. The histopathologic differential diagnosis of GA includes diseases showing the pattern of palisading granulomas such as rheumatoid nodule and necrobiosis lipoidica and also includes morphea, cutaneous T-cell lymphoma, xanthoma, and epithelioid sarcoma.

27.7 Treatment

Reassurance and clinical observation is best for localized, asymptomatic GA due its self-limiting nature. Spontaneous resolution occurs within 2 years in 50 % of patients, but there is a 40 % recurrence rate. Topical treatments include high-potency topical corticosteroids, intralesional corticosteroid injections, topical tacrolimus [7], and cryosurgery. Light and laser therapy with PUVA [8] or UVA1 therapy and CO_2 laser treatment have also been used. Systemic treatment for extensive cases includes dapsone [9], pentoxifylline, hydroxychloroquine, isotretinoin, chlorambucil, interferon gamma, cyclosporine, potassium iodide, nicotinamide, niacinamide, salicylates acids, chlorpropamide, thyroxine, and dipyridamole. Antibiotics [10] were reported with success for treatment of GA by treating underlying infections such as cefaclor, cefixime, penicillin, amoxicillin, ciprofloxacin, erythromycin, clarithromycin, and trimethoprim/sulfamethoxazole. A combination of three antibiotics (rifampin, ofloxacin, and minocycline) administered monthly for 3 months led to improvement in a series of 6 patients [11]. Case reports have reported successful treatment with TNF-α inhibitors. Adalimumab [12] and infliximab [13] were reported as being effective for generalized GA, but no randomized controlled studies have been performed to support the aforementioned results. The fact that such a wide variety of medications have been reported as treatments for GA indicates that there is no definitive treatment modality for this disorder.

References

1. Shelley ED. Granuloma annulare. In: Shelley ED, Shelley WB, editors. Advanced dermatologic therapy, vol. 2. Philadelphia: WB Saunders Ltd; 2001. p. 491–8.
2. Friedman-Birnbaum R, Haim S, Gideone O, Barzilai A. Histocompatibility antigens in granuloma annulare. Br J Dermatol. 1978;98:425–8.
3. Martin JE, Wagner AJ, Murphy GF, Pinkus GS, Wang LC. Granuloma annulare heralding angioimmunoblastic T-cell lymphoma in a patient with a history of Epstein-Barr virus-associated B-cell lymphoma. J Clin Oncol. 2009;27(31):e168–71.
4. Bassi A, Scarfi F, Galeone M, Arunachalam M, Difonzo E. Generalized granuloma annulare and non-Hodgkin's lymphoma. Acta Derm Venereol. 2013;93(4):484–5.
5. Sokumbi O, Gibson LE, Comfere NI, Peters MS. Granuloma annulare-like eruption associated with B-cell chronic lymphocytic leukemia. J Cutan Pathol. 2012;39(11):996–1003.
6. Cornejo KM, Lum CA, Izumi AK. A cutaneous interstitial granulomatous dermatitis-like eruption arising in myelodysplasia with leukemic progression. Am J Dermatopathol. 2013;35(2):e26–9.
7. Jain S, Stephens CJ. Successful treatment of disseminated granuloma annulare with topical tacrolimus. Br J Dermatol. 2004;150(5):1042–3.
8. Setterfield J, Huilgol SC, Black MM. Generalised granuloma annulare successfully treated with PUVA. Clin Exp Dermatol. 1999;24:458–60.
9. Steiner A, Pehamberger H, Wolff K. Sulfone treatment of granuloma annulare. J Am Acad Dermatol. 1985;13(6):1004–8.
10. Villahermosa LG, Fajardo Jr TT, Abalos RM, et al. Parallel assessment of 24 monthly doses of rifampin, ofloxacin, and minocycline versus two years of World Health Organization multi-drug therapy for multi-bacillary leprosy. Am J Trop Med Hyg. 2004;70(2):197–200.
11. Marcus DV, Mahmoud BH, Hamzavi IH. Granuloma annulare treated with rifampin, ofloxacin, and minocycline combination therapy. Arch Dermatol. 2009;145(7):787–9.
12. Knoell KA. Efficacy of adalimumab in the treatment of generalized granuloma annulare in monozygotic twins carrying the 8.1 ancestral haplotype. Arch Dermatol. 2009;145:610–1.
13. Murdaca G. Anti-tumor necrosis factor-alpha treatment with infliximab for disseminated granuloma annulare. Am J Clin Dermatol. 2010;11:437–9.

Part V

Connective Tissue Diseases

Cutaneous Lupus Erythematosus

28

Daniel Grabell, Kathryn A. Bowman,
and Benjamin F. Chong

Contents

D. Grabell, MBA • K.A. Bowman, BS • B.F. Chong, MD (✉)
Department of Dermatology, University of Texas Southwestern
Medical Center, 5323 Harry Hines Blvd., Dallas, TX 75390, USA
e-mail: daniel.grabell@utsouthwestern.edu;
kathryn.bowman@utsouthwestern.edu;
ben.chong@utsouthwestern.edu

28.1 Introduction

Lupus erythematosus (LE) results from dysregulation of the immune system leading to multi-organ involvement. Its clinical presentations range from life-threatening manifestations (e.g., nephritis, cerebritis) of systemic lupus erythematosus (SLE) to exclusive skin involvement. The Gilliam classification of skin lesions in LE divides them into LE-specific and LE-nonspecific skin disease (Table 28.1) [1].

28.2 Epidemiology

The age- and gender-adjusted incidence and prevalence rates of CLE have been reported as 4.30 per 100,000 and 73.24 per 100,000, respectively. CLE females outnumber males by

Table 28.1 Gilliam classification of skin lesions in LE (abbreviated version) [1]

1. LE-specific skin disease
(a) Acute cutaneous LE (ACLE)
(i) Localized ACLE – malar “butterfly” rash
(ii) Generalized ACLE – malar rash, photosensitive lupus dermatitis
(b) Subacute cutaneous LE (SCLE)
(i) Annular SCLE
(ii) Papulosquamous SCLE
(c) Chronic cutaneous LE (CCLE)
(i) Discoid LE (DLE) – the most common form of CCLE
(ii) Other less common forms – lupus panniculitis, lupus tumidus, chilblain LE
2. LE-nonspecific skin disease (examples)
(a) Photosensitivity
(b) Oral ulcers
(c) Alopecia
(d) Nail changes (e.g., periungual telangiectasia)
(e) Raynaud’s phenomenon
(f) Vasculitis
(g) Urticaria
(h) Calcinosis cutis

D. Jackson-Richards, A.G. Pandya (eds.), *Dermatology Atlas for Skin of Color*,
DOI 10.1007/978-3-642-54446-0_28, © Springer-Verlag Berlin Heidelberg 2014

almost 2:1 ratio. A cumulative incidence of progression from CLE to SLE of 19 % was reported with a mean length to progression of 8.2 years [2]. While there is no large epidemiological study of CLE patients, one quality-of-life study of 248 CLE patients reported an ethnic breakdown of 42 % Caucasian, 35 % African American, 3 % Asian, and 3 % Hispanic/Latino [3]. A cohort study showed no major differences in terms of demographical, clinical, and biological presentations between patients of African origin and Caucasian patients with cutaneous lupus [3, 4].

28.3 Etiology

Formation of CLE skin lesions likely results from multiple etiologic factors including environmental triggers (e.g., ultraviolet (UV) radiation, viruses) and genetics (e.g., HLA susceptibility genes and complement deficiencies). While the pathogenesis of CLE is not completely understood, one model proposes that UV radiation induces keratinocyte apoptosis, which leads to the translocation of blebs containing various nuclear antigens, such as Ro, La, nucleosome, and ribonucleoprotein, to the cell surface. These self-antigens subsequently can be targets of autoantibodies and dendritic cells, which can amplify the immune response by activating complement and T cells, respectively. In particular, plasmacytoid dendritic cells produce abundant amounts of type I interferons which enhance cytotoxic activity of natural killer cells and $CD8^+$ T cells, differentiation of T cells and B cells, and antibody production. UV radiation also stimulates cytokine release by keratinocytes which stimulate production of cytokines, chemokines, and adhesion molecules that recruit T cells and other leukocytes [5].

28.4 Clinical Features

CLE is divided into lupus-specific and -nonspecific lesions, with the former having histopathologic features characteristic of cutaneous lupus. According to the Gilliam classification, lupus-specific skin disease has three major categories: acute (ACLE), subacute (SCLE), and chronic cutaneous lupus erythematosus (CCLE) [1].

ACLE can occur as a generalized or localized disease. The localized form can present as bilateral, malar, transient, and erythematous patches and plaques, sparing the nasolabial folds following sun exposure (Fig. 28.1). Clinical severity ranges from mild erythema to intense edema that lasts from several hours to weeks. Dyspigmentation is more common in darker-skinned patients. Generalized ACLE is represented by multiple, erythematous confluent macules and papules in photo-exposed areas. Severe cases can involve bullae (bullous ACLE), erythema multiforme-like lesions (Rowell's syndrome) (Fig. 28.2), and widespread skin sloughing with mucous membrane involvement (TEN-like ACLE). Mimickers of ACLE include rosacea, polymorphous light eruption, seborrheic dermatitis, and dermatomyositis.

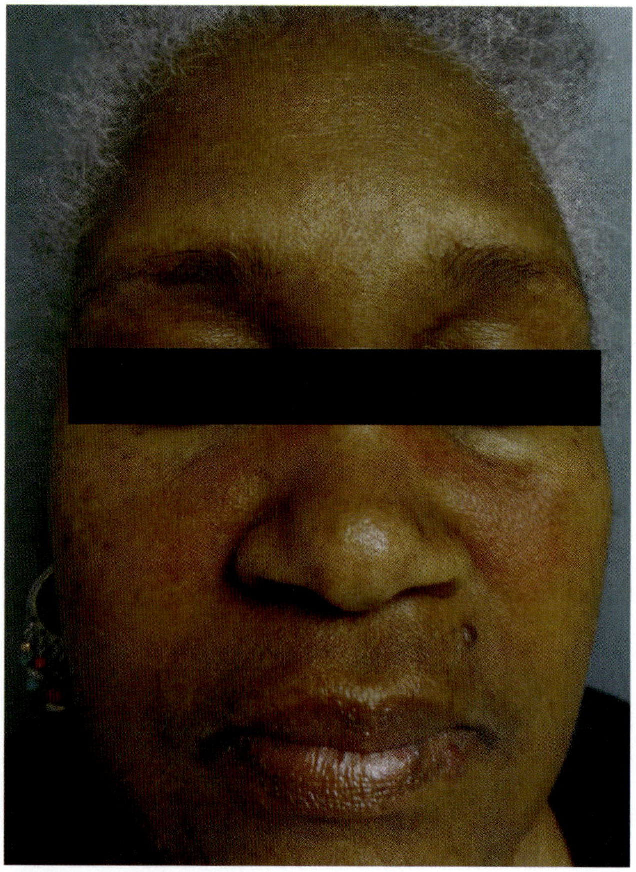

Fig. 28.1 Acute cutaneous lupus on the face of an African American female

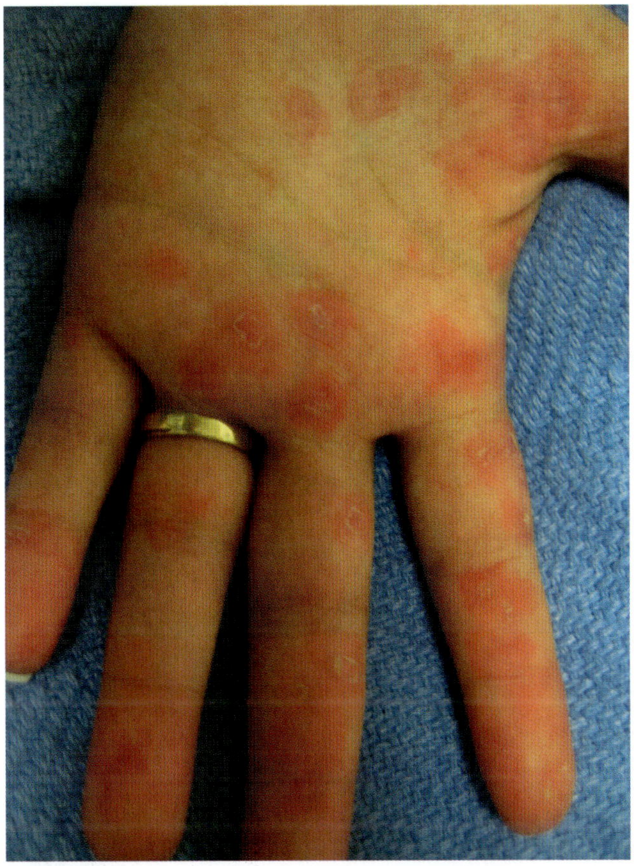

Fig. 28.2 Lesions of Rowell's syndrome on the palm of a Hispanic female

SCLE, a variant less commonly seen in darker skin types, favors the upper chest and extensor aspects of the upper extremities. Lesions typically fall into two categories, papulosquamous and annular. The papulosquamous variant is composed of erythematous papules coalescing into scaly plaques that mimic psoriasis. Annular SCLE plaques are bright red with central clearing and peripheral scale. Both types of lesions may resolve with slight atrophy and hypopigmentation. All SCLE cases need to be screened for potential offending drugs such as terbinafine, hydrochlorothiazide, and calcium channel blockers [6]. The differential diagnosis of SCLE includes tinea corporis, psoriasis, erythema annulare centrifugum, dermatomyositis, and nummular eczema.

CCLE contains several subtypes listed in Table 28.1, with the most common subtype being discoid lupus erythematosus (DLE). DLE lesions initially present as erythematous, scaly papules that become plaques with central atrophy and hypopigmentation, surrounding hyperpigmentation, and firmly adherent scale that are painful if lifted manually ("carpet tack sign") [7]. In hair-bearing areas, scarring alopecia is commonly seen (Fig. 28.3). Localized DLE can be found in sites above the neck that are either in photo-exposed (e.g., face, scalp) or photoprotected areas (e.g., ears) (Figs. 28.4, 28.5, 28.6, and 28.7). These highly visible lesions can be cosmetically disfiguring in darker skin types. Generalized DLE can include the trunk (upper more than lower) (Figs. 28.8 and 28.9) and extensor surfaces of the extremities and represent higher risk of systemic disease. Other skin diseases considered in the differential include lichen planus, lichen planopilaris, cicatricial pemphigoid, vitiligo, post-inflammatory hypopigmentation, and squamous cell carcinoma. Squamous cell carcinomas arising from CCLE have been reported in African American patients [8]. Lupus erythematosus panniculitis is a rare subtype of CCLE characterized by subcutaneous tender nodules and plaques that may adhere to overlying skin (Fig. 28.10). The lesions typically appear on the upper thighs, buttocks, breast, and face and resolve with deep atrophy. Lupus erythematosus tumidus (LET) presents in photosensitive areas with urticarial-like annular plaques with little epidermal involvement (Figs. 28.11 and 28.12).

Lupus-nonspecific lesions, some of which are listed in Table 28.1, are more often seen in SLE patients. Diffuse and linear nail dyschromia has been detected in 52 % of African Americans with SLE [9]. Oral ulcers and photosensitivity, the latter of which is less commonly seen in blacks, are included in the American College of Rheumatology diagnostic criteria for SLE.

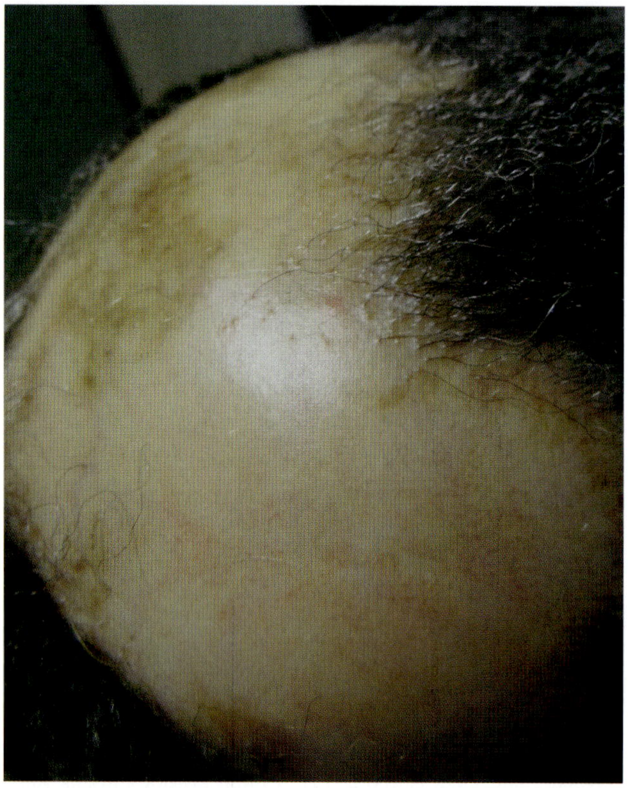

Fig. 28.3 Discoid lupus lesions with scarring alopecia on the scalp of an African American female

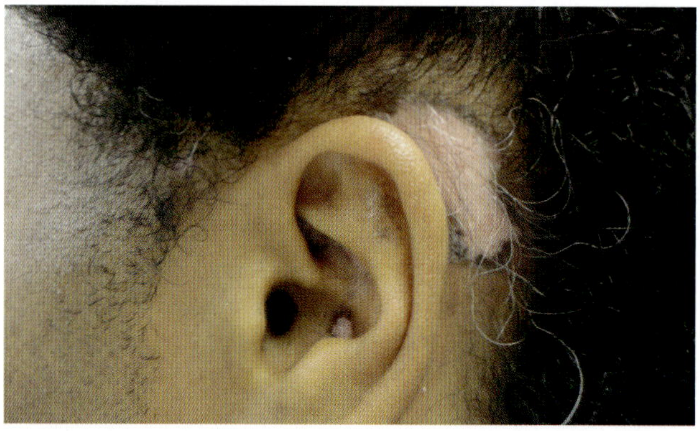

Fig. 28.4 Discoid lupus lesions on the ear and scalp in an African American male

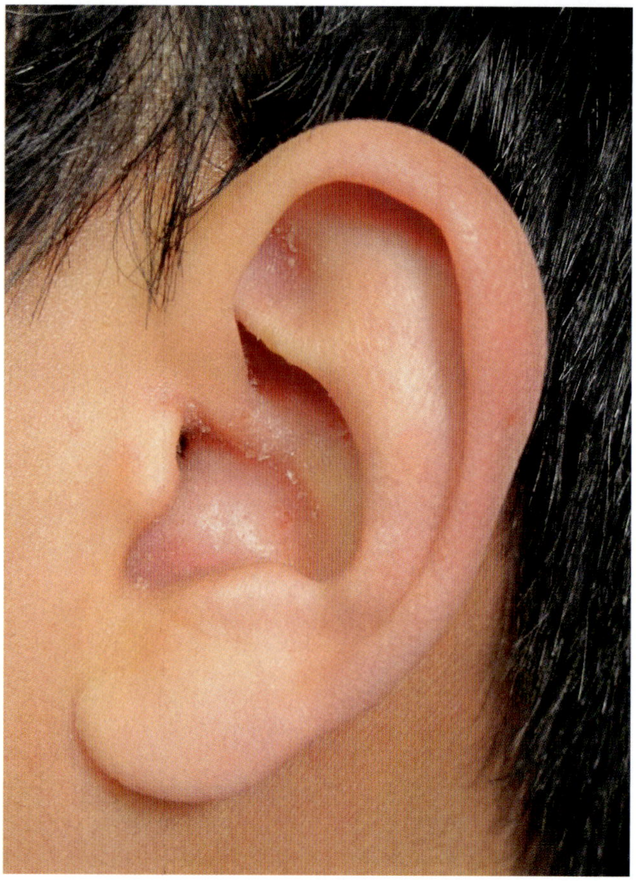

Fig. 28.5 Early discoid lupus lesions on the ear in an Asian male

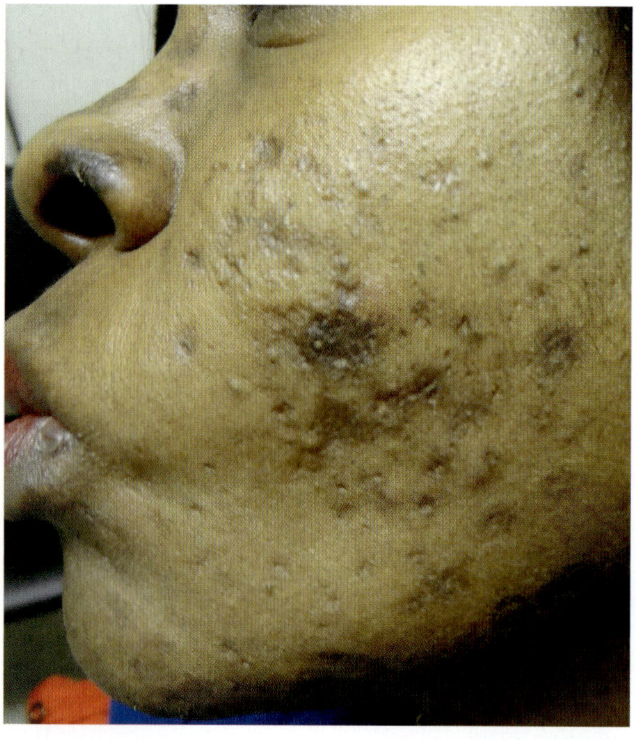

Fig. 28.6 Discoid lupus lesions with scarring on the face of an African American female

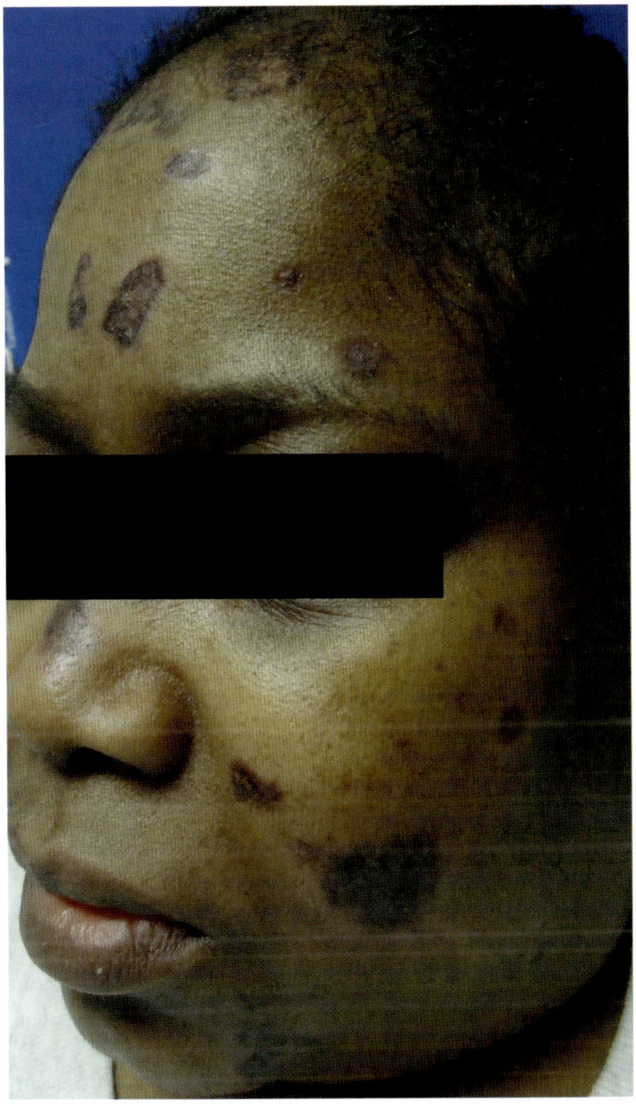

Fig. 28.7 Active discoid lupus lesions with scarring on the face of an African American female

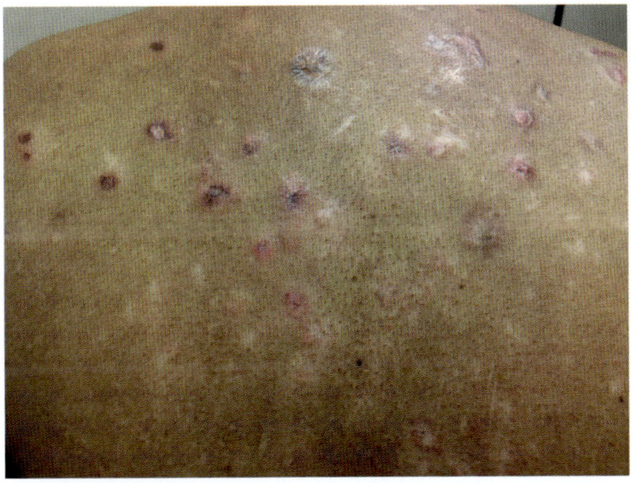

Fig. 28.8 Active discoid lupus lesions on the back of an African American female

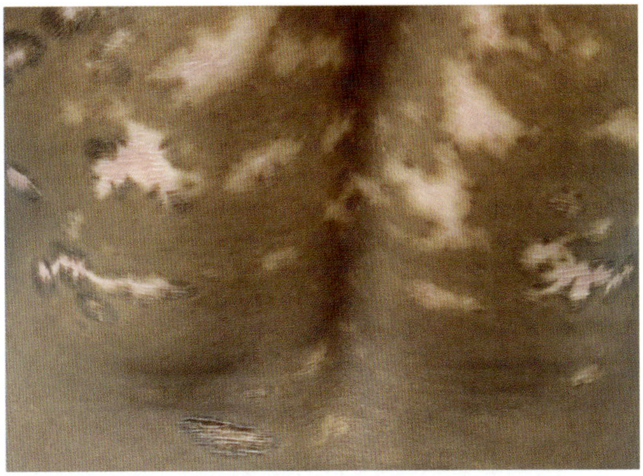

Fig. 28.9 Discoid lupus lesions on the back of an African American female

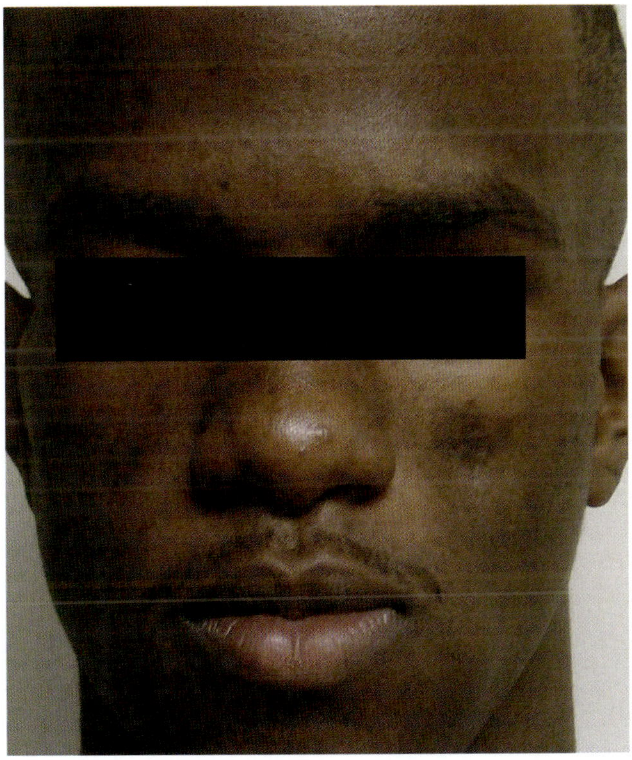

Fig. 28.10 Lupus panniculitis on the cheeks of an African male

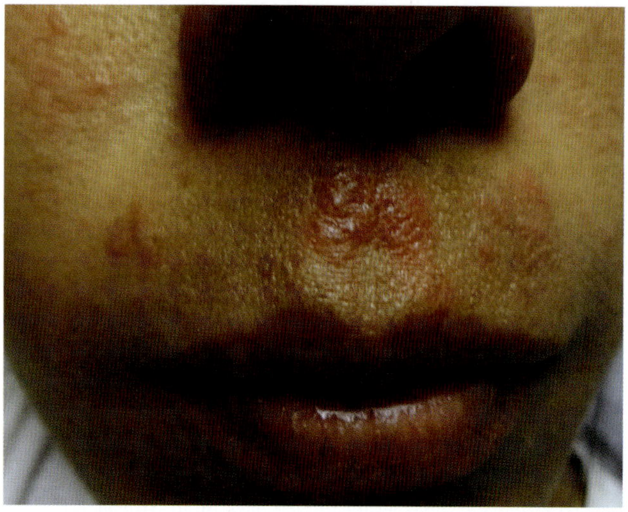

Fig. 28.11 Lupus erythematosus tumidus on the face of a Hispanic female

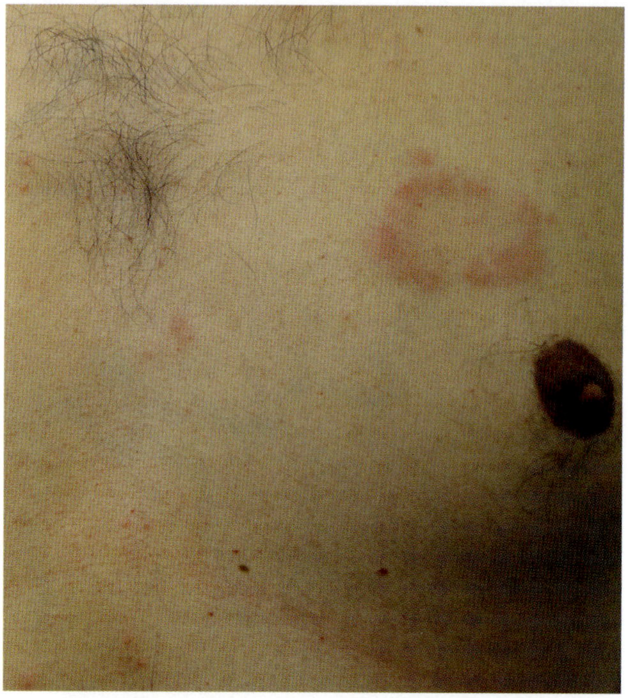

Fig. 28.12 Lupus erythematosus tumidus on the chest of a Hispanic male

28.5 Histopathology

In the early stages of CLE, neutrophils, occasional perivascular lymphocytic infiltrates, and focal vacuolar alterations of basal cells may be seen. Dense perivascular and periappendageal lymphocytic infiltrates in the papillary and reticular dermis appear in fully developed lesions. Abundant mucin deposition in the reticular dermis is also seen.

28.6 Diagnosis and Workup

The diagnosis of CLE is made after a careful history and physical exam and histological confirmation from a skin biopsy. A positive antinuclear antibody and anti-Ro antibody test would support CLE and SCLE diagnosis, respectively, but negative tests do not rule out these conditions. All CLE patients should be screened for systemic involvement through a complete review of systems. Those with signs suspicious of SLE should have blood drawn for complete blood count, renal function tests, anti-double-stranded DNA antibody, anti-Smith antibody, and complement levels and have a urinalysis ordered.

28.7 Treatment

The treatment plan for CLE patients involves discussion of photoprotection with a combination of topical and/or systemic therapies. Primary prevention is critical to the treatment of CLE. Clinicians can advise patients to avoid sun exposure during peak hours of 10 am to 3 pm, wear protective clothing, and use daily broad-spectrum sunscreen daily. While topical corticosteroids are the cornerstone in treating all CLE lesions, topical calcineurin inhibitors such as tacrolimus and pimecrolimus have been particularly helpful for long-term treatment of CLE patients because they avoid toxicity associated with topical steroids.

Patients unable to obtain adequate control of their CLE with topical agents and photoprotection should be considered for systemic agents including antimalarials and immunosuppressants. The antimalarial hydroxychloroquine (maximum dose of 6.5 mg/kg/day to avoid retinal toxicity) can be initiated for at least 2–3 months. If insufficient clinical improvement is seen, quinacrine, which requires compounding of powder into tablets or capsules, at 100 mg once daily, is added. After waiting another 2–3 months without significant change, chloroquine (maximum dose of 3 mg/kg/day to avoid retinal toxicity) can be started in place of hydroxychloroquine while quinacrine is continued. CLE patients refractory to antimalarials can progress to immunosuppressive medications. Corticosteroids (e.g., prednisone at 0.5–1 mg/kg/day) can quickly control severe flares and are tapered over several weeks to months. Methotrexate, which is often used for recalcitrant SCLE and DLE patients, can be prescribed at doses up to 25 mg/week with daily folic acid supplementation except for the day that methotrexate is taken. Mycophenolate mofetil can be an alternative to methotrexate since it requires less laboratory monitoring and is well tolerated. High doses of 2–3 grams/day are often necessary to achieve clinical improvement.

Conclusion

CLE presents in the majority of SLE patients or by itself. Diagnosis is made by clinicopathological correlation. Clinicians must evaluate CLE patients regularly for signs and symptoms seen in SLE. Treatment of CLE should be focused on preventing and controlling skin lesions through a mixture of photoprotective measures, topical medications, and/or oral immunosuppressants.

References

1. Gilliam JN, Sontheimer RD. Distinctive cutaneous subsets in the spectrum of lupus erythematosus. J Am Acad Dermatol. 1981;4(4):471–5.
2. Durosaro O, Davis MD, Reed KB, Rohlinger AL. Incidence of cutaneous lupus erythematosus, 1965–2005: a population-based study. Arch Dermatol. 2009;145(3):249–53.
3. Vasquez R, Wang D, Tran QP, et al. A multicentre, cross-sectional study on quality of life in patients with cutaneous lupus erythematosus. Br J Dermatol. 2013;168(1):145–53.
4. Deligny C, Marie DS, Clyti E, Arfi S, Couppie P. Pure cutaneous lupus erythematosus in a population of African descent in French Guiana: a retrospective population-based description. Lupus. 2012;21(13):1467–71.
5. Lin JH, Dutz JP, Sontheimer RD, Werth VP. Pathophysiology of cutaneous lupus erythematosus. Clin Rev Aller Immunol. 2007;33(1–2):85–106.
6. Lowe G, Henderson CL, Grau RH, Hansen CB, Sontheimer RD. A systematic review of drug-induced subacute cutaneous lupus erythematosus. Br J Dermatol. 2011;164(3):465–72.
7. Kuhn A. Cutaneous lupus erythematosus, vol. 1. Berlin: Springer; 2004.
8. Caruso WR, Stewart ML, Nanda VK, Quismorio Jr FP. Squamous cell carcinoma of the skin in black patients with discoid lupus erythematosus. J Rheumatol. 1987;14(1):156–9.
9. Vaughn RY, Bailey Jr JP, Field RS, et al. Diffuse nail dyschromia in black patients with systemic lupus erythematosus. J Rheumatol. 1990;17(5):640–3.
10. Mody GM, Parag KB, Nathoo BC, Pudifin DJ, Duursma J, Seedat YK. High mortality with systemic lupus erythematosus in hospitalized African blacks. Br J Rheumatol. 1994;33(12):1151–3.

Dermatomyositis

29

Kathryn A. Bowman and Benjamin F. Chong

Contents

K.A. Bowman, BS • B.F. Chong, MD (✉)
Department of Dermatology,
University of Texas Southwestern Medical Center,
5323 Harry Hines Blvd., Dallas, TX 75390-9069, USA
e-mail: kathryn.bowman@utsouthwestern.edu;
ben.chong@utsouthwestern.edu

Abbreviations

EMG	Electromyogram
ILD	Interstitial lung disease
MDA5	Melanoma differentiation-associated gene-5
MRI	Magnetic resonance imaging
NXP2	Nuclear matrix protein-2
PFTs	Pulmonary function tests
TIF1γ	Transcriptional intermediary factor-1γ

29.1 Introduction

Dermatomyositis is an idiopathic inflammatory myopathy affecting both adults and children and predominantly involving the skin and muscle. Although most dermatomyositis cases present with changes in the skin accompanied by muscle weakness and inflammation, amyopathic dermatomyositis is another form of this disorder, which represents approximately 20 % of all dermatomyositis cases. Amyopathic dermatomyositis presents with typical skin changes of dermatomyositis but without myopathic symptoms for at least 6 months. These patients may or may not have laboratory evidence of myopathy [1]. About 10 % of these patients will eventually develop muscle involvement, with this progression occurring up to 14 years after initial onset of symptoms [1].

Dermatomyositis is rarer than systemic lupus erythematosus, affecting 21 in 100,000 people annually, and it occurs three times as frequently in females as in males. Although the peak incidence is seen in adults 40–50 years old, individuals of any age may be affected, even as early as infancy [1]. Dermatomyositis affects all races, with no obvious geographical variation. However, racial variation in associated risk factors, such as an elevated risk for nasopharyngeal carcinoma in affected Asian patients [2], highlights the importance of using race as a factor in determining necessary screening for malignancy.

D. Jackson-Richards, A.G. Pandya (eds.), *Dermatology Atlas for Skin of Color*,
DOI 10.1007/978-3-642-54446-0_29, © Springer-Verlag Berlin Heidelberg 2014

29.2 Pathogenesis

Although dermatomyositis has been classically described as a humorally mediated autoimmune disorder, the etiology and pathogenesis of this disease are incompletely understood. Pathogenesis has largely been attributed to a complement-mediated microangiopathy, characterized by immune complex deposition in small vessels. However, recent evidence suggests abnormalities in cell-mediated and innate immunity as well as nonimmune mechanisms such as hypoxia [3]. A wide array of etiologic factors may play a role in the development of this disease. There is increasing evidence for the role of genetic factors, such as increased risk associated with HLA-DR3 in adult patients [4], and environmental exposures such as viral infections, suggested by increased onset of childhood disease after respiratory and gastrointestinal infections [5]. Pro-inflammatory cytokines contribute to muscle weakness without overt inflammatory changes, leading to typical muscle dysfunction.

29.3 Clinical Features

Dermatomyositis, unlike polymyositis, is associated with characteristic dermatologic lesions. Distinct skin findings include heliotrope rash, shawl sign, Gottron's sign, Gottron's papules, tendon streaking, and mechanic hands. The heliotrope rash is characterized by symmetrical violaceous, erythematous periorbital macules and plaques (Figs. 29.1 and 29.2). The shawl sign is represented by a poikilodermatous scaly patch in the upper back that often is rectangular (Fig. 29.3). Similar features can be found on the upper chest (Figs. 29.4 and 29.5) and lateral thighs ("holster sign"). Gottron's papules are violaceous or erythematous papules or plaques overlying the metacarpophalangeal and interphalangeal joints and are less commonly seen on extensor elbows and knees (Fig. 29.6 and 29.7). Linear streaking of erythematous scaly thin plaques can occur over the dorsal hands and is called tendon streaking. These may appear as hyperpigmentation, especially in patients of African descent. "Mechanic's hands," or hyperkeratosis, fissuring, and linear hyperpigmentation of radial and palmar surfaces

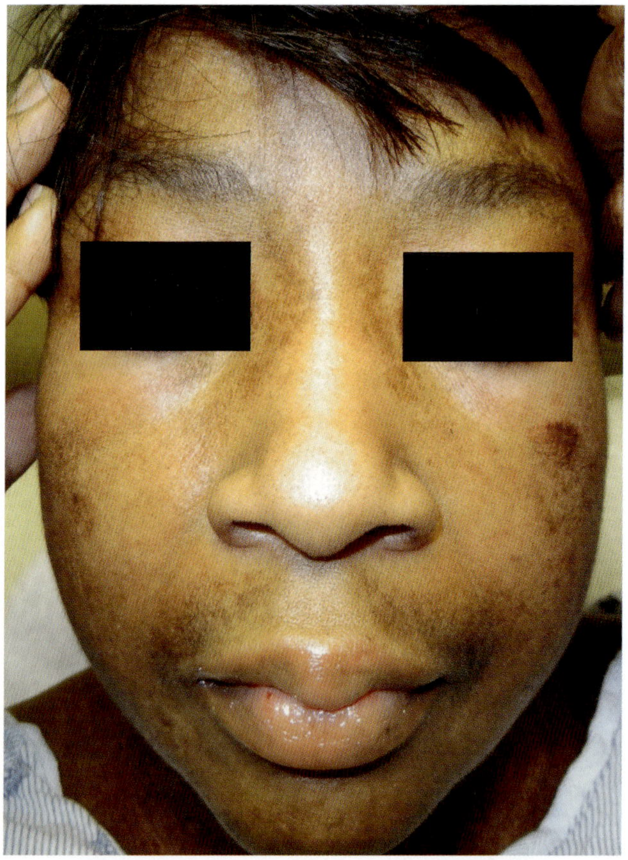

Fig. 29.1 Heliotrope rash on the face of an African American female

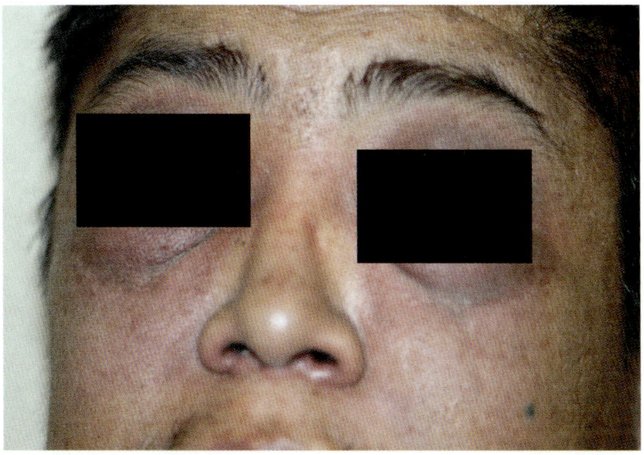

Fig. 29.2 Heliotrope rash on the face of a Hispanic male (Courtesy of Judith Dominguez Cherit, MD)

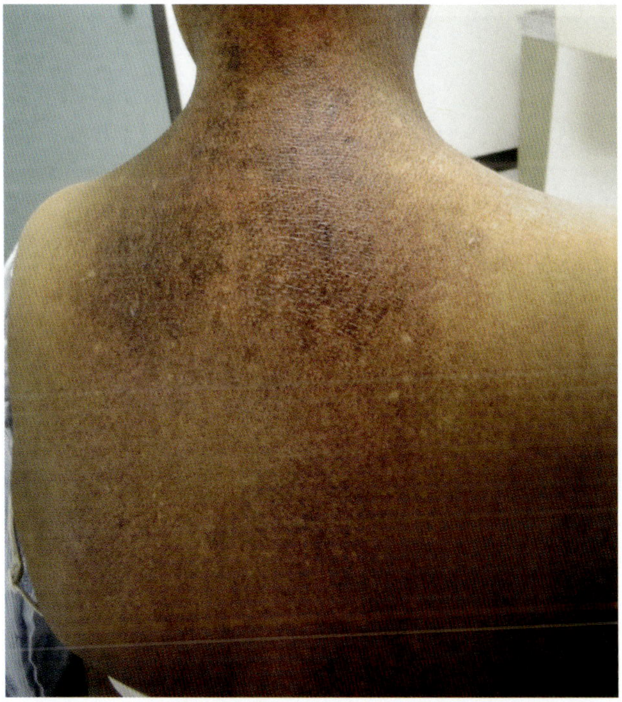

Fig. 29.3 Shawl sign on the back of an African American female

of the fingers, are more frequently observed in patients with anti-synthetase antibodies [6]. Additional nonspecific findings can be found on the scalp, which typically presents as a

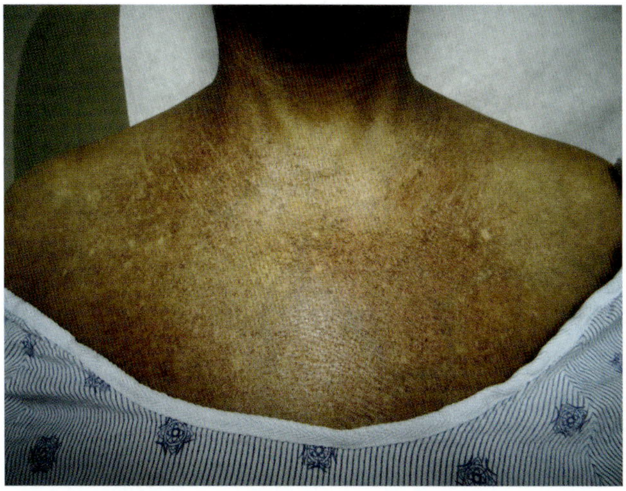

Fig. 29.4 Poikilodermatous patch on the upper chest of an African American female

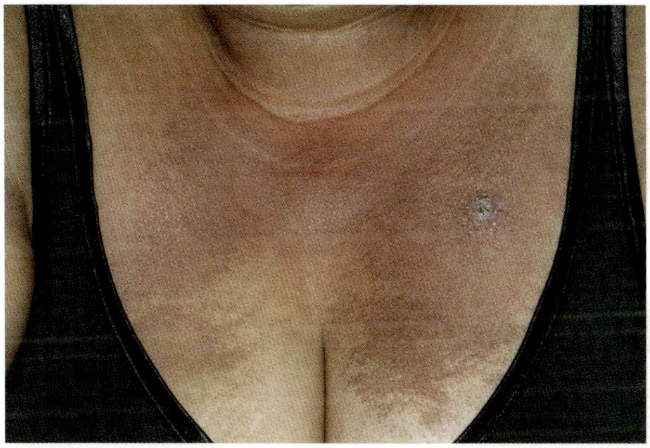

Fig. 29.5 Poikilodermatous patch on the upper chest of an African American female (Courtesy of Lu Le, MD, PhD)

violaceous, psoriasiform dermatitis, which may mimic psoriasis or seborrheic dermatitis. Although not a typical finding in adults (Fig. 29.8), calcinosis cutis occurs more often in children with dermatomyositis. More subtle findings such as periungual telangiectasias and/or cuticular hypertrophy and edema are common (Fig. 29.9). Finally, involvement of the subcutaneous fat (dermatomyositis panniculitis) rarely occurs, presenting as subcutaneous tender nodules evolving into atrophic plaques favoring the buttocks, arms, thighs, arms, and abdomen (Fig. 29.10).

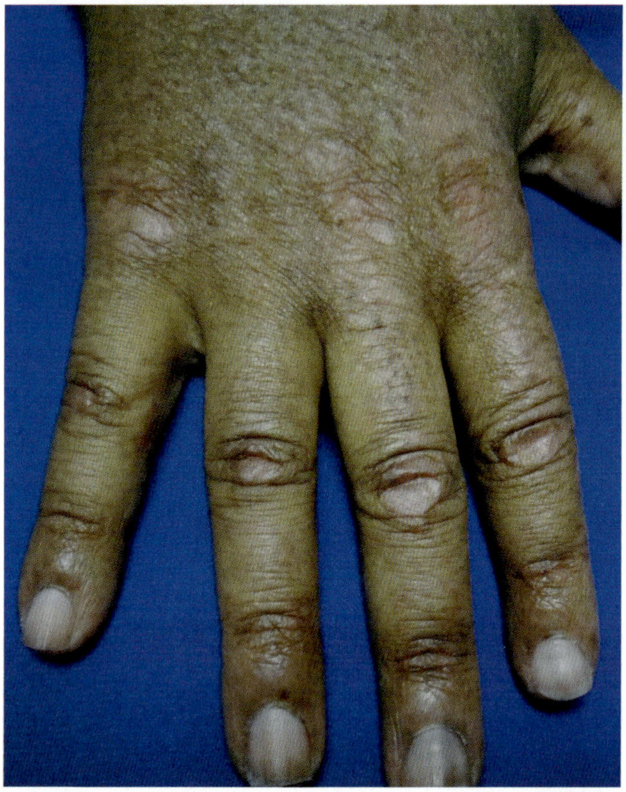

Fig. 29.6 Gottron's papules on distal and proximal interphalangeal joints of an African American female

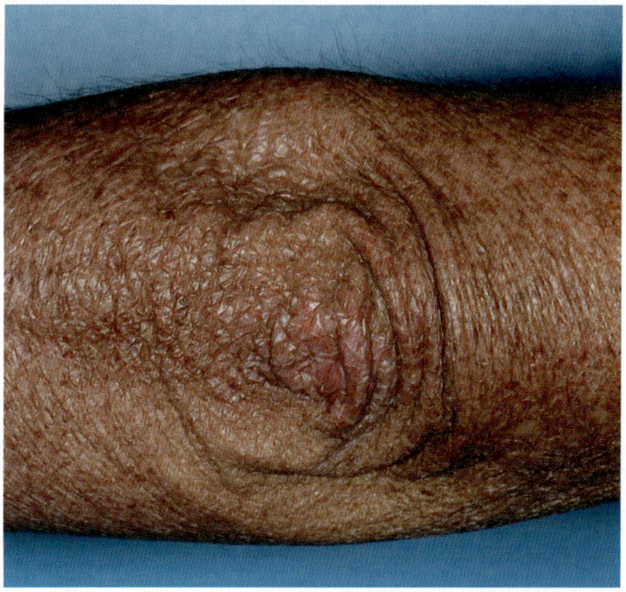

Fig. 29.7 Gottron's sign on the left elbow of a Southeast Asian female

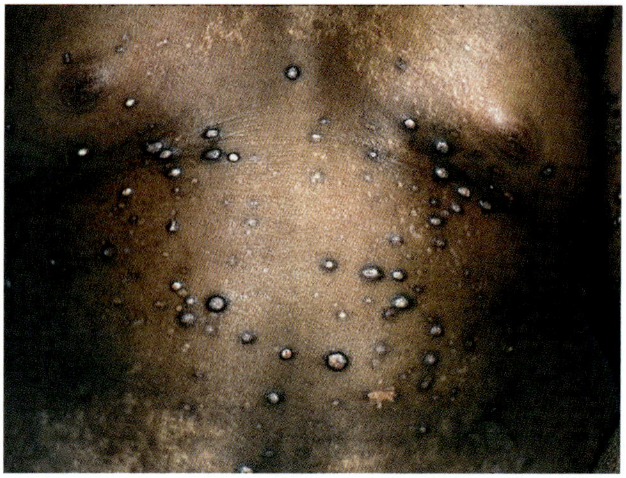

Fig. 29.8 Calcinosis cutis of the abdomen in an African American male (Courtesy of Chauncey McHargue, MD)

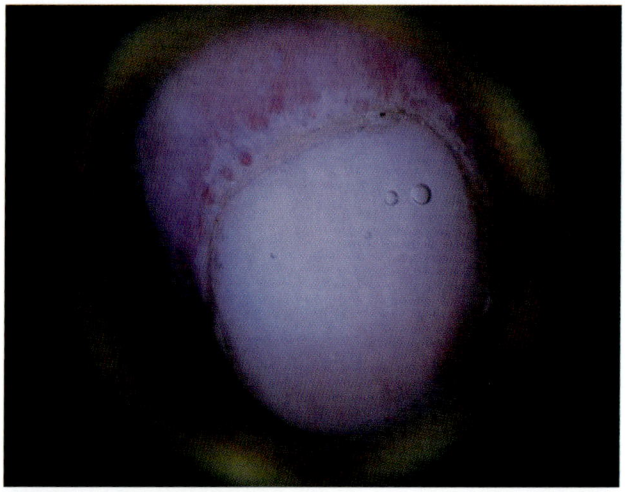

Fig. 29.9 Dilated nail capillaries seen under dermoscopy of a Hispanic patient with dermatomyositis (Courtesy of Judith Dominguez Cherit, MD)

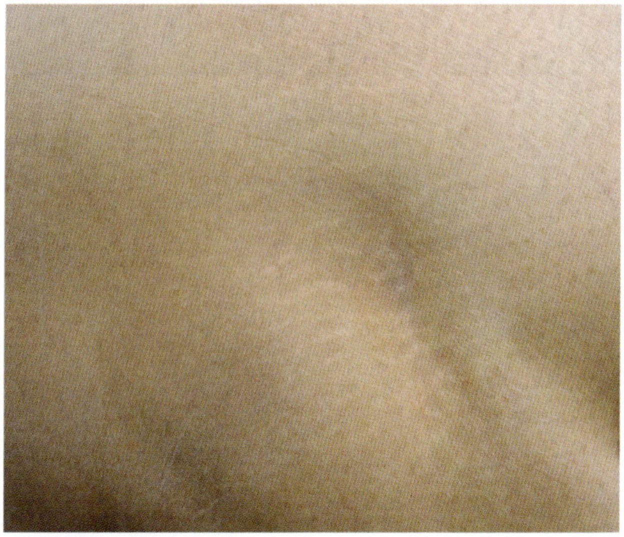

Fig. 29.10 Dermatomyositis panniculitis on buttock of a Hispanic female

In addition to these skin lesions, dermatomyositis may be associated with muscle weakness, esophageal dysmotility, arthritis, and cardiac disease, which may vary broadly in severity between patients. The onset of proximal symmetric muscle weakness is insidious, with gradual worsening over several months and without muscular atrophy. Involvement of the striated muscle of the pharynx and upper esophagus leads to dysphagia and aspiration and a corresponding increase in the incidence of aspiration pneumonia. Rheumatologic symptoms include joint swelling, especially the small joints of the hands. Cardiac disease can present as conduction defects and rhythm disturbances. In severe disease, patients may have fever, weight loss, Raynaud's phenomenon, and a nondeforming, inflammatory polyarthritis.

Dermatomyositis may be associated with several serious systemic findings, including an increased incidence of malignancy and interstitial lung disease. Cancer risk is increased three-fold in dermatomyositis patients [7]. Adenocarcinomas of the cervix, lung, ovaries, pancreas, bladder, and stomach account for 70 % of dermatomyositis-associated malignancies. This association is significantly greater than that seen in polymyositis. Of special note, the risk of nasopharyngeal carcinoma among Southeast Asians with dermatomyositis is drastically increased [2].

Lung disease, in particular interstitial pneumonitis, is common in dermatomyositis, occurring in 17–23 % of patients [8]. Interstitial lung disease (ILD) presents with nonproductive cough, dyspnea, and hypoxemia, with evidence of infiltrates or pulmonary fibrosis on imaging. Although definitive diagnosis of ILD depends on radiographic imaging, characteristic abnormalities on pulmonary function tests (PFTs) may also suggest the diagnosis. Although frequently mild and chronic, the clinical severity of ILD in dermatomyositis patients is variable and may lead to rapidly progressive respiratory deterioration. Interstitial lung disease may improve with immunosuppressive therapy; therefore, early detection and treatment is critical in order to prevent lung fibrosis [8].

29.4 Diagnosis and Differential Diagnosis

A diagnosis of dermatomyositis can be obtained by a careful medical history and examination and differentiation from similar appearing rashes such as subacute cutaneous lupus, psoriasis, lichen planus, and drug eruption (e.g., lichenoid, photodrug eruption). Measurement of serum muscle enzyme levels, including CK, aldolase, AST, and ALT, and testing for the presence of specific autoantibodies may be helpful. In dermatomyositis, up to 80 % of patients have positive antinuclear antibodies or myositis-specific autoantibodies. Some myositis-specific autoantibodies are associated with specific clinical presentations. Anti-Mi 2 antibodies, for example, are associated with a favorable prognosis, including responsiveness to steroids and a decreased incidence of malignancy [9]. Anti-transcriptional intermediary factor-1γ (TIF1-γ) (previously p155/140) has been strongly associated with coincidence of dermatomyositis and cancer [9]. Recent data has focused on two autoantibodies, antimelanoma differentiation-associated gene-5 (MDA-5) and anti-nuclear matrix protein-2 (NXP-2). Anti-MDA-5 antibodies are seen in 20–30 % of patients and are associated with rapidly progressive ILD and minimal muscle involvement, while anti-NXP-2 antibodies have been associated with juvenile dermatomyositis and calcinosis [9]. Strong associations of specific autoantibodies with distinct clinical presentations suggest that autoantibody profiles may be used as excellent clinical markers for classification of patients and potentially for prediction of clinical progression and understanding of pathogenic mechanisms.

A skin biopsy can provide histopathologic confirmation and obviate the need for muscle biopsy in a patient presenting with a typical pattern of muscle weakness and skin findings. Findings include mild atrophy of the epidermis, vacuolar changes in the basal keratinocyte layer, and perivascular lymphoid infiltrate in the dermis. Muscle tests such as electromyogram (EMG), magnetic resonance imaging (MRI), and muscle biopsy may be ordered when skin findings and biopsies are inconclusive. EMG shows increased membrane irritability in dermatomyositis and polymyositis, although similar findings may be seen in myopathies of other etiologies. Additional guidance by MRI can be used to pinpoint abnormal muscle findings and suggest high-yield biopsy sites. Biopsies should be performed on muscles found to be weak on clinical examination, typically the deltoid or quadriceps.

29.5 Treatment

For cutaneous manifestations of dermatomyositis, initial management includes strict photoprotection and topical corticosteroids or topical calcineurin inhibitors, such as tacrolimus, which reduce erythema and pruritus. However, topical therapy alone fails to control cutaneous disease in most patients, and systemic therapy is typically required.

Table 29.1 Screening recommendations for dermatomyositis patients

Disease	Recommendations
Malignancy [10]	Complete history, physical exam, chest x-ray, complete blood count with differential, serum chemistry screen, urinalysis, CA-125, transvaginal pelvic ultrasound[a], mammogram[a], abdominal/pelvic computed tomography scan[b]
Interstitial lung disease [8]	Serial PFTs, high-resolution chest computed tomography scan[c]

[a]Additional screening for women due to increased risk for ovarian cancer
[b]Optional additional imaging studies
[c]May order if diffusing capacity for carbon monoxide is less than 75 % of predicted value

First-line systemic oral therapy includes prednisone and antimalarials. Prednisone treatment often requires prolonged courses and high doses, up to 1 mg/kg/day, which is tapered over several months. Antimalarials such as hydroxychloroquine (up to 6.5 mg/kg/day) are effective for skin disease but generally do not improve associated myositis. When patients show resistance to antimalarials, methotrexate (typically up to 25 mg/week) is used as an alternative medication. While it is considered more immunosuppressive than antimalarials, methotrexate has the benefit of improving associated myositis. Folic acid supplementation is used to ameliorate side effects of methotrexate including myelosuppression and GI upset. Other second-line treatments for refractory cases include mycophenolate mofetil, a lymphocyte selective steroid-sparing immunosuppressive agent, azathioprine, and intravenous immunoglobulin. Additionally, screenings for internal malignancy and interstitial lung disease are critical aspects of the medical management of dermatomyositis patients (Table 29.1).

With several distinctive cutaneous findings, dermatomyositis patients may or may not have muscle involvement. Recognition of these signs and a diagnostic skin biopsy could obviate the need for muscle biopsy to confirm diagnosis. Regardless of their muscle status, dermatomyositis patients should be screened for malignancy and interstitial lung disease. Dermatomyositis patients typically require more than topical steroids for disease control and are usually prescribed potent oral immunosuppressants.

References

1. Bendewald MJ, et al. Incidence of dermatomyositis and clinically amyopathic dermatomyositis: a population-based study in Olmsted County, Minnesota. Arch Dermatol. 2010;146:26–30.
2. Liu WC, et al. An 11-year review of dermatomyositis in Asian patients. Ann Acad Med Singapore. 2010;39(11):843–7.
3. Nagaragu K, Lundberg I. Polymyositis and dermatomyositis: pathophysiology. Rheumatic Dis Clin North Am. 2011;37(2):159–71.
4. Werth VP, et al. Associations of tumor necrosis factor alpha and HLA polymorphisms with adult dermatomyositis: implications for a unique pathogenesis. J Invest Dermatol. 2002;119:617–20.
5. Pachman LM, et al. New-onset juvenile dermatomyositis: comparisons with a healthy cohort and children with juvenile rheumatoid arthritis. Arthritis Rheum. 1997;40:1526–33.
6. Mitra D, Lovell CL, Macleod TIF, et al. Clinical and histological features of 'mechanics hands' in a patient with antibodies to Jo-1: a case report. Clin Exp Dermatol. 1994;19:146–8.
7. Hill CL, Zhang Y, Sigurgeirsson B, et al. Frequency of specific cancer types in dermatomyositis and polymyositis: a population-based study. Lancet. 2001;357:96.
8. Morganroth PA, et al. Interstitial lung disease in classic and skin-predominant dermatomyositis: a retrospective study with screening recommendations. Arch Dermatol. 2010;146:729–38.
9. Casciola-Rosen L, Mammen AL. Myositis autoantibodies. Curr Opin Rheumatol. 2012;24:602–8.
10. Sontheimer RD. Clinically amyopathic dermatomyositis: what can we now tell our patients? Arch Dermatol. 2010;146:76–80.

Scleroderma and Morphea

30

Lauren A. Baker and Heidi T. Jacobe

Contents

L.A. Baker, BS
Department of Dermatology,
University of Texas Southwestern Medical Center,
5323 Harry Hines Blvd., Dallas, TX 75390, USA
e-mail: Lauren.Banker@utsouthwestern.edu

H.T. Jacobe, MD, MSCS (✉)
Department of Dermatology, University of Texas Southwestern
Medical Center, Dallas, TX 75390, USA

30.1 Systemic Sclerosis

30.1.1 Introduction

Systemic sclerosis (SSc), also known as scleroderma, is a chronic autoimmune disease characterized by sclerosis of the skin and visceral organs preceded by microvascular injury. Subtypes include diffuse cutaneous systemic sclerosis (dcSSc) and limited cutaneous systemic sclerosis (lcSSc), previously known as CREST (calcinosis cutis, Raynaud's phenomenon, esophageal dysmotility, sclerodactyly, and telangiectasia) syndrome, with the former portending a poorer prognosis [1].

The incidence of SSc has been stable since 1973 with a current prevalence of 240 per 1 million adults in the United States, with a marked female predominance [2]. The peak age of onset is between 30 and 50 years of age. Compared to Caucasians, African Americans have a greater age-specific incidence, disease onset at an earlier age, and more severe disease [2]. In addition, approximately two-thirds of SSc cases in African Americans are of the diffuse type compared to only one-third in Caucasians [2].

The pathogenesis of SSc involves endothelial inflammation and edema leading to a vasculopathy and recurrent tissue ischemia, crippling the ability of the immune system to repair insults. Recent studies show that the pathogenesis may specifically involve an imbalance of Th1 and Th2 cytokines in which the Th2 pathway is favored [3]. SSc has an autoimmune component implicated by the presence of concomitant autoimmune disorders and the presence of autoantibodies [3]. Recent studies support a genetic predisposition to SSc [2].

30.1.2 Clinical Features

Skin lesions begin symmetrically on the fingers, oftentimes with swelling or puffiness of the fingers that is preceded or accompanied by the onset of Raynaud's phenomenon. Lesions

D. Jackson-Richards, A.G. Pandya (eds.), *Dermatology Atlas for Skin of Color*,
DOI 10.1007/978-3-642-54446-0_30,

may progress to involve the hands, forearms, and proximal arms (Fig. 30.1). In some cases there is similar involvement of the toes and feet. As the lesions evolve, they become more sclerotic and fixed, eventually producing decreased ability to pinch or move the skin. Involvement proximal to the elbows and knees differentiates limited from diffuse disease (limited is characterized by involvement distal to the elbows). In addition, most patients with systemic sclerosis develop sclerotic plaques of the neck and upper chest. In later stages, perioral rhytides and decreased oral aperture develop.

Localized areas of depigmentation that spare the perifollicular skin, resulting in a salt-and-pepper appearance, are particularly prominent in patients with skin of color (Fig. 30.2). Microvascular changes include Raynaud's phenomenon, digital cutaneous ulcers and pitting, and capillary abnormalities in the proximal nail bed. Other changes include pterygium inversus unguis, telangiectasias, and calcinosis cutis (all are later findings).

The most common extracutaneous symptoms patients experience are related to gastrointestinal dysmotility, predominantly heartburn, and dysphagia. Patients may complain of decreased exercise tolerance and shortness of breath on exertion due to interstitial lung disease and/or pulmonary hypertension. Many patients endorse fatigue, pruritus, arthralgias, and myalgias, as polymyositis and arthritis may accompany SSc. Renal crisis with malignant hypertension is a cause of significant morbidity and mortality, particularly among those with dcSSc and RNA polymerase antibodies.

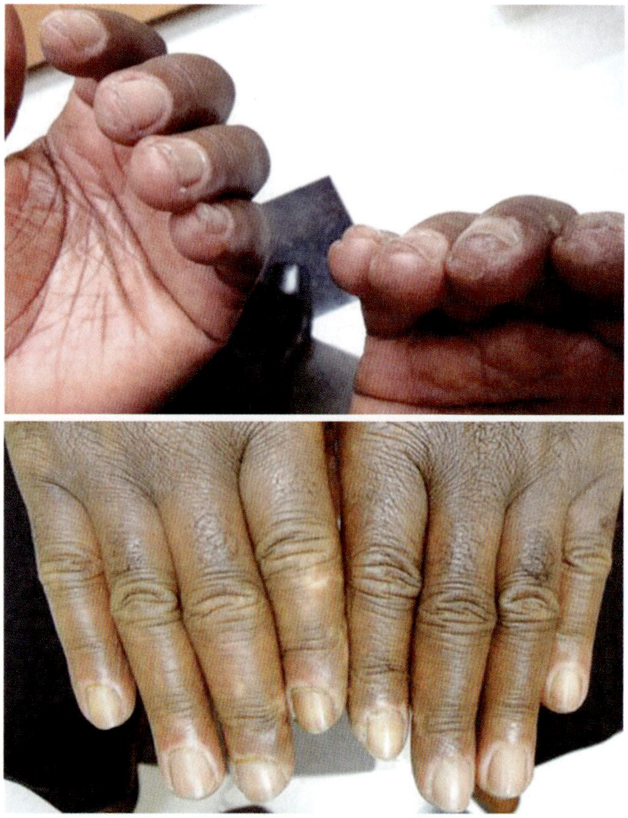

Fig. 30.1 African American female with sclerodactyly, pitted digital scars, and hypopigmentation

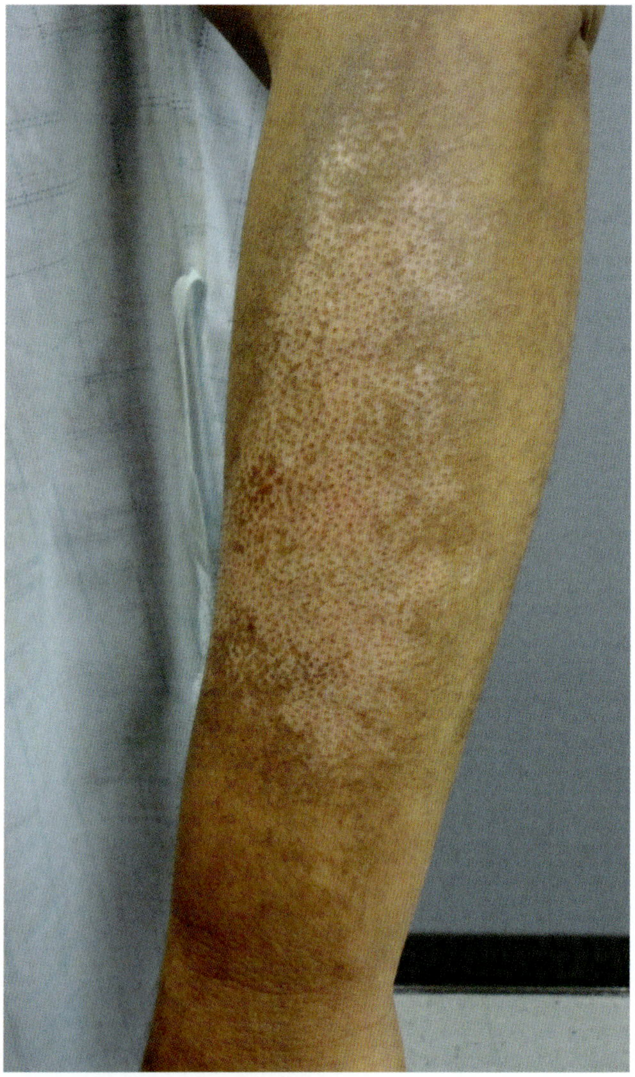

Fig. 30.2 Hispanic male with salt-and-pepper pigmentary changes on the forearm

30.1.3 Natural History and Prognosis

In the beginning stages of SSc, soft tissue swelling and arthralgia, as opposed to skin induration, in the area of involvement are prominent. Hyperpigmentation, calcinosis cutis, and telangiectasias are skin changes that occur late in the disease course. With eventual remission, the skin softens, although pigmentary changes and hand changes tend to persist. Antibodies to topoisomerase I (Scl-70) are associated with interstitial lung disease in patients with SSc and are more frequent in African Americans [1]. African Americans experience more severe disease manifestations with increased digital ulcers, pitting, and gangrene; more extensive skin, lung, renal, and gastrointestinal involvement; and higher mortality rates [2]. In comparison, Hispanic patients have more frequent musculoskeletal signs and symptoms [4].

30.1.4 Histopathologic Features

The reticular dermis is often expanded by densely packed, broad bundles of acellular collagen with loss of appendageal structures. In early lesions, inflammatory perivascular infiltrates are seen at the interface between the dermis and subcutaneous fat. Later in the disease process, fibrointimal proliferation of blood vessels is commonly seen. In general, SSc and morphea are indistinguishable based on pathological findings, necessitating clinicopathologic correlation to differentiate the disorders.

30.1.5 Diagnosis and Differential Diagnosis

The diagnosis is based on characteristic clinical findings and supported by the presence antibodies directed against antitopoisomerase I, anticentromere, or anti-RNA polymerase III (SSc hallmark antibodies, not present in all patients). Approximately 60 % of patients with SSc have one of these autoantibodies; therefore, their absence does not exclude the diagnosis. The differential diagnosis includes scleredema, scleromyxedema, diabetic sclerodactyly, myxedema, nephrogenic systemic fibrosis, amyloidosis, eosinophilic fasciitis, chronic graft-versus-host disease, drug-induced SSc (taxanes), generalized morphea, and environmental exposures.

30.1.6 Treatment

To date, no treatment has proven efficacy for SSc skin disease. However, UVA1 phototherapy may be of benefit for early skin lesions [5] as well as pruritus and salt-and-pepper pigmentary changes. Further, some studies show potential benefit of methotrexate [6]. Treatment of the internal manifestations of SSc is beyond the scope of this chapter, although referral to rheumatology, pulmonology, cardiology, and gastroenterology is essential.

30.2 Morphea

30.2.1 Introduction

Morphea, also known as localized scleroderma, is characterized by thickening and hardening of the skin and subcutaneous tissues as a result of excessive collagen deposition. Depending on the clinical presentation and depth of tissue involvement, morphea is classified as circumscribed (plaque), generalized, linear, pansclerotic, or mixed subtypes [7].

Recent studies suggest that the incidence of morphea is 0.4–2.7 per 100,000 people with a female predominance of 2.4–4.2:1 and an equal prevalence in adults and children [7]. Individuals of all races are affected by morphea; however, morphea may be more common in Caucasians, who comprise 72.7–82 % of patients (although population-based studies are lacking) [7]. The clinical presentation varies depending on age. In children, the linear subtype predominates, while in adults plaque and generalized morphea are more common. While the etiology of morphea is unknown, most evidence points to a genetic predisposition toward autoimmunity with contribution by environmental factors, including radiation. Further, although none are specific for the diagnosis, numerous autoantibodies are associated with morphea (antinuclear, anti-single-stranded DNA, and anti-histone antibodies) [8, 9]. Although prior reports have linked morphea to infectious agents, particularly Borrelia, there is no definitive evidence for an infectious etiology in the development of morphea at this time.

30.2.2 Clinical Features

Circumscribed morphea is characterized by oval plaques distributed asymmetrically on the trunk, which occasionally coalesce. Generalized morphea, which is further subdivided into coalescent plaque and pansclerotic types, initially develops on the trunk as coalescent plaques and spreads acrally, with sparing of the face, fingers, and toes (Fig. 30.3). Laxer and Zulian define coalescent plaque morphea as ≥4 plaques in at least 2 of 7 anatomic sites (head-neck, right/left upper extremity, right/left lower extremity, anterior/posterior trunk) [10]. The isomorphic pattern describes coalescent plaques on the inframammary fold, waistline, lower abdomen, and proximal thighs, while the symmetric pattern describes symmetric plaques circumferential around the breasts, umbilicus, arms, and legs. The pansclerotic type of generalized morphea is defined as circumferential involvement of the majority of the body surface area (sparing fingertips and toes), affecting the skin, subcutaneous tissue, and muscle or bone, but with no internal organ involvement [10]. Pansclerotic morphea is distinct from other morphea subtypes in that it begins as sheets of sclerosis that start on the trunk and quickly spread acrally in contiguous sheets sparing the areola, fingers, and toes (Figs. 30.4 and 30.5). Deep involvement is characteristic with concomitant disability (Fig. 30.6). Linear morphea occurs on the extremities, scalp and face (en coup de sabre), or trunk (Figs. 30.7 and 30.8). Mixed morphea describes the presence of more than one subtype, usually linear and circumscribed.

Lesions are initially erythematous with varied amounts of induration. Eventually, the center becomes white and sclerotic with an erythematous border. Lesions eventually become inactive (post-inflammatory hypo- or hyperpigmentation and dermal, subcutaneous, muscle, or bony atrophy) (Figs. 30.9 and 30.10). With scalp and nail involvement, permanent alopecia and nail dystrophy, respectively, can occur. Muscle atrophy, joint contractures, and limb-length discrepancy are seen in linear morphea and pansclerotic morphea [7]. Patients also frequently experience pruritus and pain in the affected areas.

Extracutaneous manifestations are seen in 20 % of morphea patients and include myalgia, arthralgia, fatigue, and dysphagia and dyspnea from extensive neck and trunk involvement. Ocular and neurologic involvement occurs in scalp or facial lesions or progressive hemifacial atrophy [7].

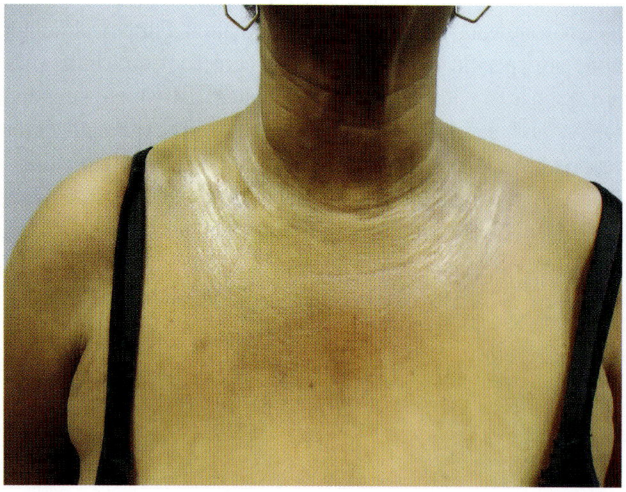

Fig. 30.3 Shiny sclerotic skin on the neck of an African American female with generalized morphea

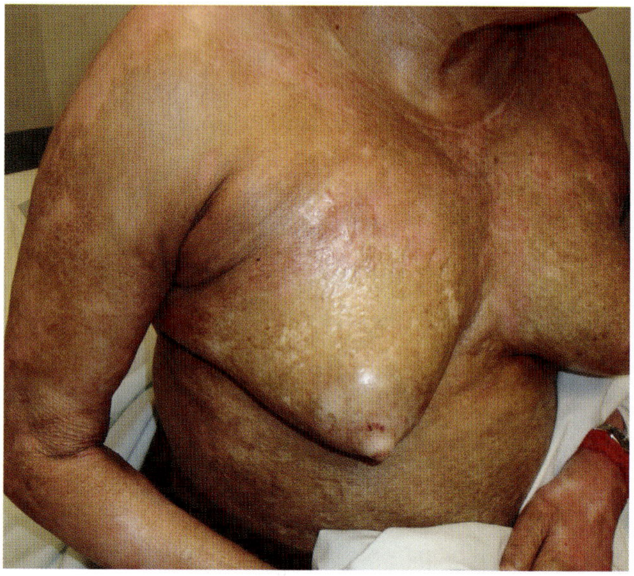

Fig. 30.4 Pansclerotic morphea in an African American female

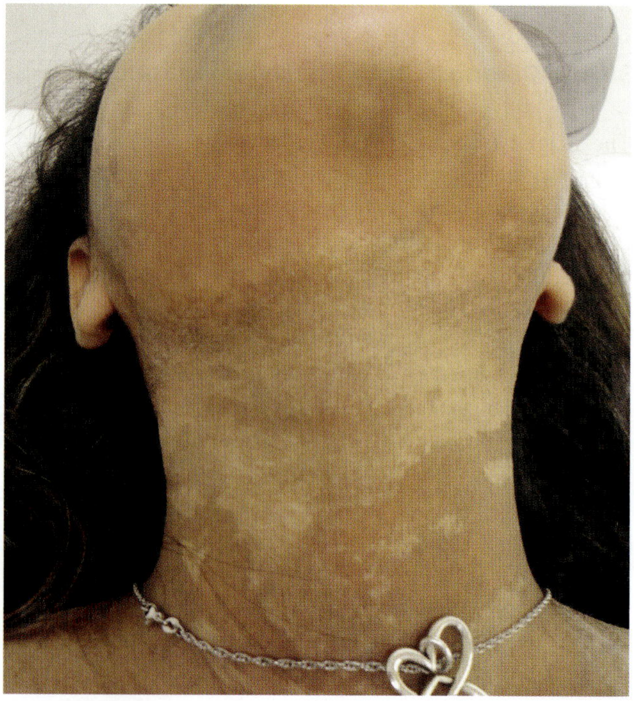

Fig. 30.5 Hispanic female with pansclerotic morphea involving the neck

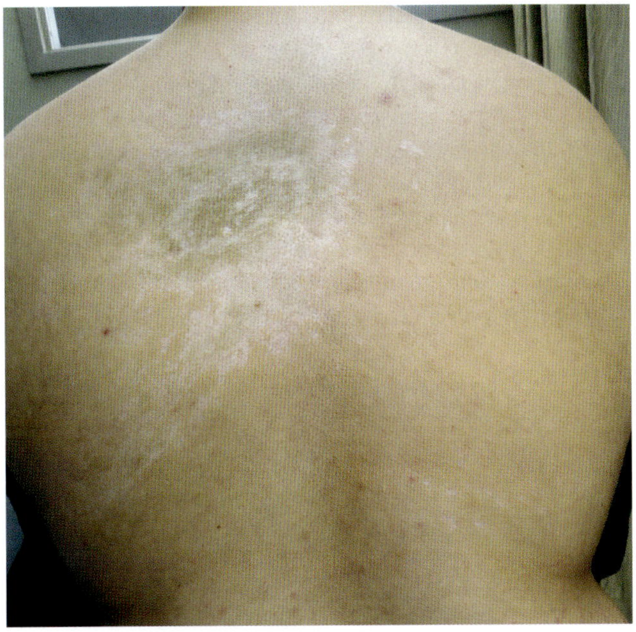

Fig. 30.6 Deep involvement on the back of a Hispanic female with circumscribed morphea profunda

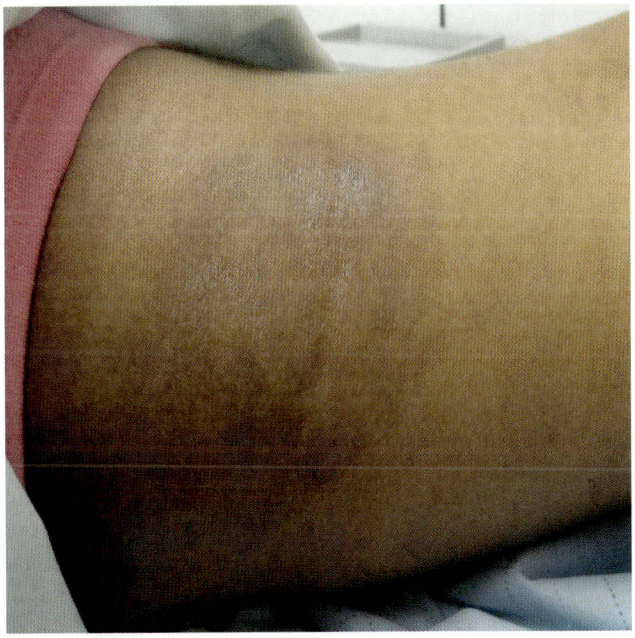

Fig. 30.7 Linear morphea in a Hispanic female

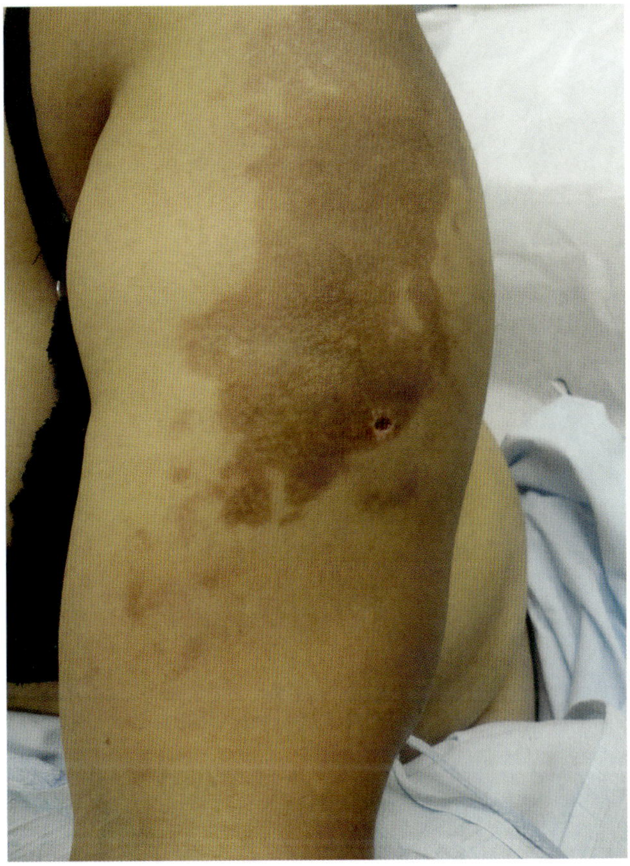

Fig. 30.8 Hyperpigmented indurated plaque on the shoulder of a Hispanic female with linear morphea

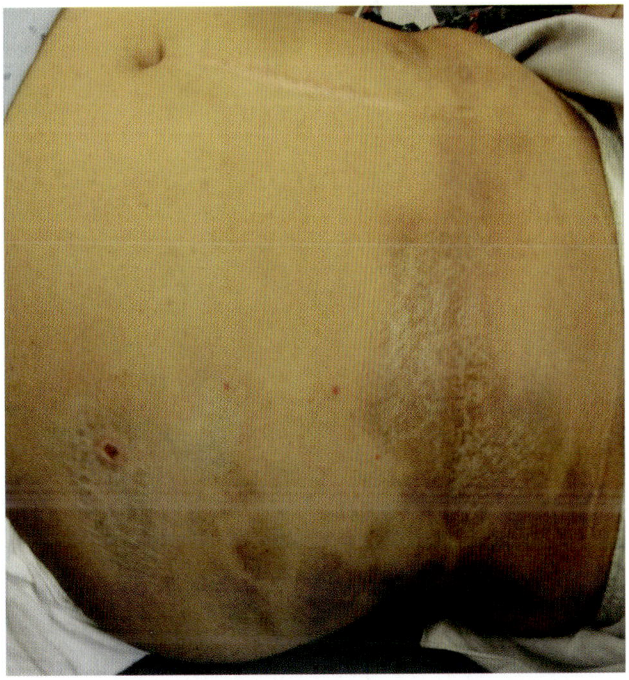

Fig. 30.9 Hypo- and hyperpigmentation and sclerosis showing an isometric pattern in a Hispanic patient with inactive morphea

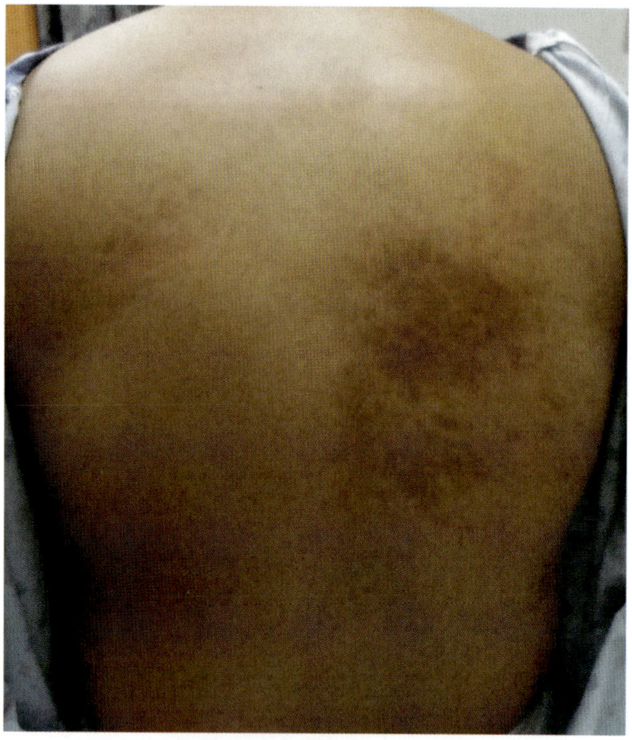

Fig. 30.10 Dermal atrophy and hyperpigmentation of a plaque in a Hispanic patient with inactive morphea

30.2.3 Natural History and Prognosis

Early morphea is subtle, resulting in frequent delay in diagnosis [11]. Newer studies suggest morphea has a remitting relapsing course with gradual accumulation of cosmetic and functional damage due to recurring episodes of new activity [12]. Disease activity generally continues for 3–6 years. Morphea produces permanent joint contractures, limb-length discrepancy, and prominent facial atrophy and treatment is warranted to prevent these sequelae (Fig. 30.11) [7].

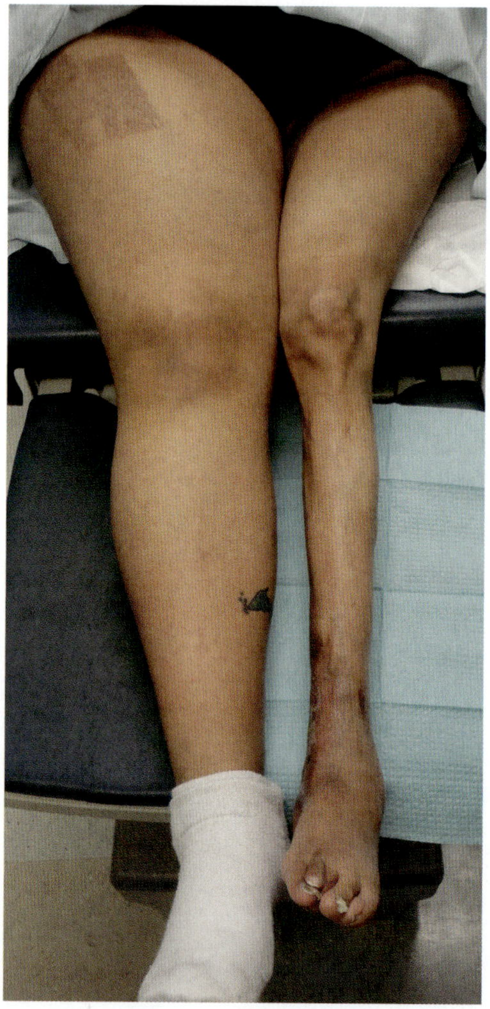

Fig. 30.11 Limb-length discrepancy in a Hispanic female with linear morphea

30.2.4 Histopathologic Features

The epidermis appears normal to atrophic with loss of rete ridges. Initially, a lymphocytic perivascular infiltrate in the reticular dermis with plasma cells and rare eosinophils predominates and in the border between the dermis and subcutes. Later, inflammation subsides and collagen bundles in the papillary and reticular dermis are notably eosinophilic, thickened, and closely packed with atrophic eccrine glands, loss of appendages, and a paucity of blood vessels [7].

30.2.5 Diagnosis and Differential Diagnosis

The diagnosis is usually made based on characteristic clinical features with biopsy to exclude other entities on the differential diagnosis. The absence of Raynaud's phenomenon, nail-fold-capillary changes, sclerodactyly, hallmark systemic sclerosis antibodies, and visceral organ involvement point to a diagnosis of morphea over SSc. Other items on the differential diagnosis include lipodermatosclerosis, chronic graft-versus-host disease, exposures (taxanes, radiation, L-tryptophan, toxic rapeseed oil, vibration), carcinoma en cuirasse, scleredema, scleromyxedema, porphyria cutanea tarda, and traumatic skin changes (intramuscular injections).

30.2.6 Treatment

Treatment during the active stage of the disease is the most efficacious [13]. Patients with limited plaque disease may benefit from topical therapy, such as moderate- to high-potency corticosteroids, tacrolimus, and calcipotriol, and/or lesion-directed phototherapy. Topical treatments, including phototherapy, are usually ineffective in cases with subcutaneous, fascial, or muscle involvement [13]. In these cases, systemic therapy with glucocorticoids or immunosuppressive drugs is preferred. Phototherapy is a good option for generalized lesions.

References

1. Mayes M. Scleroderma epidemiology. Rheum Dis Clin North Am. 1996;22:751–65.
2. Nietert PJ, Mitchell HC, Bolster MB, Shaftman SR, Tilley BC, Silver RM. Racial variation in clinical and immunological manifestations of systemic sclerosis. J Rheumatol. 2006;33:263–8.
3. Kurzinski K, Torok KS. Cytokine profiles in localized scleroderma and relationship to clinical features. Cytokine. 2011;55(2):157–64.
4. Nashid M, Khanna PP, Furst DE, Clements PJ, Maranian P, Seibold J, Postlethwaite AE, Louri JS, Mayes MD, Agrawal H, Khanna D. Gender and ethnicity differences in patients with diffuse systemic sclerosis – analysis from three large randomized clinical trials. Rheumatology. 2011;50:335–42.
5. Su O, Onsun N, Onay HK, Erdemoglu Y, Ozkaya DB, Cebeci F, Somay A. Effectiveness of medium-dose ultraviolet A1 phototherapy in localized scleroderma. Int J Dermatol. 2011;50(8):1006–13.
6. Zulian F, Vallongo C, Patrizi A, et al. A long-term follow-up study of methotrexate in juvenile localized scleroderma (morphea). J Am Acad Dermatol. 2012;67(6):1151–6.
7. Fett N, Werth VP. Update on morphea: part I. Epidemiology, clinical presentation, and pathogenesis. J Am Acad Dermatol. 2011;64(2):217–28.
8. Leitenberger JJ, Cayce RL, Haley RW, Adams-Huet B, Bergstresser PR, Jacobe HT. Distinct autoimmune syndromes in morphea: a review of 245 adult and pediatric cases. Arch Dermatol. 2009;145(5):545–50.
9. Dharamsi JW, Victor S, Aguwa N, Ahn C, Arnett F, Mayes M, Jacobe H. Morphea in adults and children (MAC) cohort III: the prevalence and clinical significance of autoantibodies in morphea: a prospective case-control study. JAMA Dermatol. 2013;149(10):1159–65.
10. Laxer RM, Zulian F. Localized scleroderma. Curr Opin Rheumatol. 2006;18(6):606–13.
11. Johnson W, Jacobe H. Morphea in adults and children cohort II: patients with morphea experience delay in diagnosis and large variation in treatment. J Am Acad Dermatol. 2012;67(5):881–9.
12. Saxton-Daniels S, Jacobe HT. An evaluation of long-term outcomes in adults with pediatric-onset morphea. Arch Dermatol. 2012;146(9):1044–5.
13. Zwischenberger BA, Jacobe HT. A systematic review of morphea treatments and therapeutic algorithm. J Am Acad Dermatol. 2011;65(5):925–41.

Part VI

Infectious Diseases

Bacterial Skin Infections

31

Katherine Omueti Ayoade
and Arturo Ricardo Dominguez

Contents

K.O. Ayoade, MD, PhD • A.R. Dominguez, MD, BS (✉)
Department of Dermatology, University of Texas Southwestern
Medical Center, 5323 Harry Hines Blvd., Dallas, TX 75390, USA
e-mail: katherine.ayoade@utsouthwestern.edu

31.1 Introduction

The skin, the largest human organ, is a barrier that is an important innate defense against skin infections. In addition to the protective physical barrier, the skin has natural flora composed of microorganisms that prevent skin infection. The type of bacterial infection that develops in the skin depends on the type of bacteria and the depth and location of infection in the skin once the barrier has been breached (Table 31.1).

31.2 Impetigo

31.2.1 Epidemiology

Impetigo is a highly contagious superficial skin infection most commonly observed in children aged 2–5 years [1, 2]. It spreads rapidly via direct person-to-person contact. Contact with fomites has also been implicated in spread of the disease [3]. There is no sex predilection, and all races are susceptible [2].

Impetigo presents as bullous and non-bullous forms. The non-bullous type accounts for 70 % of cases of impetigo [1, 3].

D. Jackson-Richards, A.G. Pandya (eds.), *Dermatology Atlas for Skin of Color*,
DOI 10.1007/978-3-642-54446-0_31, © Springer-Verlag Berlin Heidelberg 2014

Table 31.1 Clinical definitions

Condition	Clinical definition
Impetigo	Superficial infection of the skin, typically at the stratum corneum level of the epidermis
Non-bullous impetigo	Vesicles and pustules that rupture rapidly leading to honey-colored plaques. *S. aureus* is the most common cause or in combination with *streptococci*, beta hemolytic, group A subtype
Bullous impetigo	*Localized* superficial flaccid bullae that rupture easily. Bullae formed due to cleavage of desmoglein-1 protein by exfoliative toxins A and B of *S. aureus*
Staphylococcal Scalded Skin Syndrome	*Generalized* formation of bullous impetigo during which painful denuded skin progresses to flaccid bullae and extensive superficial desquamation and flaccid bullae
Ecthyma	An *ulcerative staphylococcal* or *streptococcal* skin infection where the pathology extends from the epidermis into the dermis
Erysipelas	A bacterial infection of the dermis and upper subcutaneous tissue that can be differentiated from cellulitis by its well-demarcated edges. Clinically it presents as a fiery red, tender, painful well-defined plaque commonly on the lower extremities. Commonly caused by streptococcal species, usually *S. pyogenes*
Folliculitis	Inflammation of the outer canal of the hair follicle after physical or chemical injury or infection (bacterial, viral, fungal, parasite)
Furuncles	Usually develop from existing folliculitis when infection progresses more deeply and to the surrounding tissue
Carbuncles	Infection of a group of adjoining hair follicles
Cellulitis	Infection of the subcutaneous tissues with involvement of the dermis, relative sparing of the epidermis

31.2.2 Etiology

The most frequently isolated pathogen is *S. aureus* followed by *S. pyogenes* [1, 2].

31.2.3 Clinical Features

Non-bullous impetigo begins as small erythematous macules that rapidly progress to vesicles and pustules, ultimately leading to honey-colored crusted plaques typically on the exposed surface of the skin, the face, around the nose and mouth, and the extremities (Figs. 31.1, 31.2, 31.3, and 31.4) [2]. Acute post-streptococcal glomerulonephritis can result after infection with certain stains of *S. pyogenes*. This risk is unaltered by treatment with antibiotics. Impetigo can progress to ecthyma or cellulitis. Bullous lesions appear initially as superficial vesicles that rapidly enlarge to form flaccid bullae filled with clear yellow fluid, which later becomes darker, more turbid, and sometimes purulent. The bullae may rupture, often leaving a thin brown crust resembling lacquer (Fig. 31.5) [2].

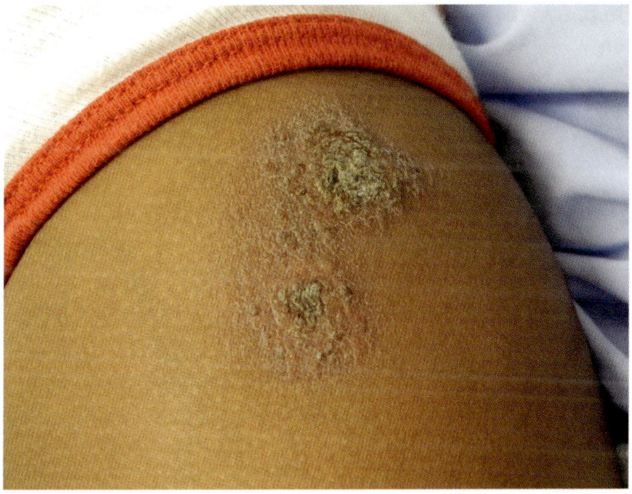

Fig. 31.1 Impetigo on the thigh of a Hispanic boy

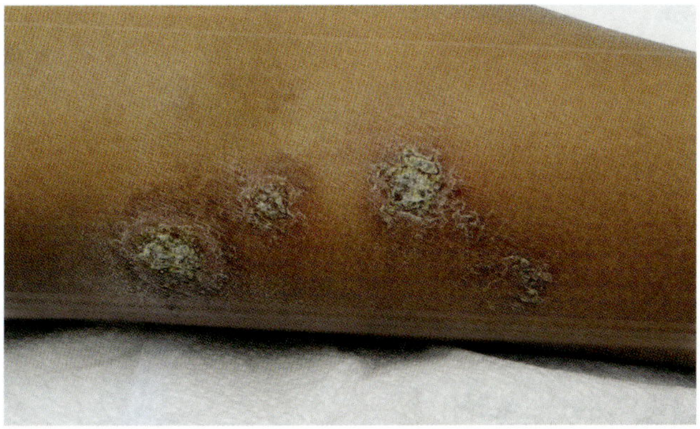

Fig. 31.2 Impetigo on the calf of a Hispanic boy

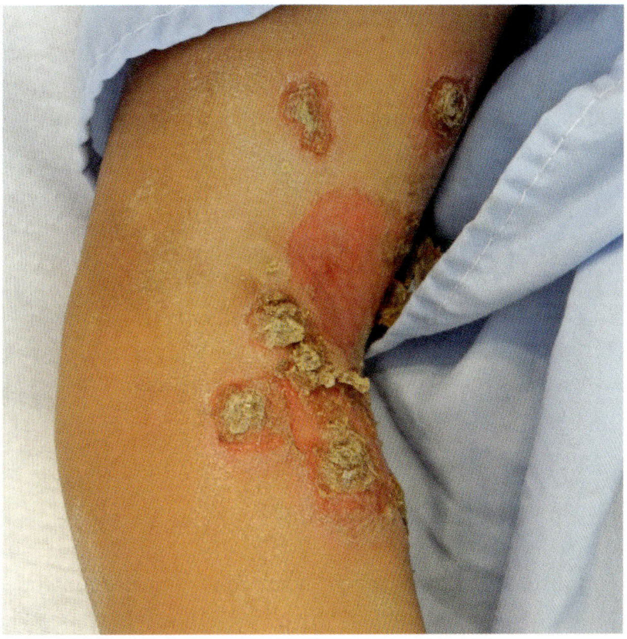

Fig. 31.3 Impetigo on the antecubital fossa of a Hispanic girl

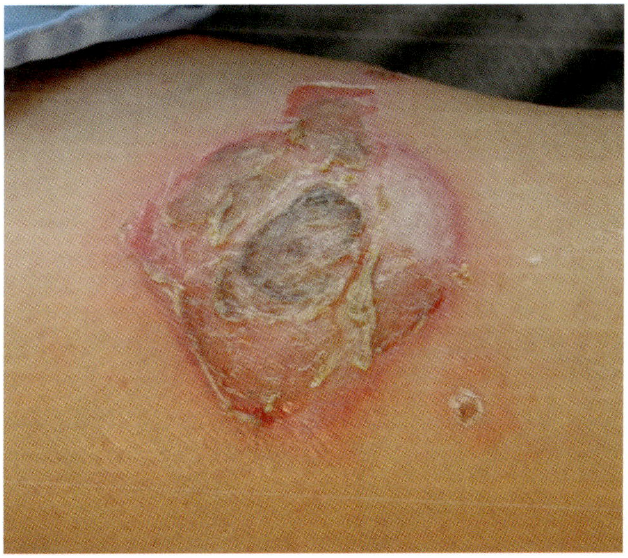

Fig. 31.4 Impetigo on the arm of a Hispanic girl

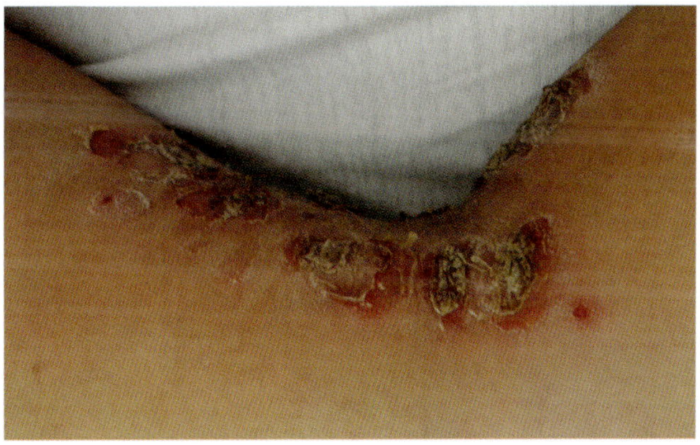

Fig. 31.5 Impetigo with collapsed bullae on the arm of a Hispanic girl

31.2.4 Natural History and Prognosis

Non-bullous impetigo resolves without treatment or scarring within 2–3 weeks. Untreated patients with bullous impetigo heal in 3–6 weeks [3].

31.2.5 Histopathological Features

Non-bullous impetigo histological findings include neutrophils as well as chains or clusters of *S. pyogenes* or *S. aureus* in the stratum corneum. There is also superficial necrosis and crusting [4].

31.2.6 Differential Diagnosis

Skin diseases that can mimic non-bullous impetigo include insect bites, herpes simplex virus (HSV) infection, varicella, pemphigus foliaceus, and scabies [3]. The differential diagnosis for bullous impetigo includes bullous insect bites, thermal burns, HSV infections, bullous erythema multiforme, SJS, and autoimmune blistering dermatoses such as linear IgA disease and bullous pemphigoid [3].

31.2.7 Diagnosis

The diagnosis of impetigo is made clinically. Exudate may be sent for culture and sensitivity to guide therapy.

31.2.8 Treatment

Systemic therapies include dicloxacillin, cephalexin and other cephalosporins, erythromycin, clindamycin, and amoxicillin/clavulanate. Topical treatment, in particular mupirocin 2 % ointment, may be used in patients with a limited number of lesions. [2]

31.3 Staphylococcal Scalded Skin Syndrome

31.3.1 Epidemiology

The term Staphylococcal Scalded Skin Syndrome (SSSS) was introduced in 1970 by Melish and Glasgow after demonstrating in an animal model that SSSS was caused by a staphylococcal toxin that they called exfoliative toxin [5]. SSSS typically affects infants and children less than 6 years of age. Although SSSS is rarely seen in adults [3, 5], it can occur in those with serious underlying conditions such as immunodeficiency, renal failure, or malignancy [6]. Men are more often affected than women [5].

31.3.2 Etiology

Most cases of SSSS are caused by phage group II strains (types 3A, 3C, 55, 71) of *S. aureus*, which use these exfoliative toxins (ETs) to disrupt the barrier of the human epidermis to survive and proliferate [3]. Specifically, the exfoliative toxins ETA (chromosomally encoded) and ETB (plasmid encoded) cleave desmoglein-1 at the granular layer of the epidermis, which creates an intraepidermal cleft leading to a sterile flaccid bullae [3].

31.3.3 Clinical Features

Patients, particularly children, may present with fever, erythema, and edema, which rapidly develops into superficial blisters that rupture on the slightest pressure, leaving areas of denuded skin (Figs. 31.6, 31.7, 31.8, and 31.9) [6].

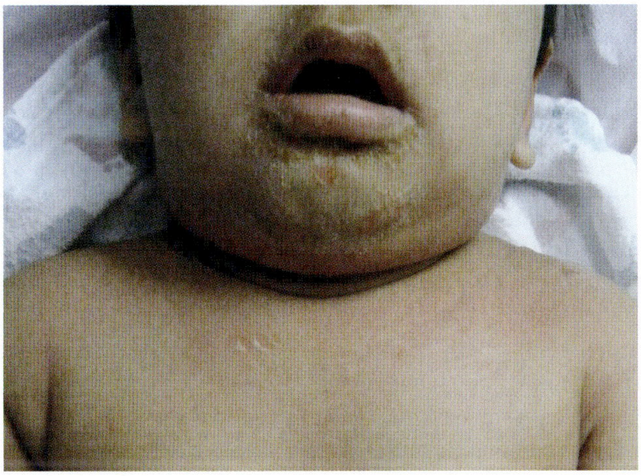

Fig. 31.6 SSSS with yellow crusting around the mouth and erythema of the chest of a Hispanic male infant

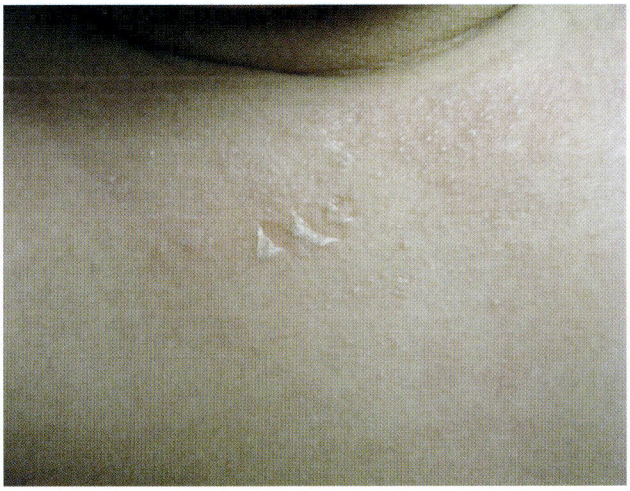

Fig. 31.7 SSSS close-up showing superficial exfoliation on the chest of a Hispanic male infant

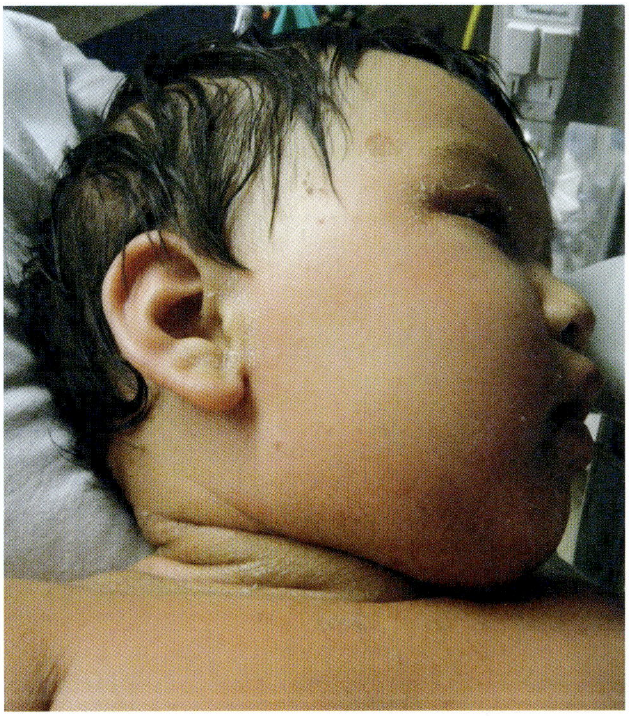

Fig. 31.8 SSSS of the face, neck, and chest, showing erythroderma and exfoliation of a Hispanic male infant

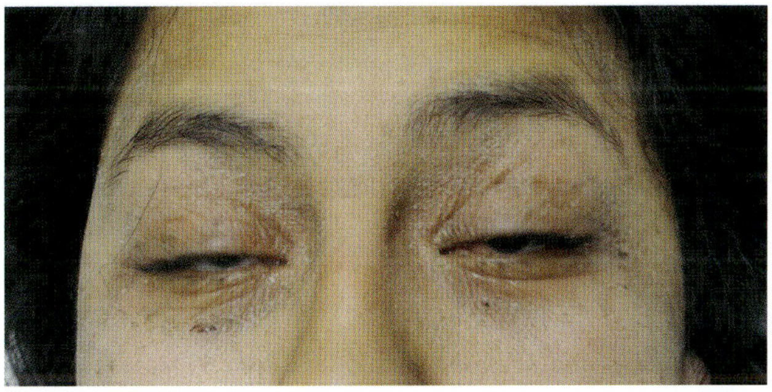

Fig. 31.9 SSSS of the eyelids and upper face, showing erythema and exfoliation of a Hispanic female

31.3.4 Histopathological Features

Biopsy specimens may demonstrate intraepidermal cleavage within the stratum granulosum or high in the stratum spinosum [5]. A small number of acantholytic cells are sometimes observed beneath the bullae, but the basal layer remains intact [5]. A few lymphocytes are present around the superficial dilated dermal vessels [5].

31.3.5 Natural History and Prognosis

Because the condition is toxin mediated, exfoliation scaling and desquamation continue for 3–5 days [3, 6]. Lesional skin heals without scarring [3]. With proper treatment, SSSS resolves in 1–2 weeks, usually without sequelae [3]. The prognosis of the disease is good in children, and the mortality rate is low if they are treated. In adult cases of SSSS, however, mortality rates are high, despite appropriate antibiotic therapy [5].

31.3.6 Diagnosis

Diagnosis of SSSS is clinical. If confirmation is required, a biopsy of the lesion remains the most useful investigation [6]. Isolating *S. aureus* from skin lesions does not aid in diagnosis, as it is neither sensitive nor specific. One of the main characteristics of SSSS in adults is the frequent isolation of *S. aureus* from blood cultures [5]. Blood cultures are positive in <5 % of pediatric patients compared with >50 % in adults [6].

31.3.7 Differential Diagnosis

The differential diagnosis of SSSS includes sunburn, drug reaction, Kawasaki disease, extensive bullous impetigo, and less often a viral exanthem, toxic shock syndrome (TSS), GVHD, and pemphigus foliaceus [3]. In cases of localized SSSS in adults, the distinction from bullous impetigo is sometimes difficult. Mucous membranes are generally preserved in SSSS, whereas they are often involved in toxic epidermal necrolysis (TEN); pustules are observed in SSSS but not in TEN. The Nikolsky sign is present in seemingly uninvolved skin in SSSS but not in TEN [5].

31.3.8 Treatment

Patients with extensive lesions should be treated with intravenous anti-staphylococcal antibacterial agents and carefully assessed for pain, temperature, and hydration status, particularly young infants [6]. Severe cases should also be given systemic antibiotics to cover for possible secondary gram-negative bacterial infection, and transfer to an intensive care unit specializing in burns may be useful [6].

31.4 Ecthyma

31.4.1 Etiology

A deeply ulcerated form of impetigo is known as ecthyma [2]. Group A beta hemolytic *Streptococci* (GAS) and *S. aureus* are the major cause of this infection.

31.4.2 Clinical Features

Ecthyma typically presents as shallow, punched out ulcers on extremities, at sites of abrasions, insect bites, or previous trauma (Fig. 31.10) [7].

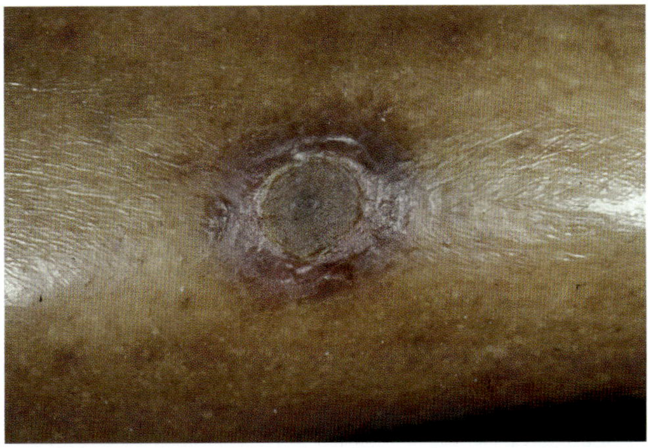

Fig. 31.10 Ecthyma on the legs of an African American male

31.4.3 Natural History and Prognosis

Unlike impetigo, ecthyma is painful and frequently leaves a prominent scar after healing [8]. Treatment of *Streptococcal* pyoderma will not prevent the subsequent development of post-streptococcal glomerulonephritis [7].

31.4.4 Treatment

Mupirocin 2 % ointment may be used on limited local areas. A 7–10-day treatment course of oral antimicrobial therapy is recommended for GAS ecthyma.

31.5 Erysipelas

31.5.1 Epidemiology/Etiology

Erysipelas is commonly caused by *streptococcal* species, usually *S. pyogenes* [2].

31.5.2 Clinical Features

Classically, erysipelas is a fiery red, tender, painful plaque with well-demarcated edges (Fig. 31.11) [2]. Regional lymphadenopathy is normally present, with or without lymphatic streaking. Pustules, vesicles, bullae, and small areas of hemorrhagic necrosis may also form [3]. Although historically erysipelas was thought to have a predilection for the face, recent articles have reported that as many as 85 % of cases now occur on the legs and feet. Development of erysipelas on the trunk or extremities is often associated with a surgical incision or wound. In neonates, infection can originate at the umbilical stump or at the circumcision site [7].

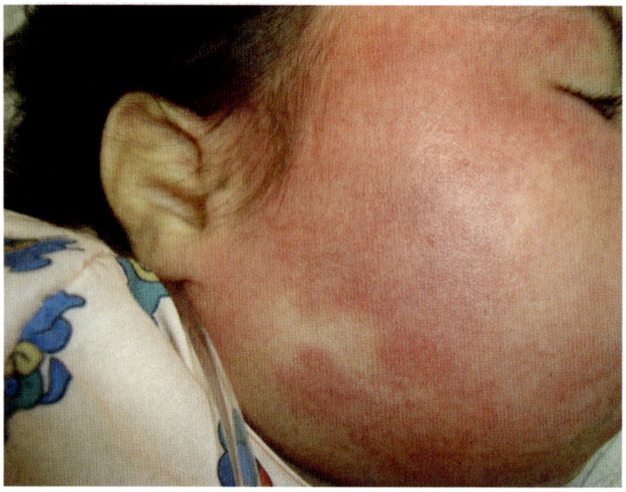

Fig. 31.11 Erysipelas on the cheek of a Hispanic female infant

31.5.3 Histopathological Features

Biopsy specimens reveal diffuse edema of the dermis and a dermal neutrophilic infiltrate. Involvement of the lymph vessels (dilation), dermal foci of suppurative necrosis, and a dermal–epidermal separation are commonly seen. There is no primary necrotizing vasculitis, thrombosis, or leukocytoclasis [3].

31.5.4 Diagnosis and Differential Diagnosis

The diagnosis of erysipelas is primarily made clinically. The differential diagnosis includes cellulitis, contact dermatitis, and necrotizing fasciitis. Blood cultures are positive in <5 % of cases [3].

31.5.5 Treatment

Penicillin, oral or parenteral, is the treatment of choice for erysipelas [2]. Other suitable agents include dicloxacillin, cephalexin, clindamycin, or erythromycin, unless *streptococci* or *staphylococci* resistant to these agents are common in the community [2].

31.6 Folliculitis, Furuncles, and Carbuncles

Furuncles (or "boils") are infections of the hair follicle, usually caused by *S. aureus,* in which suppuration extends through the dermis into the subcutaneous tissue, where formation of a small abscess occurs [2]. They differ therefore from folliculitis, in which inflammation is more superficial and pus is present only in the upper dermis and epidermis [2]. When the infection extends to involve several adjacent follicles, producing a coalescent inflammatory mass with pus draining from multiple follicular orifices, the lesion is called a carbuncle [2].

31.6.1 Epidemiology

Obesity, malnutrition, diabetes, immunosuppression, hyperhidrosis, dermatitis lesions, maceration, and friction predispose to development of furuncles and carbuncles [6].

31.6.2 Etiology

S. aureus is the most common cause of folliculitis, furuncles, and carbuncles [6]. Patients with acne vulgaris, who are treated with long-term broad-spectrum antibacterial agents, may develop folliculitis due to gram-negative organisms, such as *Klebsiella* spp., *Enterobacter* spp., *E. coli*, and *P. aeruginosa.* These infections often present as superficial pustules over the nose, cheeks, and chin, while *Proteus* spp. may cause deeper nodular folliculitis over the face and trunk [6].

31.6.3 Clinical Features

The lesions of superficial folliculitis are small, discrete pustules over an erythematous base located at the ostium of the pilosebaceous canals (Fig. 31.12) [6]. The scalp, buttocks, and extremities are the most common sites [6]. Furuncles are painful, erythematous papules with walled-off purulent material arising from the hair follicle [6]. The lesion eventually develops into a fluctuant mass that opens to the skin surface to release its purulent contents (Fig. 31.13) [6]. Carbuncles refer to infection of a group of adjoining follicles that form large, swollen, tender masses with multiple drainage points and inflammation of the surrounding connective tissue [6]. Furuncles and carbuncles occur in hair-bearing areas of the face, axillae, buttocks, and groin, particularly in areas of skin exposed to friction [6].

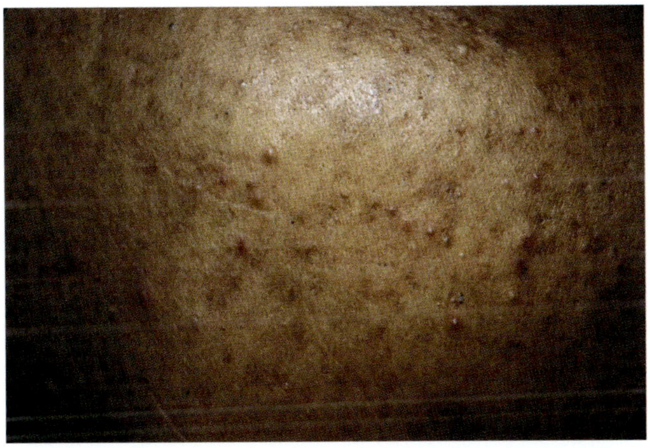

Fig. 31.12 Folliculitis on the back of an African American male

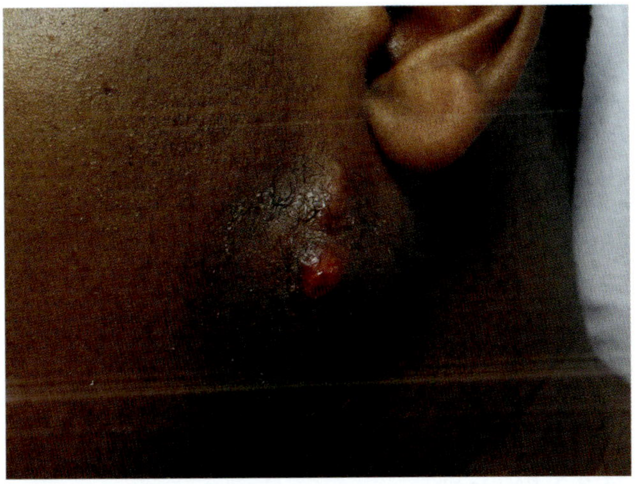

Fig. 31.13 Furunculosis on the cheek of an AA male

31.6.4 Histopathological Features

Suppurative inflammation in or around a follicle is the most common histological change seen in folliculitis [4].

31.6.5 Diagnosis and Differential Diagnosis

The differential diagnosis includes acne, rosacea, pustular drug eruptions, and necrotizing fasciitis [4, 6]. The causative organism can usually be identified by gram stain and culture of the purulent fluid extracted from the infected lesions [6].

31.6.6 Treatment

Localized lesions usually only require topical antibacterial cleansers such as chlorhexidine or topical antibacterial ointments such as mupirocin. Frequent use of hot, moist compresses may facilitate drainage of the lesions. More severe and recurrent cases require systemic antistaphylococcal antibacterial agents, and efforts should be made to eliminate staphylococcal carriage [6]. For persons with nasal colonization, one approach is the application of mupirocin ointment twice daily in the anterior nares for the first 5 days each month [2]. Large or deep nodular lesions may also require incision and drainage. Any loculations in carbuncles should be broken and the wound packed to encourage further drainage. In severe cases, parenteral antibiotics may be required [6].

31.7 Cellulitis

31.7.1 Epidemiology

Cellulitis is an acute infection of the dermis and subcutaneous tissue [9]. It is a common cause of outpatient medical visits and inpatient hospital admissions accounting for 10 % of the infectious disease related US hospitalizations in 1998–2006 [9]. Traumas to the skin including piercing, IV drug use, or "skin popping" are important risk factors [9].

31.7.2 Etiology

Streptococci are usually the cause of bacterial cellulitis without an underlying abscess. *S. aureus* is a possible culprit in cases with abscess or history of penetrating trauma. Gram-negative organisms can also cause lower extremity cellulitis in patients with underlying chronic medical conditions, such as diabetes and chronic kidney disease.

31.7.3 Clinical Features

Cellulitis typically presents with erythema, pain, warmth, and edema. Typically, the borders of cellulitis are smooth and ill defined (Fig. 31.14) [9]. In severe cases, vesicles, bullae, pustules, and necrosis may be present [9]. Cellulitis is typically unilateral, as opposed to bilateral involvement in stasis dermatitis, a condition that often mimics cellulitis. The presence of pain distinguishes cellulitis from another mimicker, contact dermatitis or an eczematous dermatitis in which the patient usually complains of pruritus [9].

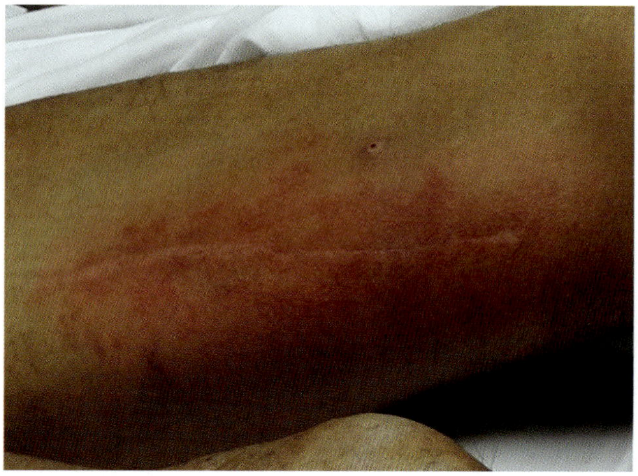

Fig. 31.14 Cellulitis on the leg surrounding a vein graft harvesting scar of a Hispanic male

31.7.4 Histopathological Features

A skin biopsy of standard cellulitis usually demonstrates subepidermal edema with diffuse infiltration of neutrophils without abscesses. There is often vascular lymphatic dilatation and secondary panniculitis [9].

31.7.5 Diagnosis and Differential Diagnosis

The differential diagnosis includes stasis dermatitis, acute lipodermatosclerosis, lymphedema, contact dermatitis, deep vein thrombosis (DVT), panniculitis, and erythema migrans. Diagnosis is made clinically. Supporting laboratory information includes a complete blood count with differential that may show a slightly elevated WBC count. Cultures of bullae, pustules, and ulcers should be performed and may provide useful information if positive. Needle aspirates and punch biopsies are usually not helpful. When there is clinical doubt, a skin biopsy may be helpful in distinguishing true cellulitis from noninfectious causes or to rule out atypical nonbacterial infectious causes of cellulitis, such as fungi or mycobacteria [9].

31.7.6 Treatment

Therapy for cellulitis should include an antibiotic active against streptococci. Many clinicians choose an agent that is also effective against *S. aureus,* although this organism rarely causes cellulitis unless associated with an underlying abscess or penetrating trauma [2]. Suitable agents include dicloxacillin, cephalexin, clindamycin, or erythromycin, unless streptococci or staphylococci resistant to these agents are common in the community [2, 3].

31.8 Necrotizing Fasciitis

31.8.1 Epidemiology

Necrotizing fasciitis (NF) is a relatively rare subcutaneous infection that tracks along fascial planes [2]. Risk factors for the development of NF include diabetes mellitus, peripheral vascular disease, intravenous drug use, obesity, and malnutrition [10].

31.8.2 Etiology

Various aerobic and anaerobic pathogens can cause necrotizing soft-tissue infections (NSTI) either alone or in combination and tend to be different from the pathogens that cause non-necrotizing soft-tissue infections [11].

31.8.3 Clinical Features

Patients initially present with nonspecific symptoms such as pain and high fever as well as local edema and erythema on exam. The affected area is initially red, hot, shiny, swollen without sharp margins, and exquisitely tender. The process progresses over several days with the skin color changing to characteristic blue-gray ill-defined patches as early as 36 h after onset. Vesicles, bullae, and skin necrosis may also be seen. The presence of marked systemic toxicity and severe pain out of proportion to the local findings should suggest the possibility of NF [10]. In cellulitis or erysipelas, the subcutaneous tissues can be palpated and are yielding to touch. But in fasciitis, the underlying tissues are firm, and the fascial planes and muscle groups cannot be discerned by palpation [2].

31.8.4 Diagnosis

The "finger test" is a bedside procedure whereby a 2-cm incision is made down to the deep fascia under local anesthesia and gentle probing with the index finger is performed. Lack of bleeding, presence of characteristic "dishwater pus," and lack of tissue resistance to blunt finger are features of necrotizing fasciitis [11]. Lab findings such as C-reactive protein >150 mg/L, WBC >25,000 cells/mm [3], hyponatremia, hyperglycemia, anemia, and acute kidney injury may be suggestive as well [12].

31.8.5 Differential Diagnosis

The differential diagnosis of NF includes cellulitis, pyomyositis, phlebitis, bursitis, and arthritis [3]. Clinical clues that differentiate NF from cellulitis include severe pain, rapidly spreading tense edema, foul-smelling discharge, and gray-blue discoloration [3]. The presence of hemorrhagic bullae or epidermal necrosis may indicate the presence of a serious soft-tissue infection.

31.8.6 Treatment

Once diagnosis is confirmed, early debridement is indicated and must not be delayed. A broad-spectrum antibiotic should also be initiated at the earliest opportunity to cover gram-positive, gram-negative, and anaerobic organisms. Mortality has been found to be significantly lower with early and aggressive debridement [11]. Most patients with necrotizing fasciitis should return to the operating room 24–36 h after the first debridement and daily thereafter until the surgical team finds no further need for debridement [2]. Acceptable antibiotic regimens include ampicillin–sulbactam or piperacillin–tazobactam plus clindamycin plus ciprofloxacin and vancomycin. Other options are carbapenems such as imipenem/cilastatin or meropenem plus metronidazole or clindamycin plus vancomycin. Clindamycin is added to reduce toxin production and has also been shown to decrease cytokine production. IVIG use is controversial and has been used in some cases of streptococcal and clostridium-induced infections. It is believed IVIG has neutralizing antibodies against streptococcal antigens and clostridial toxins [11].

References

1. Bangert S, Levy M, Hebert AA. Bacterial resistance and impetigo treatment trends: a review. Pediatr Dermatol. 2012;29(3):243–8.
2. Stevens DL, Bisno AL, Chambers HF, et al. Practice guidelines for the diagnosis and management of skin and soft-tissue infections. Clin Infect Dis. 2005;41(10):1373–406.
3. Halpern AV, Heymann WR. Bacterial diseases. In: Bolognia JL, Jorizzo JL, Rapini RP, editors. Dermatology, vol. 1. 2nd ed. St. Louis: Mosby; 2008. p. 1075–106.
4. Elston D. Bacterial, spirochete and protozoan infections. In: Elston DM, Ferringer T, Ko CJ, Peckham S, High WA, DiCaudo DJ, editors. Dermatopathology. Philadelphia: Saunders Elsevier; 2009. p. 261–73.
5. Cribier B, Piemont Y, Grosshans E. Staphylococcal scalded skin syndrome in adults. A clinical review illustrated with a new case. J Am Acad Dermatol. 1994;30(2 Pt 2):319–24.
6. Ladhani S, Garbash M. Staphylococcal skin infections in children: rational drug therapy recommendations. Paediatr Drugs. 2005; 7(2):77–102.
7. Martin JM, Green M. Group A Streptococcus. Semin Pediatr Infect Dis. 2006;17(3):140–8.
8. Wasserzug O, Valinsky L, Klement E, et al. A cluster of ecthyma outbreaks caused by a single clone of invasive and highly infective Streptococcus pyogenes. Clin Infect Dis. 2009;48(9):1213–9.
9. Bailey E, Kroshinsky D. Cellulitis: diagnosis and management. Dermatol Ther. 2011;24(2):229–39.
10. Chapnick EK, Abter EI. Necrotizing soft-tissue infections. Infect Dis Clin North Am. 1996;10(4):835–55.
11. Mullangi PK, Khardori NM. Necrotizing soft-tissue infections. Med Clin North Am. 2012;96(6):1193–202.
12. Wong CH, Khin LW, Heng KS, Tan KC, Low CO. The LRINEC (Laboratory Risk Indicator for Necrotizing Fasciitis) score: a tool for distinguishing necrotizing fasciitis from other soft tissue infections. Crit Care Med. 2004;32(7):1535–41.

Tinea Corporis, Tinea Versicolor, and Candidiasis

32

Diane Jackson-Richards

Contents

32.1 Etiology

Dermatophytoses or "tinea," tinea versicolor (pityriasis versicolor), and candidiasis are the three most common types of superficial fungal infections. Dermatophytes infect the skin, hair, and nails, require keratin for growth, and do not infect mucosal surfaces. Dermatophytes are named by the involved body part. Tinea corporis is a fungal infection of the body, tinea capitis involves the hair and scalp, tinea pedis involves the foot, and tinea unguium or onychomycosis involves the nails. Dermatophytes are further subdivided by the mode of transmission, of which there are three types. Anthropophilic dermatophytes have human to human transmission, geophilic have soil to animal or human transmission, and zoophilic have animal to human transmission. Transmission of these infections can occur from direct skin to skin contact or by indirect contact with fomites, such as hair brushes, hats, and beddings.

Tinea versicolor or pityriasis versicolor is a superficial, noninflammatory mycosis of the skin, first described by Eichstedt in 1846. *Malassezia globosa* is felt to be the causative organism. *Malassezia furfur* was the species originally thought to cause tinea versicolor. A recent study by Lyakhovitsky et al. [1] examined samples taken from the skin of tinea versicolor patients and used polymerase chain reaction multiplication to define the species of *Malassezia* organisms. *M. globosa* was found in 97.3 % of patients, and *M. restricta* was associated with *M. globosa* in 1.3 %. *Malassezia* organisms in small quantities are normal flora on human skin. Under conditions of warmer temperatures and higher humidity, there is overgrowth of the mycelial form producing this common skin disorder. It is felt that these lipophilic yeasts metabolize surface lipids on the skin, producing dicarboxylic acids that in turn inhibit melanocytes.

D. Jackson-Richards, MD
Department of Dermatology, Multicultural Dermatology Center,
Henry Ford Hospital, 3031 West Grand Blvd.,
Detroit, MI 48202, USA
e-mail: djackso1@hfhs.org

D. Jackson-Richards, A.G. Pandya (eds.), *Dermatology Atlas for Skin of Color*,
DOI 10.1007/978-3-642-54446-0_32, © Springer-Verlag Berlin Heidelberg 2014

32.2 Epidemiology

Superficial mycoses or fungal infections are the most common type of skin infections affecting 20–25 % of people worldwide [2]. The prevalence of superficial fungal infections is increasing, and the causative organisms have shifted or changed over the past several decades. The changes in causative organisms seen in various geographic locations have been influenced by migration as well as changes in socioeconomic conditions and lifestyle [3, 8]. *Trichophyton rubrum* is the most common dermatophyte worldwide and the most common cause of tinea corporis in the United States [4]. *T. rubrum* is the most frequently isolated organism as the cause of tinea pedis, tinea cruris (groin), and onychomycosis worldwide. Tinea pedis and onychomycosis are felt to be increasing in many parts of the world due to increased urbanization, use of communal bathing facilities, and wearing of occlusive footwear [3]. A study by Vena et al. looked at the frequency of dermatophyte infections in an outpatient clinic in Italy from 2005 to 2010. Their data showed onychomycosis to be the highest of dermatophyte infections at 39.2 % followed by tinea corporis, 22.7 % and tinea pedis 20.4 % [5]. This parallels other studies that report incidence of tinea pedis at 30 % in Mexico and 27 % in Singapore. This is in contrast to India and rural Africa where the incidence of tinea pedis is low due to lack of occlusive footwear. Tinea infections of the feet, nails, and scalp may act as a reservoir and cause tinea corporis through autoinoculation.

Despite the predominance of tinea versicolor in warmer, tropical environments, tinea versicolor occurs worldwide, even in more temperate climates. There is no age, sex, or racial predilection. Tinea versicolor may occur at any age but is more common in adolescents and young adults.

32.3 Clinical Features

Trichophyton rubrum is the most frequent cause of tinea corporis in North America; however, it can also be caused by *Trichophyton tonsurans*, *Trichophyton mentagrophytes*, *Epidermophyton floccosum*, and *Microsporum canis*. *M. canis* is a zoophilic fungus and is usually acquired by exposure to cats or dogs. Classic tinea corporis presents as a single or few, well-demarcated erythematous, circular, or annular scaly plaques (Fig. 32.1). Often there is central clearing giving rise to an expanding ring-like lesion. The raised border may be papular, pustular, or vesicular. Pruritus is a common complaint. If lesions have inadvertently been treated with topical corticosteroids, lesions may show less inflammation and no pruritus. As with many skin conditions, tinea corporis lesions may be less erythematous and more hyperpigmented in patients with darker skin type compared to Caucasians. Tinea occurs in all areas of the body. Facial lesions are referred to as tinea faciei (Fig. 32.2), tinea on the palms is tinea manuum, and tinea on the feet is tinea pedis. Tinea on the dorsum of the hands presents as any other tinea lesion on the body, but here there is usually lack of erythema and diffuse fine scale. A clue to tinea manum is the presence of fingernail involvement. Often tinea manuum is unilateral and associated with bilateral tinea pedis and referred to as "two-foot one-hand syndrome."

Tinea pedis is caused by the same organisms that cause tinea corporis. The usual presentation is diffuse scaling with hyperkeratosis and fissuring of the soles. Vesicles may be present and pruritus is variable. This presentation is often referred to as moccasin-type tinea pedis as it involves the areas of the foot that a moccasin shoe would cover (Figs. 32.3 and 32.4). Another common finding is maceration of the interdigital web spaces, particularly the third and fourth spaces. Tinea unguium or onychomycosis is infection of the fingernails or toenails with dermatophytes or non-dermatophyte molds. Toenail involvement is much more common than fingernail involvement (Fig. 32.5). Onychomycosis presents as hyperkeratosis of the nail bed with yellowing, thickening, and onycholysis of the nail plate.

Tinea cruris is a dermatophyte infection of the inguinal folds. Typically there are thin erythematous plaques extending from the inguinal fold onto the upper, inner thigh. Fine scaling is seen at the advancing border. Instead of erythema, there may be just hyperpigmentation seen in darker-skinned individuals (Fig. 32.6). Pruritus and burning are common symptoms. Although this infection occurs in both males and females, it is more common in males because of the warm, moist environment of the scrotum and because associated onychomycosis is more common in men.

Cutaneous candidiasis is most often caused by *Candida albicans* and usually presents in warm, moist body folds. It appears as erythematous, eroded plaques with satellite pustules near the border of the lesion. Commonly involved areas are the inframammary skin, fold of pannus on the lower abdomen, inguinal folds, and diaper area in infants (Fig. 32.7). The nail bed and periungual areas are common sites also. Mucocutaneous candidiasis presents as a thick white exudate in the mouth as oral thrush or a vulvovaginitis or balanitis. Candidiasis is often seen when patients are being treated with corticosteroids or systemic antibiotics.

Malassezia organisms are lipophilic, and skin lesions of tinea versicolor typically occur on the upper chest and back and less commonly on the face. The lesions present as round or oval macules that coalesce into larger patches. On close examination, fine scaling may be seen thereby categorizing the lesions as thin plaques. Classically lesions are hypopigmented but can be brown or hyperpigmented as well (Figs. 32.8, 32.9, 32.10, and 32.11). Metabolites of skin lipids by *Malassezia* inhibit melanocytes, but many individuals present with hyperpigmented or pink lesions that may be a result of a mild inflammatory response. Tinea versicolor is usually asymptomatic. Along with the characteristic clinical appearance, KOH preparations show diagnostic yeasts and hyphae classically referred to as a "spaghetti and meatballs" pattern. Wood's light examination of the skin produces yellow fluorescence.

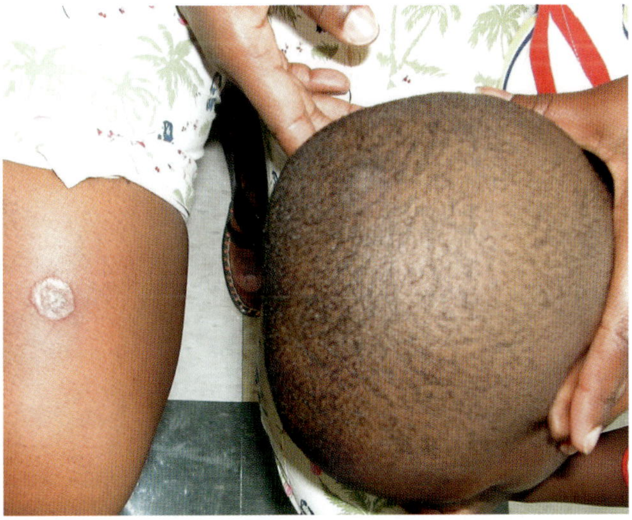

Fig. 32.1 Tinea capitis in an African American boy and tinea corporis in his mother (Courtesy of Dr. Tor Shwayder)

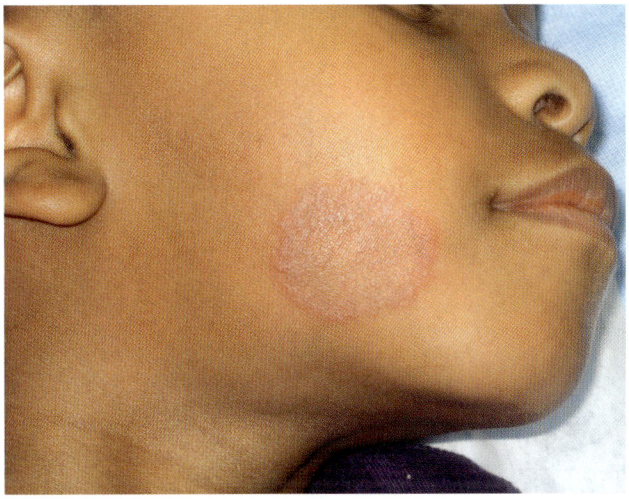

Fig. 32.2 Tinea faciei in a young African American girl

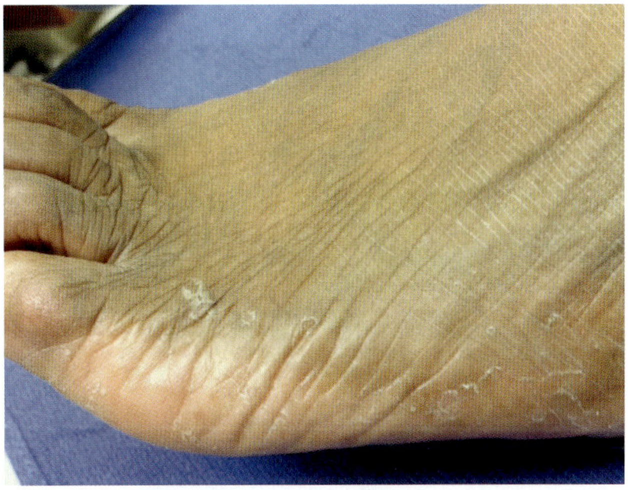

Fig. 32.3 Tinea pedis in an African American female (Courtesy of Dr. Tor Shwayder)

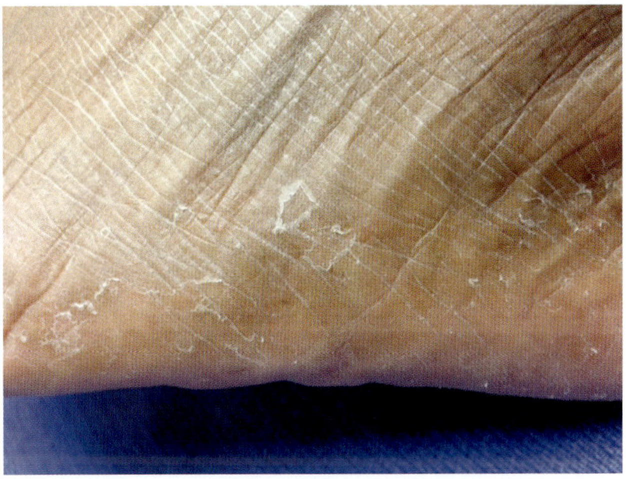

Fig. 32.4 Tinea pedis in an African American female

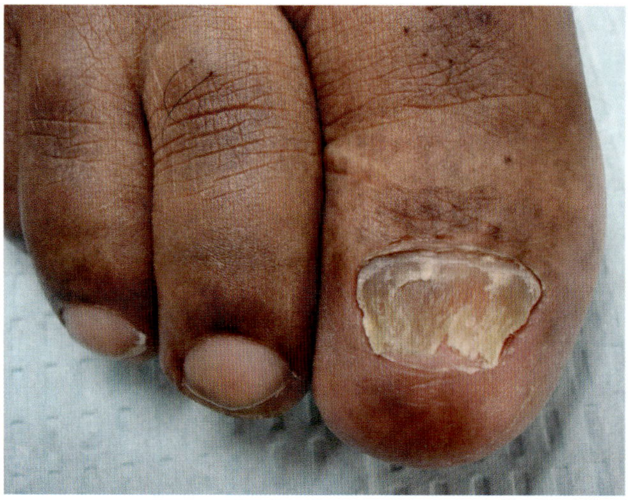

Fig. 32.5 Tinea unguium (onychomycosis) in an African American male

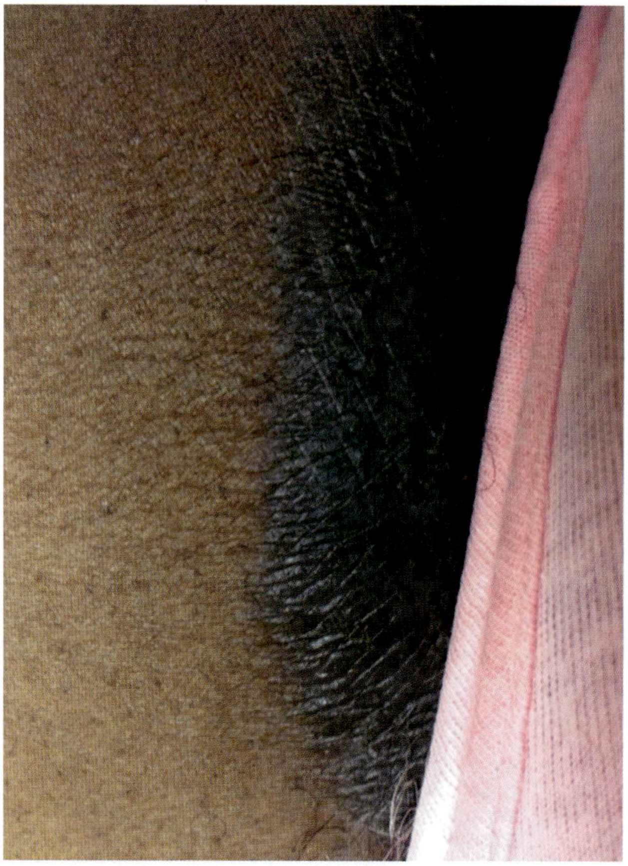

Fig. 32.6 Tinea cruris in an African American female

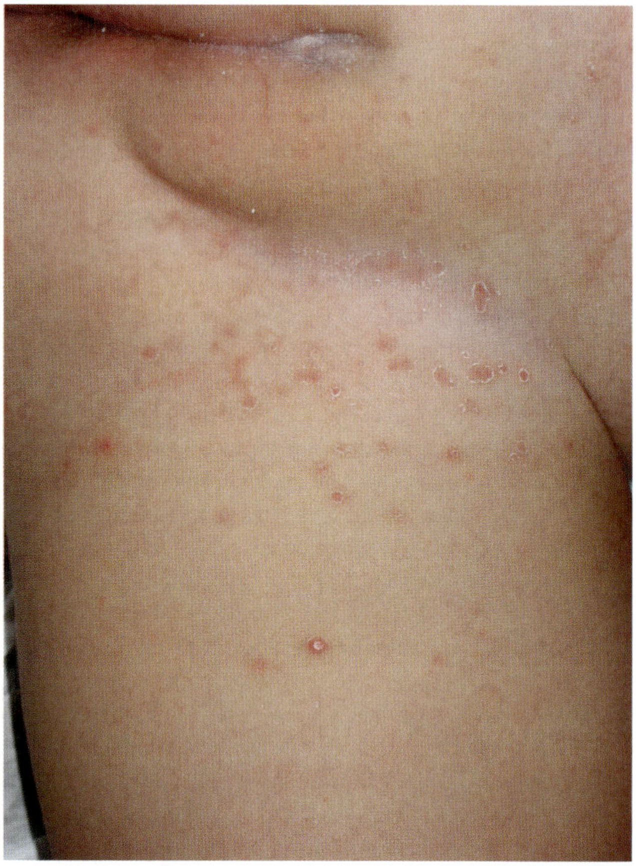

Fig. 32.7 *Candida* diaper dermatitis (Courtesy of Dr. Tor Shwayder)

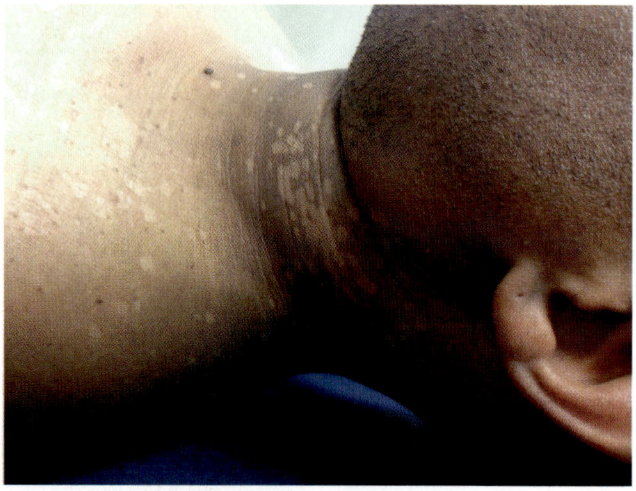

Fig. 32.8 Tinea versicolor in an African American male

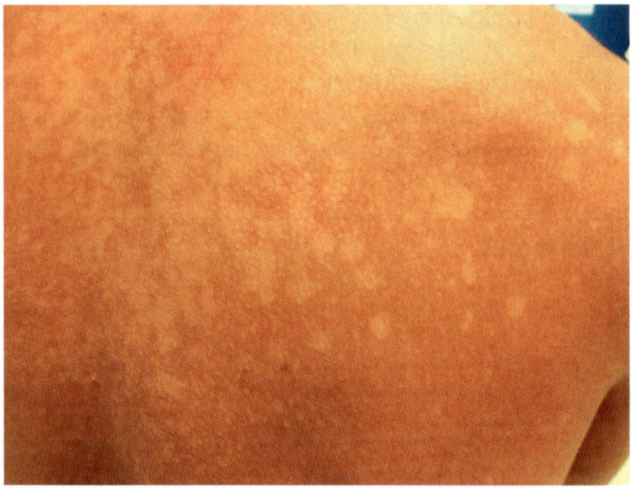

Fig. 32.9 Tinea versicolor in an African American male

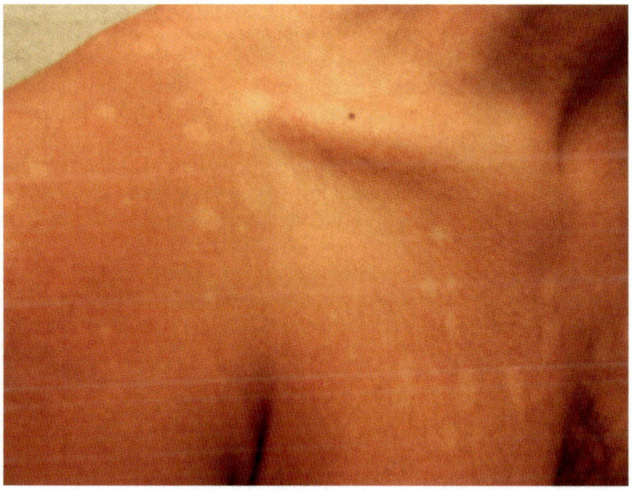

Fig. 32.10 Tinea versicolor in an African American male

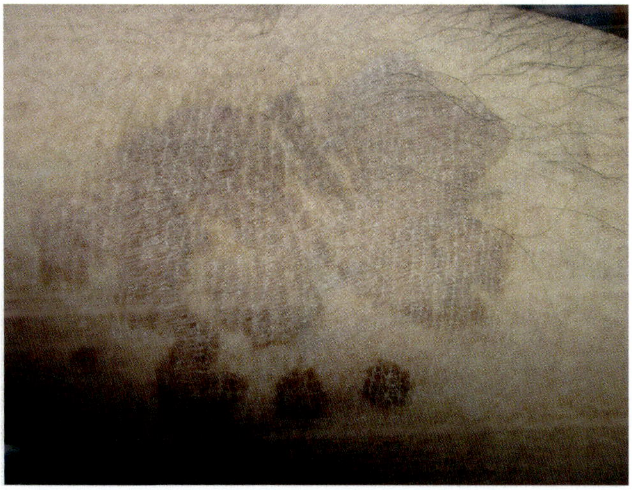

Fig. 32.11 Tinea versicolor on the arm of a South Asian male

32.4 Diagnosis and Differential Diagnosis

Fungal cultures of skin or nail scrapings are the best way to confirm a fungal infection, but results may take 7–14 days to come back. Microscopic confirmation by potassium hydroxide (KOH) preparation is a simple test to perform and gives immediate confirmation at the bedside. After gently scraping the involved skin area with a blade, fine scales are placed on a glass slide with 10–20 % KOH and a coverslip. Microscopic examination should reveal branching hyphae or budding yeast.

Pityriasis rosea, nummular dermatitis, and granuloma annulare all can be confused with tinea corporis. A negative KOH preparation helps to rule out these conditions. In addition granuloma annulare lacks epidermal changes such as scaling or vesicles [4]. Tinea pedis can be misdiagnosed as dyshidrotic eczema or psoriasis, both of which would have a negative KOH. Tinea cruris appears similar to erythrasma, intertrigo, psoriasis, and Hailey-Hailey. Erythrasma, which is caused by a corynebacterium, has a coral-pink fluorescence on Wood's lamp examination. A history of trauma and psoriasis should be ruled out when considering onychomycosis.

The hypopigmentation of tinea versicolor can be confused with pityriasis alba or any other post-inflammatory response in darker skin such as seborrheic dermatitis [4]. The possibility of vitiligo might be considered, but vitiligo usually presents with depigmentation rather than hypopigmentation. Tinea versicolor might also be confused with secondary syphilis or pityriasis rosea.

32.5 Histopathologic Features

Since superficial fungal infections can be diagnosed with KOH preparations and fungal cultures, biopsies are not commonly performed. Histopathology shows spongiosis with parakeratosis and PAS-positive hyphae in the stratum corneum. Since the clinical presentation along with KOH preparations are diagnostic, biopsies of tinea versicolor are rarely done. When performed, biopsy of tinea versicolor shows yeast and hyphae in the stratum corneum

32.6 Treatment

Most dermatophytoses such as tinea corporis, tinea cruris, and tinea pedis can be treated with topical antifungal agents. Tinea capitis requires systemic antifungals because the organisms are in the hair follicle root [4, 7]. Topical agents do not penetrate the nail plate well enough to provide adequate treatment for onychomycosis. If tinea corporis is very extensive, systemic antifungals may provide better resolution than topicals alone. Imidazoles are safe, fungistatic drugs that cure most dermatophyte infections in 2–6 weeks. Allylamines are fungicidal and are very effective for most dermatophytes. Allylamines often provide higher cure rates with just once-daily applications compared to the azoles which are applied twice daily [4]. A study by Rotta et al. performed an extensive review of many studies that compared topical antifungal treatments. In general, allylamines performed better than azoles for a mycological cure and a sustained cure [6]. Although *Candida* can be treated with nystatin, it is ineffective on dermatophytes. *Candida* does respond to topical and oral azoles. Topical antifungals combined with corticosteroids are less effective, and overuse of these agents can cause atrophy of the skin, especially in intertriginous areas.

There are many antifungal treatments that are effective for tinea versicolor; however, it often recurs, and the length of treatment needed for complete clearing has not been established. Topical treatments consist of imidazoles and non-imidazoles. Daily ketoconazole, selenium sulfide, and zinc pyrithione shampoos applied to the affected skin for 5–10 min then washed off for 2–4 weeks is effective. Unfortunately, shampoos can be drying to the skin. Topical ketoconazole, econazole, miconazole, clotrimazole, and ciclopirox creams applied one to two times daily for 2–4 weeks are also commonly used effective treatments. Oral imidazoles, including ketoconazole, 200 mg/day for 10 days; itraconazole, 200 mg/day for 7 days; or fluconazole, 300 mg/week for 2–4 weeks, have been studied in clinical trials. Since the oral imidazoles inhibit cytochrome P450, caution must be used to avoid drug-drug interactions. There are also reports of ketoconazole and itraconazole causing elevation of liver enzymes, GI upset, and fatigue. Itraconazole has been associated with hepatotoxicity and congestive heart failure [9].

References

1. Lyakhovitsky A, Shemer A, Amichai B. Molecular analysis of Malassezia species isolated from Israeli patients with pityriasis versicolor. Int J Dermatol. 2013;52:231–3.
2. Havlickova B, Czaika VA, Friedrich M. Epidemiological trends in skin mycoses worldwide. Mycoses. 2008;51 Suppl 4:2–15.
3. Ameen M. Epidemiology of superficial fungal infections. Clin Dermatol. 2010;28:197–201.
4. Kelly BP. Superficial fungal infections. Pediatr Rev. 2012;33:e22.
5. Vena GA, et al. Epidemiology of dermatophytoses: retrospective analysis from 2005 to 2010 and comparison with previous data from 1975. New Microbiol. 2012;35:207–13.
6. Rotta I, et al. Efficacy of topical antifungal drugs in different dermatomycoses: a systematic review with meta-analysis. Rev Assoc Med Bras. 2012;58(3):308–18.
7. Lorch Dauk KC, Comrov E, Blumer JL, et al. Tinea capitis: predictive value of symptoms and time to cure with griseofulvin treatment. Clin Pediatr. 2010;49(3):280–6.
8. Borman AM, Campbell CK, Fraser M, Johnson EM. Analysis of the dermatophyte species isolated in the British Isles between 1980 and 2005 and review of worldwide dermatophyte trends over the last three decades. Med Mycol. 2007;45:131–41.
9. Hu SW, Bigby M. Evidence based review to determine efficacy of topical of systemic agents in the treatment and prevention of pityriasis versicolor. Arch Dermatol. 2010;42:1–18.

Tinea Capitis

33

Mio Nakamura and Raechele Cochran Gathers

Contents

M. Nakamura, BS
Wayne State University, School of Medicine,
320 E. Canfield, Detroit, MI 48201, USA

Department of Dermatology,
Multicultural Dermatology Center, Henry Ford Hospital,
3031 West Grand Boulevard, Suite 800, Detroit, MI 48202, USA
e-mail: mnakamur@med.wayne.edu

R.C. Gathers, MD (✉)
Department of Dermatology, Multicultural Dermatology Center,
Henry Ford Hospital,
3031 West Grand Boulevard, Suite 800, Detroit, MI 48202, USA
e-mail: rgather1@hfhs.org

33.1 Introduction

The most common pediatric dermatophyte infection worldwide is that of the scalp. The incidence of tinea capitis is highest in 3- to 7-year-old children, although a recent retrospective study has found 47 % of tinea capitis occurring in individuals 13 and older [1]. In the same study, tinea capitis disproportionately affected the black population with black individuals comprising 87 % of all patients diagnosed with tinea capitis in a dermatology clinic during a 15-year period. It routinely affects individuals who are otherwise healthy, but there is increased susceptibility in immunocompromised individuals. The growth and transmission of the fungi are favored in warm, humid, and overcrowded environments. Incidence appears to correlate with low socioeconomic status, large family size, poor hygiene, and frequent person-to-person contact. The incidence of tinea capitis is increasing worldwide and has had considerable shifts in the causative organisms over the past 50 years. This infection is especially prevalent in Afro-Caribbean and African American children.

Tinea capitis is the most common superficial fungal infection in North America and in the United States. It affects 3–8 % of children in urban areas, especially those of African or Afro-Caribbean descent. Over the past 50 years, the epidemiology of tinea capitis has changed more than other tinea infections. *Microsporum canis* and *Microsporum audouinii* have been eradicated and replaced by *Trichophyton tonsurans* as the cause of tinea capitis in 95 % of the cases in the United States and Canada [2, 6]. Although *M. canis* is still the most predominant cause of tinea capitis in Europe, Mexico, South America, and China, trends are changing. The United Kingdom now reports 83 % of tinea capitis cases being caused by *T. tonsurans*, and cities like Paris and Amsterdam are showing similar trends [7]. *Microsporum audouinii* is the most prevalent organism in Africa; however, *T. violaceum* and *T. soudanense* are common organisms in Asia and Africa.

The dermatophytes causing tinea capitis are from the *Microsporum* and *Trichophyton* groups. *M. canis* is the most

D. Jackson-Richards, A.G. Pandya (eds.), *Dermatology Atlas for Skin of Color*,
DOI 10.1007/978-3-642-54446-0_33, © Springer-Verlag Berlin Heidelberg 2014

common cause worldwide. *M. canis* can be carried by pets in the household and is therefore difficult to eradicate. There has been an increasing incidence of *T. tonsurans*, which now comprises 95 % of all tinea capitis in the United States and Canada. Its rates are increasing similarly in Europe as well [2]. *T. soudanense* and *T. violaceum* are major causes of tinea capitis in parts of Africa.

Dermatophytes cause infection by entering keratinized tissues. The dermatophyte hyphae penetrate hair cuticles and grow downward into the hair, invading newly formed keratin, which becomes visible at the skin surface after 12–14 days of inoculation. The hair becomes brittle, causing breakage by 3–4 weeks.

33.2 Clinical Features

There are several clinical presentations of tinea capitis, including gray patch, moth eaten, black dot, diffuse scale, pustular, and kerion. The gray patch (Fig. 33.1) and moth-eaten (Fig. 33.2) presentations consist of areas of alopecia with superficial scaling, with scaling being more prominent in the gray patch presentation. The black dot presentation is seen due to breakage of hair shafts, leaving tiny black dots in the affected areas. Tinea capitis presenting with diffuse scale mimics generalized dandruff. The slight erythema of the scalp in the above presentations is difficult to appreciate on darker-skinned individuals. The presence of comma and corkscrew hairs on dermoscopy may be a reliable sign of tinea capitis in such patients [3]. Pustular tinea capitis often implies a superficial bacterial infection (Fig. 33.3). A kerion represents a delayed hypersensitivity reaction and granuloma formation due to immune reaction to the dermatophyte and is often mistaken for a bacterial abscess (Figs. 33.4 and 33.5). A kerion can be painful with associated adenopathy (Fig. 33.6) and can also leave scarring alopecia. In a study consisting of predominantly black children, scaling of the scalp presenting with adenopathy had a positive predictive value of 97 % for tinea capitis [4]. In another study, Hispanic children presenting with scalp hyperkeratosis were more likely than not to have tinea capitis [5]. There have been several case reports of erythema nodosum associated with kerions, which usually occurs at the height of infection or shortly after induction of therapy. It is thought to be due to delayed hypersensitivity to systemically absorbed fungal antigens, antigen release induced by treatment, or a large antigen load from the primary inflammatory response [6].

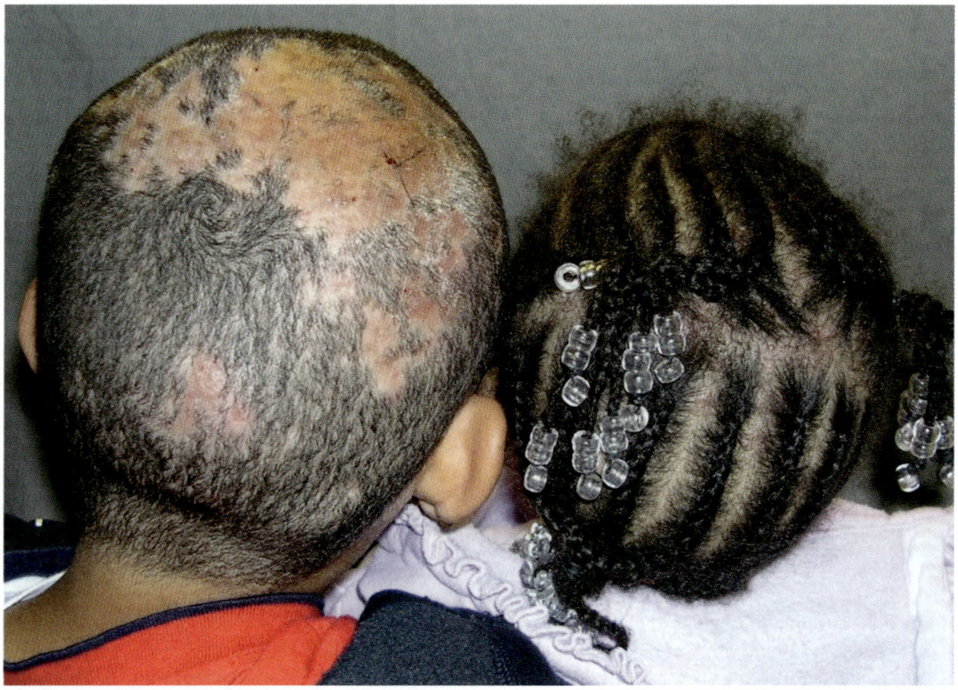

Fig. 33.1 A 12-year-old black male with *gray* patch tinea capitis (*left*) with his sister who also had a positive culture (*right*) (Photo courtesy of Dr. Tor Shwayder)

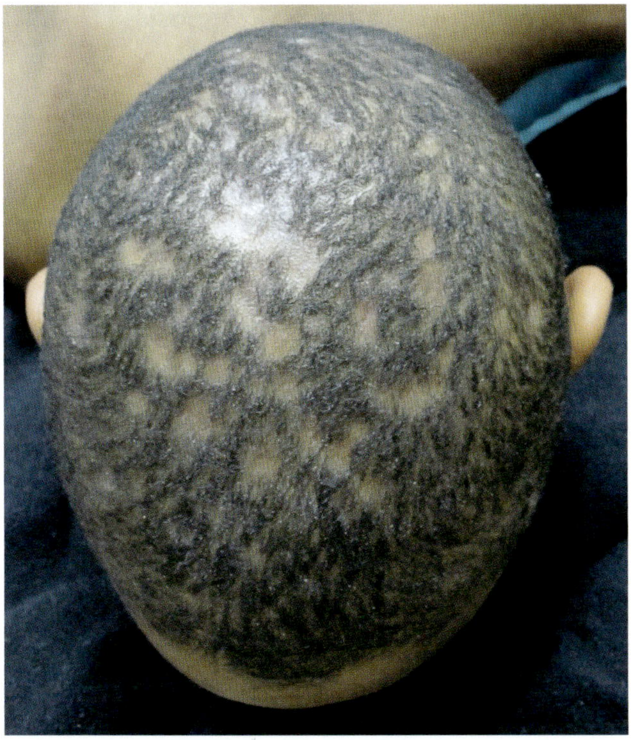

Fig. 33.2 A 6-year-old black male with moth-eaten tinea capitis (Photo courtesy of Dr. Tor Shwayder)

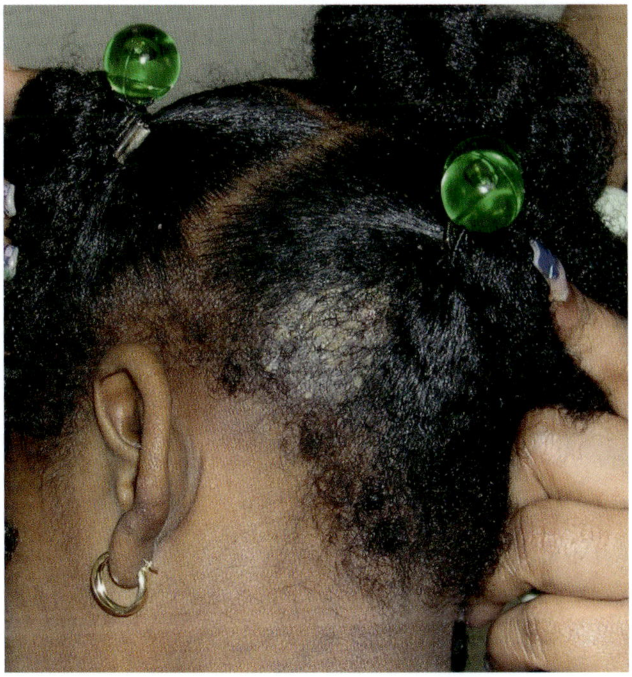

Fig. 33.3 A 5-year-old black female with pustular tinea capitis (Photo courtesy of Dr. Tor Shwayder)

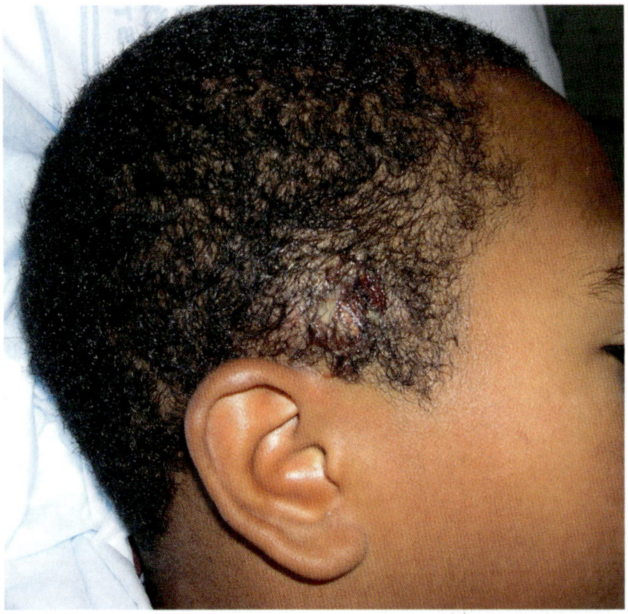

Fig. 33.4 An 11-year-old black male with a kerion (Photo courtesy of Dr. Tor Shwayder)

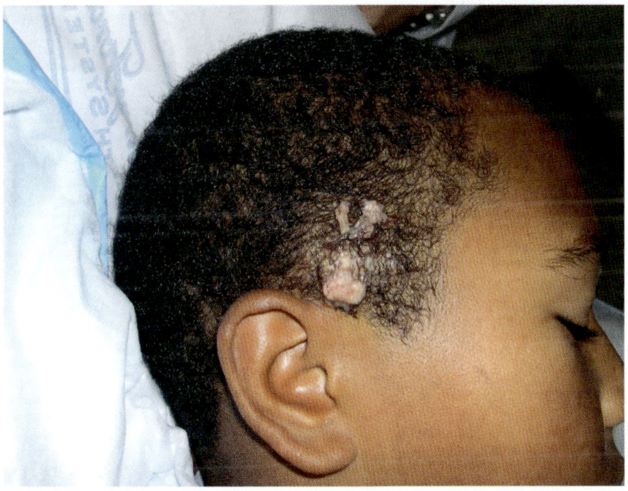

Fig. 33.5 Same patient as Fig. 33.4 with expressed contents of the kerion (Photo courtesy of Dr. Tor Shwayder)

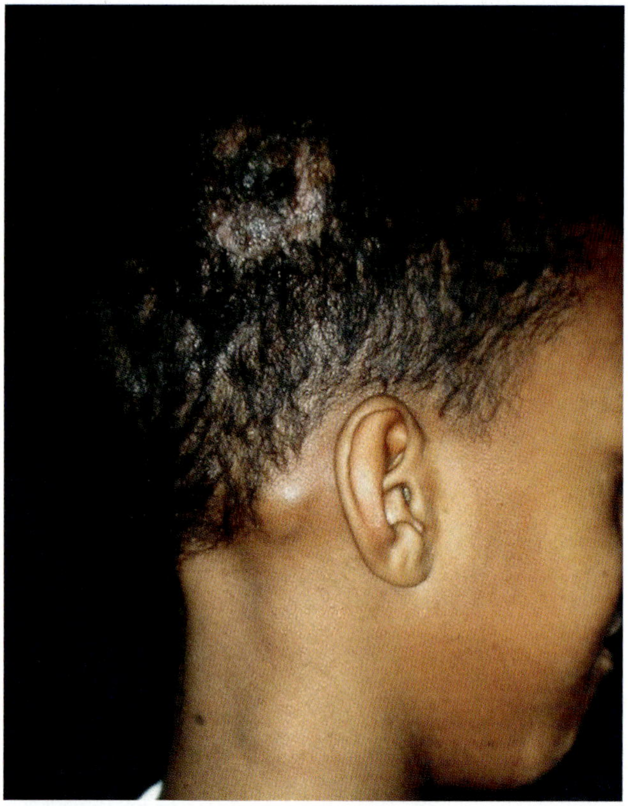

Fig. 33.6 Tinea capitis with lymphadenopathy (Photo courtesy of Dr. Tor Shwayder)

33.3 Natural History and Prognosis

With early diagnosis and appropriate treatment, transmission and permanent sequelae of tinea capitis, including scarring and alopecia, can be avoided.

33.4 Histopathological Features

Dermatophytes are usually visible within and around the hair shaft and can be elucidated by using periodic acid-Schiff or methenamine silver stains. Multinucleated giant cells with surrounding chronic inflammatory infiltrate are sometimes present along the degenerated hair follicles. A mild perivascular lymphocytic infiltrate may be present in the dermis. Kerions may have perifollicular dermal mononuclear infiltrate, follicular pustules, interfollicular neutrophilic infiltrate, and chronic inflammatory infiltrate.

33.5 Diagnosis and Differential Diagnosis

The diagnosis of tinea capitis must be confirmed by microscopic visualization of branching hyphae, culture, or polymerase chain reaction (PCR). Samples can be collected using scalp brushings or swabbing in cases of pustular tinea capitis and kerions. Potassium hydroxide preparation and fluorescent stains such as calcofluor of the skin and hair are both rapid but can have false-negative results, especially in early disease. Cultures are more time consuming, requiring at least 6 weeks of incubation to establish negative results, but are more sensitive and can give antifungal susceptibilities. Although expensive, PCR is useful when the patient has been pretreated with antifungals. Wood's lamp can be used to detect infection with *Microsporum* spp. which fluoresce bright green.

Differential diagnoses of tinea capitis include seborrheic dermatitis and psoriasis when presenting with erythema and hyperkeratosis of the scalp. Alopecia areata may be considered for tinea capitis presenting with patchy hair loss. Dermoscopy may be useful to distinguish tinea capitis from alopecia areata. Pustular tinea capitis can look like impetigo, which begins as vesicles that evolve into erosions with superficial honey crusting, and is difficult to distinguish from a primary bacterial infection due to possible bacterial superinfection of the primary dermatophyte infection. Bacterial abscess should be considered in the differential diagnosis for a kerion.

33.6 Treatment

Tinea capitis requires treatment with oral antifungals to appropriately penetrate the hair shaft and eradicate disease. Griseofulvin and terbinafine are common treatment options. Azole antifungals are off-label therapies for tinea capitis. In a prospective, non-blinded, cross-sectional study, griseofulvin was found to be the most effective treatment option with a cure rate of 96 %. The cure rates for terbinafine and fluconazole were 88 and 84 %, repsectively [7]. Other studies have suggested that griseofulvin is the most efficacious for *Microsporum* spp. and terbinafine appears to the most efficacious for *T. Tonsurans* [8].

In the United States, griseofulvin, given at a dose of 20–25 mg/kg/day for 8 weeks, remains the mainstay of therapy with low risk of adverse effects. However, there are reports of resistance developing toward griseofulvin as well as issues with compliance due to the long duration of therapy. The main side effects of griseofulvin are gastrointestinal symptoms. Terbinafine is given at 250 mg daily for 4 weeks and is the mainstay of therapy in European countries. The shorter course makes this therapy more convenient, and it can be used in pregnancy. However, terbinafine can cause liver toxicity, and patients should be monitored for the occurrence of this rare side effect. Gastrointestinal side effects can also occur with terbinafine. Azoles are administered at 6–8 mg/kg/week. Caution must be taken with patients on multiple medications due to cytochrome P450 metabolism of azoles.

There have been debates over the management for kerions. Some argue in favor of intralesional corticosteroids to decrease the host inflammatory response. A recent retrospective study showed successful cure rates of kerions with oral antifungals alone and no evidence that intralesional corticosteroids help clear the infection [9]. There is also questionable data for advocating the use of prophylactic ketoconazole shampoo for kerions [10].

In addition to medical therapy, the individual's social settings should be considered. Reinfection can occur through carrier pets, clothing, bedding, toys, combs, and phones. In some infections, especially with *T. tonsurans*, some recommend treatment for all household members. Lastly, patient education and close follow-up should be stressed in every patient.

References

1. Chapman JC, Daniel 3rd CR, Daniel JG, Daniel MP, Sullivan S, Howell D, Elewski BE, Thames LC. Tinea capitis caused by dermatophytes: a 15-year retrospective study from a Mississippi Dermatology Clinic. Cutis. 2011;88(5):230–3.
2. Alshawa K, Lacroix C, Benderfouche M, Mingui A, Derouin F, Feuilhade CM. Increasing incidence of Trichophyton tonsurans in Paris, France: a 15-year retrospective study. Br J Dermatol. 2012;166(5):1149–50.
3. Hughes R, Chiaverini C, Bahadoran P, Lacour JP. Corkscrew hair: a new dermoscopic sign for diagnosis of tinea capitis in black children. Arch Dermatol. 2011;147(3):355–6.
4. Hubbard TW. The predictive value of symptoms in diagnosing childhood tinea capitis. Arch Pediatr Adolesc Med. 1999;153(1):1150–3.
5. Coley MK, Bhanusali DG, Silverberg JI, Alexis AF, Silverberg NB. Scalp hyperkeratosis and alopecia in children of color. J Drugs Dermatol. 2011;10(5):511–6.
6. Zaraa I, Trojjet S, El Guellali N, et al. Childhood erythema nodosum associated with kerion celsi: a case report and review of literature. Pediatr Dermatol. 2012;29(4):479–82.
7. Grover C, Arora P, Manchanda V. Comparative evaluation of griseofulvin, terbinafine, and fluconazole in the treatment of tinea capitis. Int J Dermatol. 2012;51(4):455–8.
8. Elewski BE, Cacerest HW, DeLeon L, et al. Terbinafine hydrochloride oral granules vs. oral griseofulvin suspension in children with tinea capitis: results of two randomized, investigator-blinded, multicenter, international, controlled trials. J Am Acad Dermatol. 2008;59(1):41–54.
9. Proudfoot LE, Higgins EM, Morris-Jones R. A retrospective study of the management of pediatric kerion in Trichophyton tonsurans infection. Pediatr Dermatol. 2011;28(6):655–7.
10. Bookstaver PB, Watson HJ, Winters SD, Carlson AL, Schulz RM. Prophylactic ketoconazole shampoo for tinea capitis in a high-risk pediatric population. J Pediatr Pharmacol Ther. 2011;16(3):199–203.

Human Papillomavirus (HPV)

34

Amanda Strickland and Gabriela Blanco

Contents

A. Strickland, BS
Department of Dermatology,
University of Texas Southwestern Medical Center,
5323 Harry Hines Boulevard, Dallas, TX 75235, USA
e-mail: amanda.strickland@utsouthwestern.edu

G. Blanco, MD (✉)
Department of Dermatology,
University of Texas Southwestern Medical Center,
5323 Harry Hines Blvd., Dallas, TX 75390, USA
e-mail: gabriela.m.blanco@gmail.com

34.1 Epidemiology

Human papillomavirus (HPV) causes warts in humans. It can occur on any part of the skin or mucous membranes but is commonly found on the hands, face, feet, and genital tract of both males and females. There are four main subgroups of warts: common warts, flat warts, plantar warts, and condyloma acuminata (genital warts). It is estimated that common warts are found in 3.5 % of adults and up to 33 % of primary schoolchildren [1]. The incidence of warts increases in immunosuppressed patients.

Transmission of HPV requires viral inoculation in basal epithelial cells. This is usually caused by microinjuries through skin-skin contact, microabrasions, or sexual intercourse [1]. While genital HPV infection most often occurs by intimate contact with an infected person, most cases of HPV transmission are not sexually transmitted. There is usually direct or indirect skin contact, and autoinoculation has been reported [2]. Cutaneous warts are very frequent in children, and among patients in larger households, many of the cohabitants may present with warts as well.

Human papillomavirus is also sexually transmitted and is considered the most common sexually transmitted infection in the United States [3]. HPV is associated with five key risk factors: sexual activity, number of current and lifetime sexual partners, sexual history of the partner(s), immune health, and age of coitarche. It is estimated that 20 million people are currently infected in the United States, and 6.2 million more acquire the virus each year [4]. HPV is widespread among the general population, especially among sexually active young adults; the Centers for Disease Control and Prevention estimates that at least 80 % of women will acquire HPV by age 50. While most strains of the virus involve a transient infection that may or may not involve a wart that will spontaneously regress (termed low-risk strains), certain strains are more oncogenic and persist with clinically significant symptoms (termed high-risk strains). It is well established that the virus is a necessary but insufficient cause of lower genital tract neoplasia. Infected women are at risk of developing

D. Jackson-Richards, A.G. Pandya (eds.), *Dermatology Atlas for Skin of Color*,
DOI 10.1007/978-3-642-54446-0_34, © Springer-Verlag Berlin Heidelberg 2014

cervical cancer, the second most common cause of cancer and cancer-related mortality for women worldwide. Men are much less likely to be diagnosed with genital malignancies after having genital warts for unclear reasons [5, 6].

34.2 Etiology

HPV is a non-enveloped virus with an icosahedral protein capsid containing DNA. The virus does not have an envelope, which makes it resistant to many forms of sterilization, such as heat [2]. HPV exclusively infects epithelial cells, though the specific anatomical locations or type of epithelial cell infected may vary by virus strain [4, 7]. Common warts are usually caused by HPV types 1, 2, and 4 [1]. Flat warts, also known as plane warts, are most commonly caused by HPV 3 and 10. Plantar warts are more often associated with HPV 1 and HPV 4. Condylomata are usually sexually transmitted and are most commonly caused by HPV 6, 11, 16, and 18. Types 6 and 11 are considered less oncogenic, while types 16 and 18 are considered high-risk HPV types with greater risk for malignant transformation.

34.3 Clinical Features

34.3.1 Distribution and Arrangement

Common warts (verrucae vulgaris) frequently involve the hands, especially the fingers, but can occur anywhere. Flat warts are generally located on the face, neck, hands, wrists, elbows, or knees and are more common in children. They are usually found in groups of multiple warts. Plantar warts are usually on the heel of the foot or other pressure points on the plantar surface. Condylomata, or genital warts, are usually multiple and may be found anywhere along the anogenital tract, including the vulva, vagina, cervix, scrotum, penis (glans, meatus, shaft), and anal area [1]. Condylomata may also be found in the oropharyngeal tract in rare cases.

34.3.2 Morphology of Lesions

Common warts are usually small, dome-shaped flesh-colored or pink papules with a hyperkeratotic or verrucous surface (Figs. 34.1 and 34.2) They may also appear filiform (Fig. 34.3), especially in certain locations, like periorificial skin [1]. Flat warts are flat-topped, smooth-surfaced papules that often match the patient's skin color (Figs. 34.4 and 34.5). Plantar warts frequently present as a painful, endophytic papules and plaques with a central depression and are surrounded by gentle slopes, resembling an anthill (Fig. 34.6). A clue in identifying warts is that they interrupt normal dermatoglyphic lines on the palmar and plantar surfaces. Condylomata (condyloma acuminatum), or genital warts, present as exophytic papillomas (Figs. 34.7, 34.8,

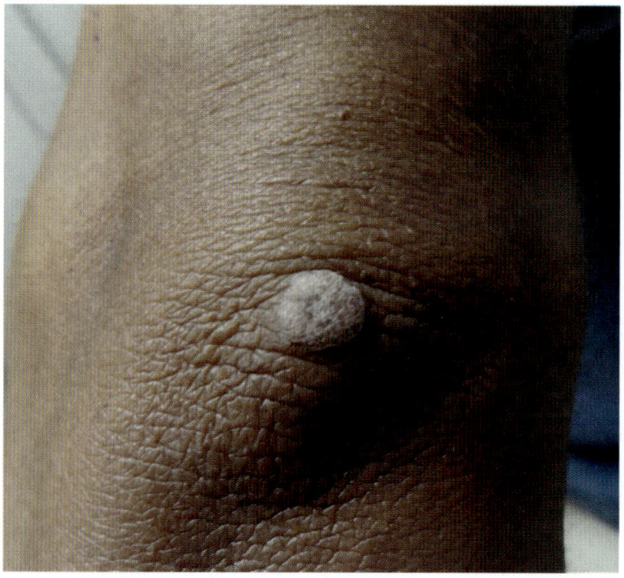

Fig. 34.1 Common wart on the elbow of a Hispanic male

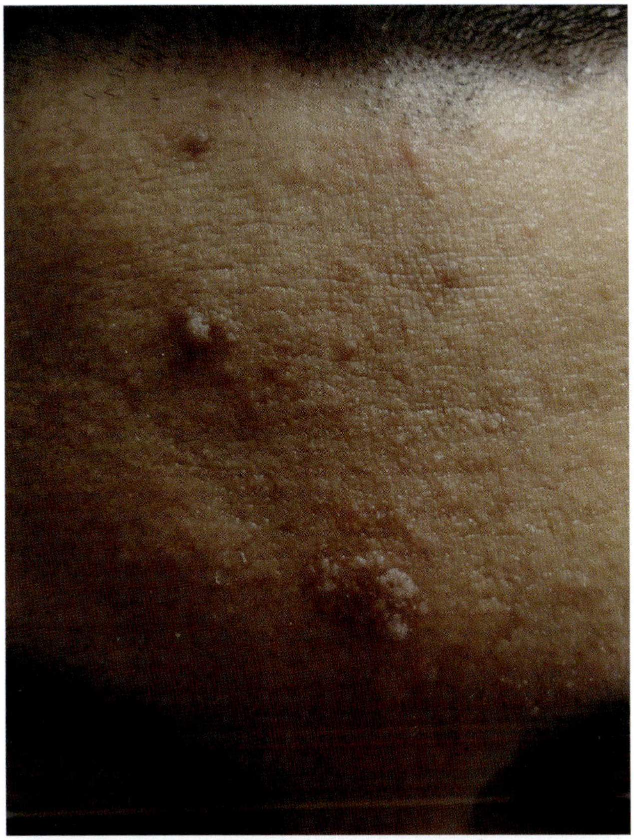

Fig. 34.2 Common warts on the forehead of a Hispanic male

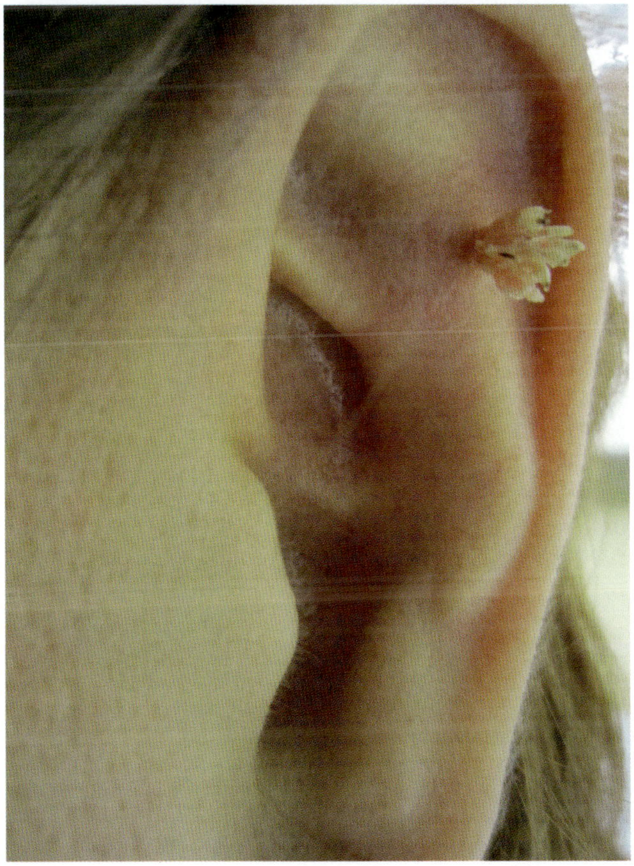

Fig. 34.3 Filiform wart on the ear with fingerlike projections showing thrombosed capillaries

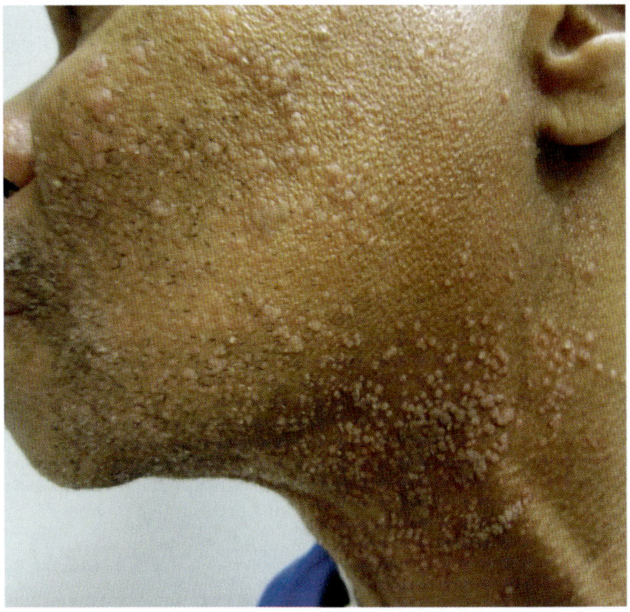

Fig. 34.4 Flat warts on the face and neck of an AA male with HIV infection

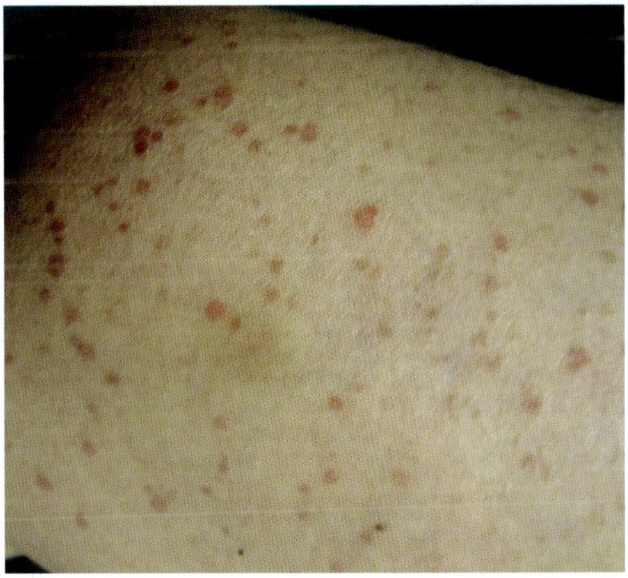

Fig. 34.5 Flat warts on the thigh of a Hispanic male with HIV infection

34.9, and 34.10) [1]. Mosaic warts are plaques composed of several individual small warts coalescing together and are especially recalcitrant to therapy (Fig. 34.11). Cutaneous warts often contain thrombosed capillaries which appear as small black points scattered over the surface of the lesion.

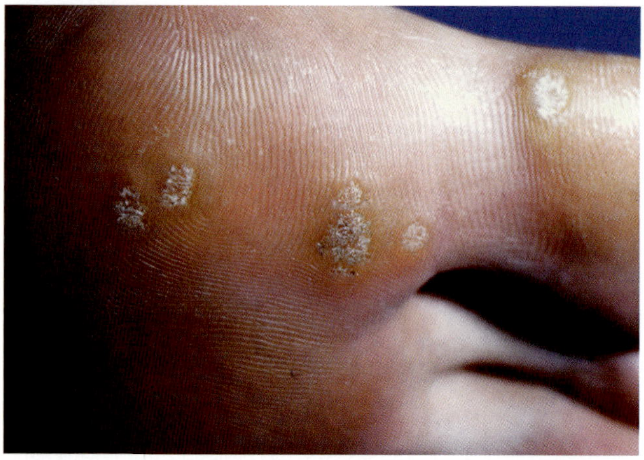

Fig. 34.6 Plantar warts on the great toe and foot of a Hispanic male showing an endophytic papule interrupting dermatoglyphic lines

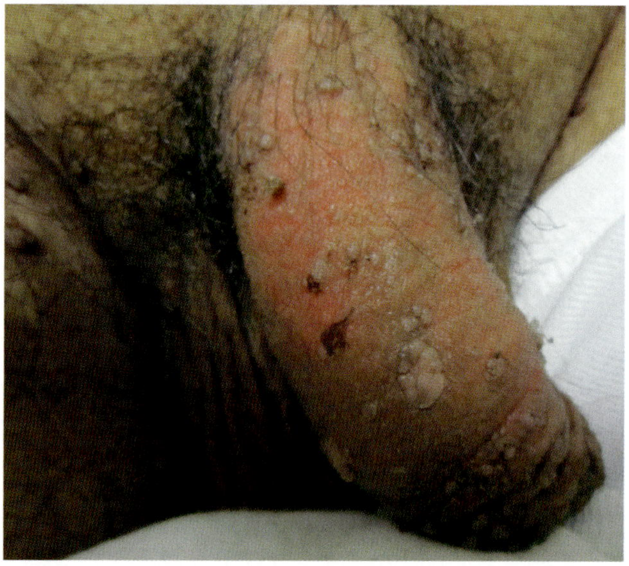

Fig. 34.7 Condyloma acuminata on the penis of a Hispanic male

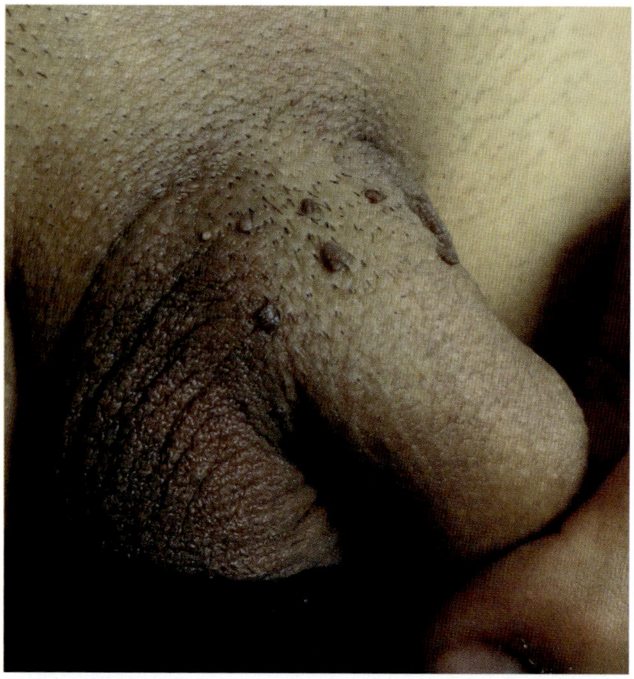

Fig. 34.8 Condyloma acuminata on the penis of a Hispanic male

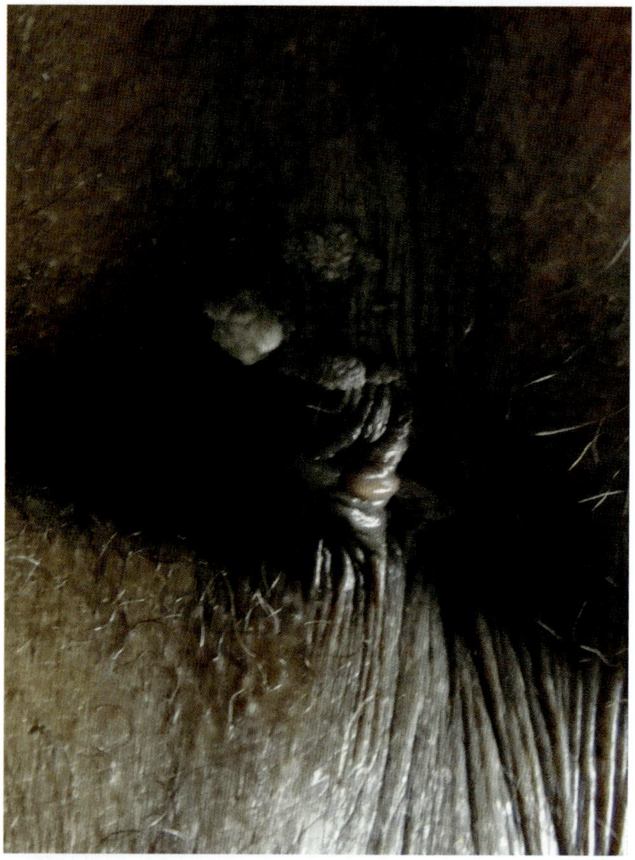

Fig. 34.9 Multiple anogenital warts on the perianal skin of an AA female with HIV infection

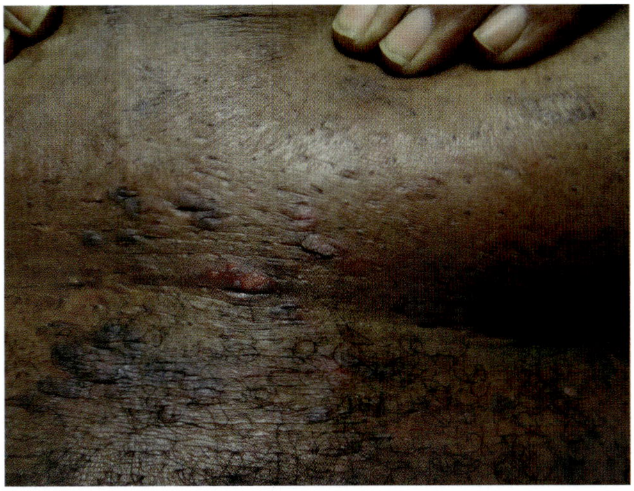

Fig. 34.10 Multiple warts on the abdomen of an AA female with HIV infection

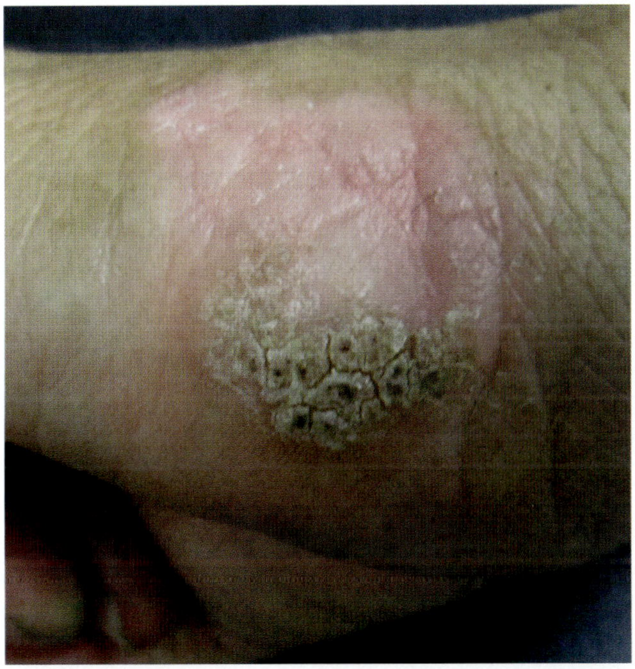

Fig. 34.11 Partially treated mosaic wart on the hand made up of individual small warts

34.4 Associated Symptoms

HPV infections are usually asymptomatic. Pain may or may not be present depending on the location of the wart and HPV type. Genital warts may occasionally cause irritation, pruritus, dysuria, bleeding, or dyspareunia [8]. Plantar warts that occur in pressure point areas can be very painful.

34.5 Systemic Findings

Systemic findings are not usually associated with HPV, except that an immunosuppressed status causes patients to be at higher risk for HPV infection.

34.6 Natural History and Prognosis

Many people infected with HPV are asymptomatic because the immune system tends to eliminate the virus before a wart can form. If a wart does form, the natural history is spontaneous resolution. Lesion regression tends to take place between weeks 8 and 12, and the epithelium resumes a normal appearance by 16 weeks, but many warts last much longer [7]. Reported clearance rates in children are 23 % at 2 months, 30 % at 3 months, 65–78 % at 2 years, and 90 % over 5 years [9]. Immunocompromised patients, such as organ transplant or HIV-infected patients, have a greater predisposition for the development of warts. Because of their impaired immune system, these patients usually have a greater number of warts, which are more challenging to treat and thus have a more protracted course. The distribution, morphology and other findings of warts vary depending on the strain of HPV.

Because most HPV infections go unnoticed or present as benign warts that regress on their own, the prognosis is generally positive. However, HPV in the cervix must be checked with periodic screenings to ensure that neoplasia does not develop.

34.7 Brief Description of Histopathologic Features

Warts have many epidermal changes including parakeratosis and the presence of koilocytes, superficial vacuolated keratinocytes, found in the granular layer [1]. There is also varying degrees of hyperkeratosis, parakeratosis, papillomatosis, acanthosis, and hypergranulosis, depending on the clinical appearance of the warts. Dilated capillaries are found in the dermis.

34.8 Diagnosis and Differential Diagnosis

Diagnosis is usually made by inspection of the affected areas. Condyloma acuminata can also be diagnosed via colposcopy or Pap smear. A biopsy is recommended when the lesions look atypical [8]. DNA testing for the HPV type is usually not indicated because of marginal cost-effectiveness. Differential diagnoses include seborrheic keratosis, actinic keratosis, psoriasis, acrokeratosis verruciformis, angiokeratomas, and Fordyce spots [8]. Other non-HPV-induced cancers can be considered in the differential, including amelanotic melanoma, Bowen's disease, and Paget's disease.

34.9 Treatment

There is no specific antiviral treatment for HPV. Most therapies focus on the local destruction or removal of the wart or induction of cytotoxicity of the infected epithelial cells. Because most warts tend to regress on their own after several months, treatment is usually symptom based [8]. Cryotherapy and curettage is commonly employed, as is treatment with topical creams and gels such as salicylic acid and other keratolytic creams. Cryotherapy in skin of color can lead to prominent hypopigmentation, which is usually transient but can be permanent (Fig. 34.12). It is not clear whether removing the wart reduces infectivity of the patient. Warts in immunosuppressed patients tend to resolve when the immune system is reconstituted, such as with HAART for HIV-positive patients. Plantar warts tend to be more recalcitrant to treatment but usually resolve on their own, though the time course may be longer for adults than children.

It is very difficult to prevent warts, but the best method is generally to avoid skin contact with an infected person. This includes avoiding moist environments where an infected person's skin has had contact, such as in a pool or gym. This also includes sexual intercourse with an individual infected

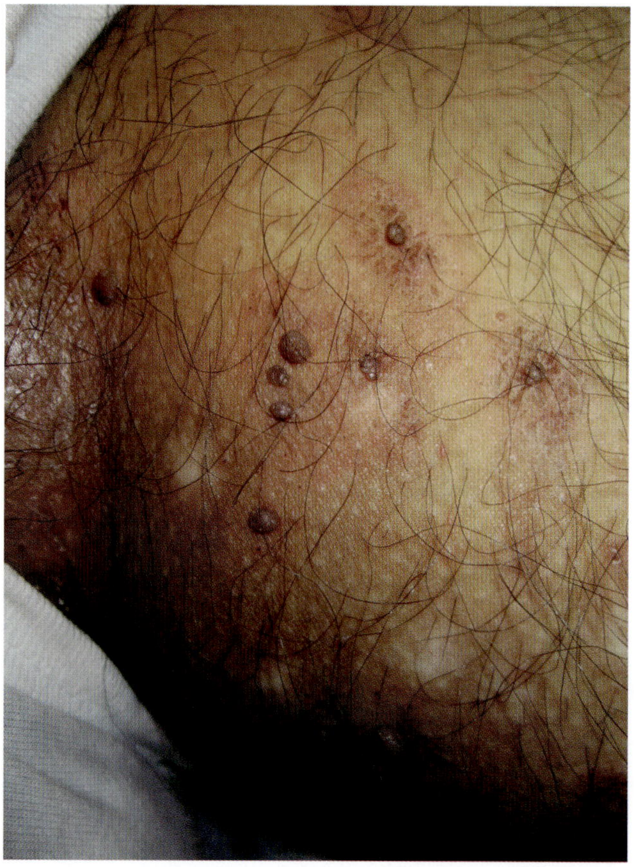

Fig. 34.12 Condyloma acuminata on the thigh of a Hispanic patient with hypopigmentation after cryotherapy

with HPV. Regular Pap smears and limiting sexual partners are important protective measures for genital warts, with a mutually monogamous relationship with a low-risk partner giving the lowest risk. An effective vaccine is available for girls and boys aged 9–26 that protects against the four most common HPV types causing genital warts (HPV types 6, 11, 16, 18), including the two that cause over 90 % of cervical cancers (HPV types 16 and 18).

References

1. Cardoso JC, Calonje E. Cutaneous manifestations of human papillomaviruses: a review. Acta Dermatovenerol Alp Panonica Adriat. 2011;20(3):145–54.
2. Bolognia J, Jorizzo JL, Schaffer J. Dermatology. 3rd ed. Philadelphia: Elsevier; 2012.
3. Dunne EF, Unger ER, Sternberg M, et al. Prevalence of HPV infection among females in the United States. JAMA. 2007;297(8):813–9.
4. Dunne EF, Markowitz LE. Genital human papillomavirus infection. Clin Infect Dis. 2006;43(5):624–9.
5. Giuliano AR, Anic G, Nyitray AG. Epidemiology and pathology of HPV disease in males. Gynecol Oncol. 2010;117(2 Suppl):S15–9.
6. Dunne EF, Nielson CM, Stone KM, Markowitz LE, Giuliano AR. Prevalence of HPV infection among men: a systematic review of the literature. J Infect Dis. 2006;194(8):1044–57.
7. Doorbar J. The papillomavirus life cycle. J Clin Virol. 2005;32 Suppl 1:S7–15.
8. Forcier M, Musacchio N. An overview of human papillomavirus infection for the dermatologist: disease, diagnosis, management, and prevention. Dermatol Ther. 2010;23(5):458–76.
9. James WD, Berger T, Elston D. Andrews' diseases of the skin: clinical dermatology. 11th ed. Philadelphia: Saunders Elsevier; 2011.

Herpes Simplex and Varicella Zoster

35

Sharif Currimbhoy and Arturo Ricardo Dominguez

Contents

S. Currimbhoy, BS • A.R. Dominguez, MD, BS (✉)
Department of Dermatology,
University of Texas Southwestern Medical Center,
5939 Harry Hines Blvd., Dallas, TX 75235, USA
e-mail: arturo.dominguez@utsouthwestern.edu

35.1 Introduction

Herpes simplex virus (HSV) is the causative agent of a recurrent cutaneous infection characterized clinically by painful, erythematous vesicles and ulcers. Transmission occurs via direct skin contact with a lesion or infected secretions. Herpes simplex virus type 1 (HSV-1) causes mainly oral and perioral lesions, while herpes simplex type 2 (HSV-2) typically causes genital infection [1–3]. Herpes simplex type 1 affects 70–80 % of adults and is commonly acquired during childhood by nonsexual transmission [4]. Infections with herpes simplex type 2 is mainly acquired via sexual contact with a symptomatic or asymptomatic individual. Genital herpes affects approximately 50 million persons in the USA and about one in four adults over the age of 30 [1–3]. There is a major disparity of HSV-2 infections in African Americans with an estimated prevalence of 40.3 % with genital herpes compared to 13.7 % of Caucasians [5]. This large discrepancy in prevalence has been proposed to be due to high transmission rates in undiagnosed African Americans because of poor access to care, screening practices, and healthcare quality [5].

Reactivation of the varicella zoster virus (VZV) causes herpes zoster, also known as shingles. Herpes zoster presents clinically with an intensely painful vesicular rash along a dermatome [6, 7]. Each year there are one million cases of herpes zoster with an annual rate of 3–4 cases per 1,000 people [6]. Herpes zoster outbreaks are much more common in older and immunocompromised persons due to reduction in immunity to the virus [6, 7]. By age 85, individuals who are previously unvaccinated for herpes zoster have a 50 % chance of having a shingles episode [6].

D. Jackson-Richards, A.G. Pandya (eds.), *Dermatology Atlas for Skin of Color*,
DOI 10.1007/978-3-642-54446-0_35, © Springer-Verlag Berlin Heidelberg 2014

35.2 Clinical Features

The incubation period after infection with HSV is between 2 and 14 days [2–4]. The initial eruption is often preceded by burning, itching, tingling, or painful sensations that can occur hours to days before the appearance of skin lesions [2, 3]. The rash of herpes simplex is characterized by small grouped vesicles on an erythematous base that eventually form painful superficial ulcers with fluid and overlying crust (Figs. 35.1, 35.2, 35.3, 35.4, and 35.5). In contrast to cutaneous lesions, ulcerations in mucosal areas tend to remain moist and do not form a crust. Infections with HSV-1 tend to affect the oral and perioral regions, although it is possible for lesions to be spread to the genital region. HSV-1 primarily affects the

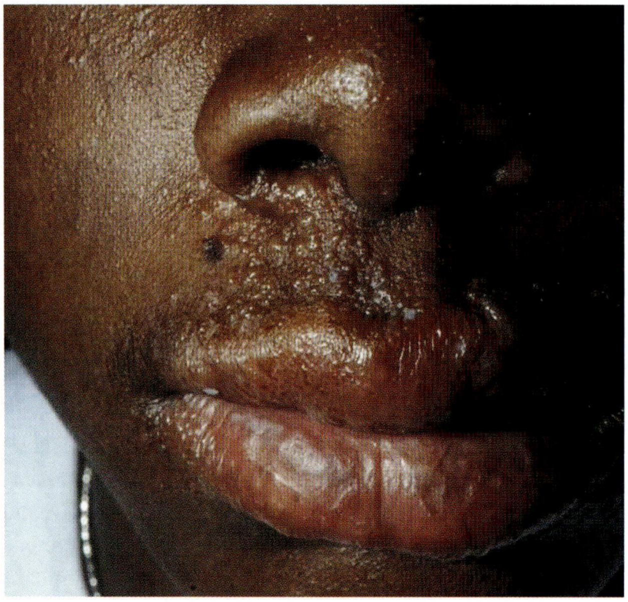

Fig. 35.1 Grouped vesicles on the lips and nose due to labial herpes in an African American male

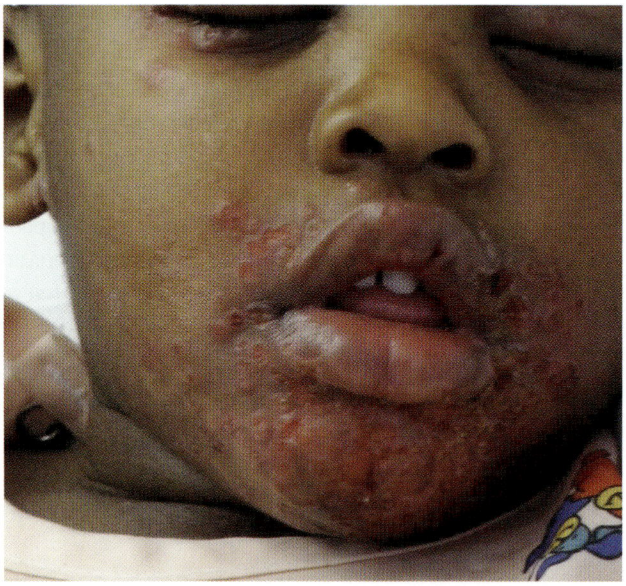

Fig. 35.2 Perioral herpes simplex in an African American boy

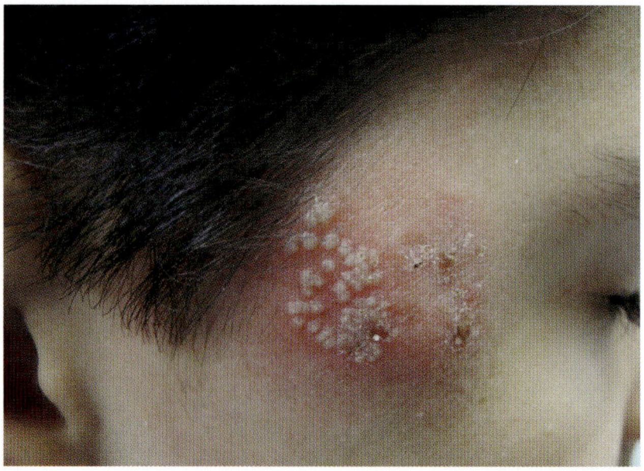

Fig. 35.3 Localized herpes simplex on the temple of a Hispanic boy

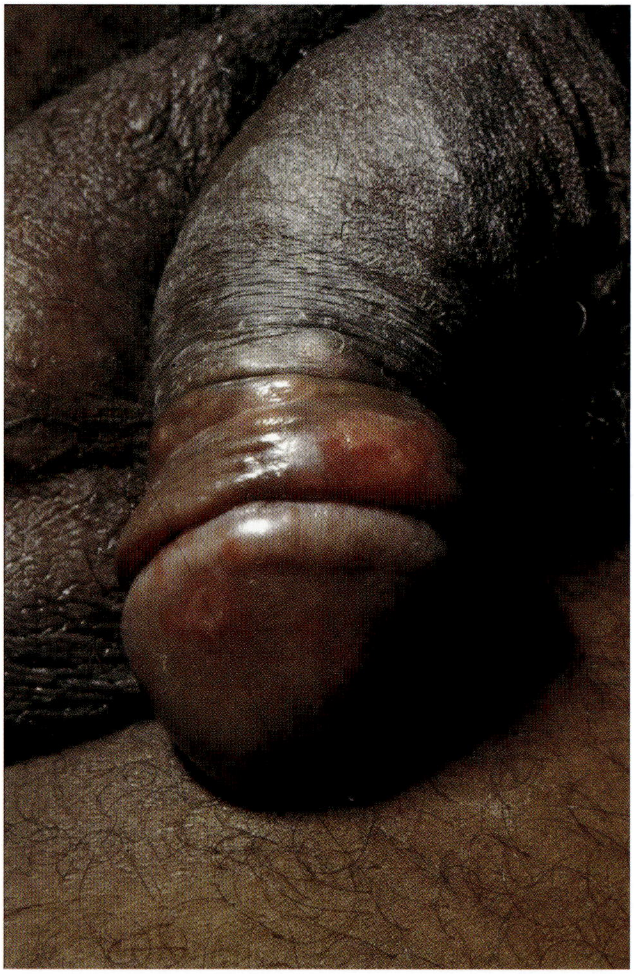

Fig. 35.4 Genital herpes simplex of the penis in an African American male

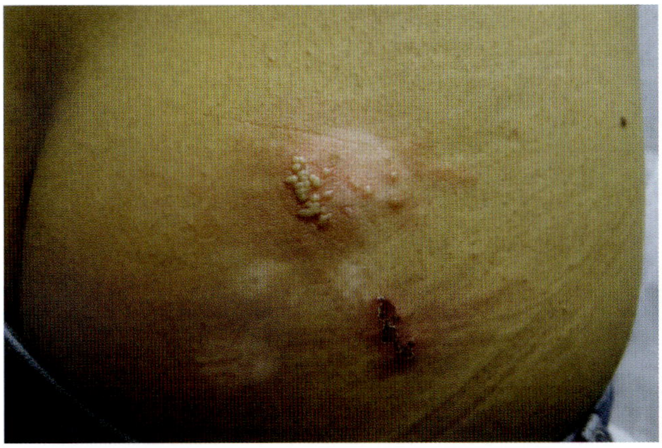

Fig. 35.5 Grouped vesicles on the buttock due to herpes simplex in a Hispanic female

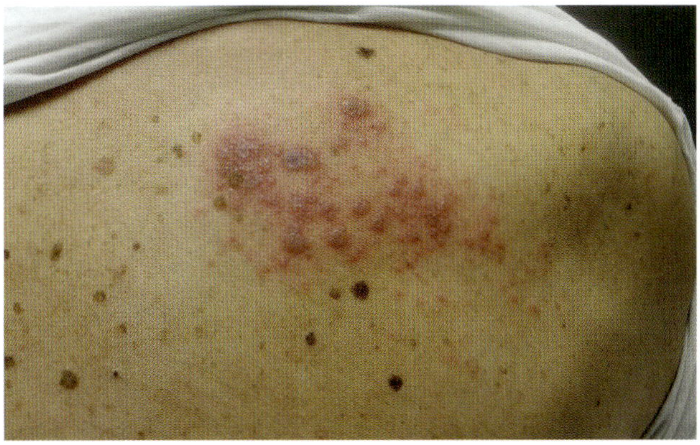

Fig. 35.6 Unilateral vesicles along a dermatome on the upper back due to herpes zoster in a Hispanic male

keratinized oral mucosal surfaces including the cutaneous lip, dorsal and lateral tongue, gingiva, and hard palate. The rash of HSV-2 typically affects the shaft and glans of the penis in men and the labia and urethral meatus in women. Outbreaks in women tend to be more extensive and severe [3]. Systemic findings such as fatigue, fever, malaise, and tender lymphadenopathy are common, especially with initial infection [2, 3]. The lesions of HSV-1 and HSV-2 typically resolve after 10–14 days, although the virus still remains present in a dormant state in the local nerve root ganglia.

Herpes zoster presents similarly to herpes simplex, with grouped vesicles on an erythematous base; however, lesions typically present unilaterally along a single dermatome and do not typically cross the midline (Figs. 35.6 and 35.7) [6, 7]. However, it is not uncommon for herpes zoster to involve multiple continuous dermatomes. Disseminated zoster is defined as disease involving greater than 20 individual vesicles or erosions occurring outside of contiguous dermatomes. Involvement of the trigeminal V-1 distribution from the eye to the tip of the nose is termed herpes zoster ophthalmicus and can present with conjunctivitis, keratitis, and anterior uveitis [7]. Ramsay-Hunt syndrome or herpes zoster oticus involves the external ear canal that can lead to unilateral facial weakness or Bell's palsy due to involvement of the peripheral facial nerve (Fig. 35.8). Herpes zoster ophthalmicus and oticus are considered emergencies, and referral to an ophthalmologist or otolaryngologist may be necessary. Individuals with zoster are typically more elderly or immunocompromised and present with an intensely painful, burning sensation located along a dermatome, most commonly the thoracic, trigeminal, lumbar, and cervical regions [6]. Lesions are typically self-resolving after 7–14 days, but residual neuropathic dysesthesias can remain for weeks to months after resolution of the lesions [6, 7].

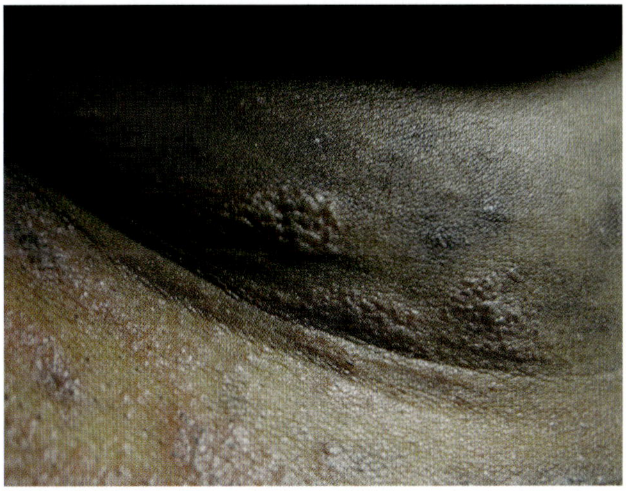

Fig. 35.7 Grouped vesicles on the neck due to herpes zoster in an African American female

Primary varicella zoster infection, or chicken pox, is typically seen in children, but may be seen in adults, often immigrants or minorities who are unvaccinated or cannot remember having primary varicella as child. The lesions typically appear with numerous erythematous vesicles that present initially on the trunk and spread to involve the extremities and face (Figs. 35.9, 35.10, and 35.11). Lesions are typically seen in all stages of development with active vesicles and pustules, superficial erosions, and crusted lesions all present concurrently [10].

In darker-skinned patients, the base of the herpetic lesions may not display the typical red erythema and only hyperpigmentation may be present beneath and around vesicles. Additionally in patients with skin of color, lesions may leave behind a residual post-inflammatory hyperpigmentation which can last for months to years after resolution of the rash [8].

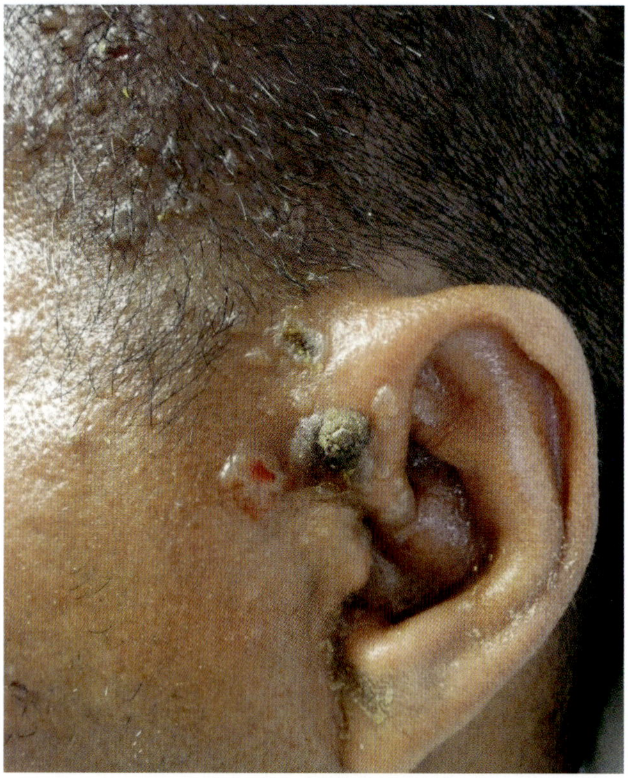

Fig. 35.8 Unilateral vesicles on the scalp and ear in a Hispanic male with Ramsay-Hunt syndrome

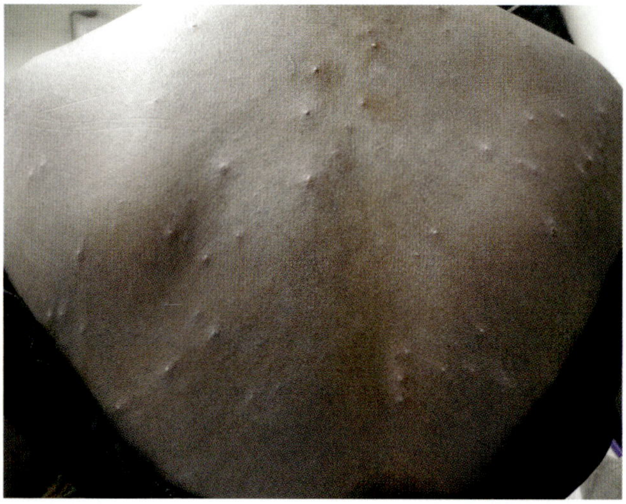

Fig. 35.9 Primary varicella infection on the back of an African American female

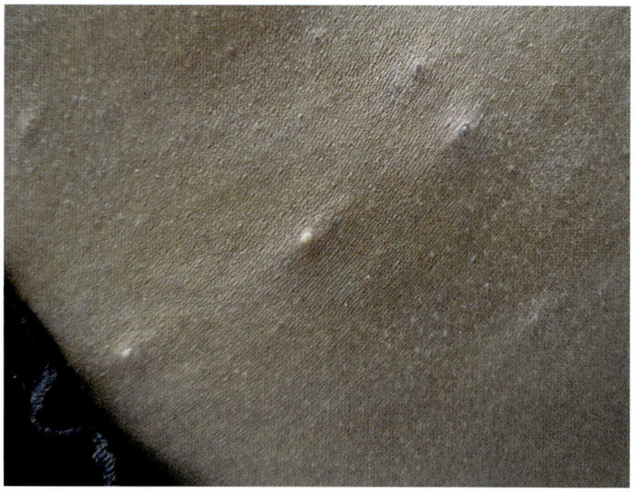

Fig. 35.10 Close-up of vesicles due to primary varicella infection on the back of an African American female

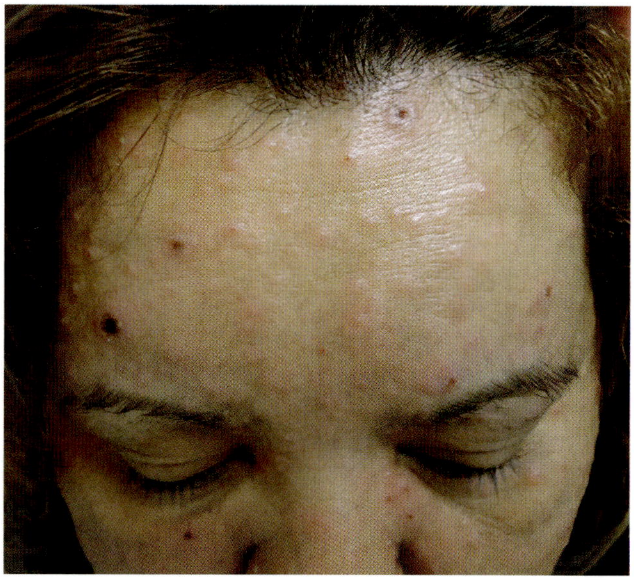

Fig. 35.11 Primary varicella infection on the face of a Hispanic female

35.3 Diagnosis and Differential Diagnosis

Diagnosis of HSV or VZV infections can often be made solely by the characteristic clinical examination. A Tzanck smear or viral culture can be performed by swabbing the base of an active lesion and can help confirm the diagnosis and differentiate the viral type between HSV-1 and HSV-2, although sensitivity is low [10]. Polymerase chain reaction testing (PCR) is the preferred modality to help confirm the presence of viral DNA and has a sensitivity of 95 % [3]. Direct Fluorescent Antibody Stain (DFA) for VZV and HSV is sensitive as well. Viral culture for VZV is neither sensitive nor cost-effective and has fallen out of favor. Other techniques used to test for the presence and typing of HSV include serologic studies which screen for the presence of antibodies to HSV-1 and HSV-2 [3, 6].

The differential diagnosis for HSV-1, or oral lesions, includes aphthous stomatitis and autoimmune bullous diseases such as pemphigus vulgaris and impetigo. The differential for HSV-2, or genital lesions, includes other sexually transmitted infections that can cause genital ulcers such as syphilis and chancroid. The differential diagnosis for herpes zoster includes herpes simplex, allergic contact dermatitis, cellulitis, and folliculitis [10].

35.4 Histopathological Features

A biopsy is not required for the diagnosis of HSV or VZV. Lesion evaluation with Tzanck smear shows characteristic multinucleated giant cells seen under microscopy [6] (Fig. 35.3). If biopsy is obtained, presence of intraepidermal blistering with ballooning of keratinocytes and presence of multinucleated giant cells may be seen with surrounding necrosis of epithelium [11]. Pathology of herpes zoster may additionally reveal the presence of a vasculitis with swelling and necrosis of endothelial cells, a feature not seen with infection with HSV [11].

35.5 Natural History and Prognosis

The vesicular rashes of HSV and VZV are self-limiting and typically resolve within 7–14 days after initial symptoms in immunocompetent patients [2, 3, 6, 7]. Infection with HSV is present indefinitely and recurrent episodes are common; however, the frequency and severity of outbreaks decrease over time in the majority of immunocompetent patients [2]. Inciting factors for an episode include stress, local trauma, and UV radiation. Asymptomatic shedding can occur between HSV-2 outbreaks, and transmission to an unaffected partner can be decreased by as much as 60 % with the use of condoms during intercourse [2]. Transmission rates of HSV-2 are highest among African Americans most likely due to the combination of higher prevalence and a low proportion of diagnosis of infection compared to Caucasians [5].

Herpes zoster typically resolves within 7–10 days, although as mentioned previously, painful postherpetic neuralgia may result due to damage of sensory nerves [7].

35.6 Treatment

Initial treatment for episodic HSV includes oral antivirals such as acyclovir, valaciclovir, and famciclovir for a 7–10-day course [2, 3]. Therapy should be administered promptly after the initial signs of an outbreak, and, if given early (within 72 h) in the disease course, the duration of symptoms can be shortened by 2–3 days and the time to healing by 4 days [2, 3]. For patients with persistent or frequent episodes of herpes simplex, suppressive therapy can be administered with daily antivirals to decrease recurrences by 70–80 % [3]. Suppressive therapy can also reduce the transmission of HSV-2 to an unaffected partner by 48 % between outbreaks when asymptomatic viral shedding still occurs [2]. Disseminated herpes simplex infection, seen more commonly in immunocompromised patients, requires intravenous dosing of acyclovir at a dose of 10 mg/kg [4]. Hospitalized patients with disseminated infection should be placed in airbone and contact precautions.

Treatment of herpes zoster consists of a 7–10-day course of antiviral therapy with acyclovir, valaciclovir, or famciclovir [7, 9]. Addition of analgesics are recommended for the alleviation of the severe pain associated with the rash and include tramadol, oxycodone, and gabapentin [7]. Herpes zoster ophthalmicus and oticus are emergencies, and consultation with an ophthalmologist or otolaryngologist may be necessary. Live attenuated vaccination is recommended for persons 60 years of age and older to prevent the occurrence of herpes zoster and decrease the chance of postherpetic neuralgia [9].

References

1. Xu F, Sternberg MR, Kottiri BJ, et al. Trends in herpes simplex virus type 1 and type 2 seroprevalence in the United States. JAMA. 2006;296(8):964–73.
2. Kimberlin DW, Rouse DJ. Clinical practice. Genital herpes. N Engl J Med. 2004;350(19):1970–7.
3. Beauman JG. Genital herpes: a review. Am Fam Physician. 2005; 72(8):1527–34.
4. Arduino PG, Porter SR. Oral and perioral herpes simplex virus type 1 (HSV-1) infection: review of its management. Oral Dis. 2006;12(3):254–70.
5. Pouget ER, Kershaw TS, Blankenship KM, Ickovics JR, Niccolai LM. Racial/ethnic disparities in undiagnosed infection with herpes simplex virus type 2. Sex Transm Dis. 2010;37(9):538–43.
6. Cohen JI. Clinical practice: herpes zoster. N Engl J Med. 2013; 369(3):255–63.

7. Sengupta S. Cutaneous herpes zoster. Curr Infect Dis Rep. 2013;15(5):432–9.
8. Davis EC, Callender VD. Postinflammatory hyperpigmentation: a review of the epidemiology, clinical features, and treatment options in skin of color. J Clin Aesthet Dermatol. 2010;3(7):20–31.
9. Sen P, Barton SE. Genital herpes and its management. BMJ. 2007;334(7602):1048–52.
10. Habif TP, Campbell JL, Shane Chapman M, et al. Skin disease, diagnosis and treatment. Edinburgh: Saunders; 2011.
11. Leinweber B, Kerl H, Cerroni L. Histopathologic features of cutaneous herpes virus infections (herpes simplex, herpes varicella/zoster): a broad spectrum of presentations with common pseudolymphomatous aspects. Am J Surg Pathol. 2006;30(1):50–8.

Syphilis

36

Kathryn Kinser and Arturo Ricardo Dominguez

Contents

36.1 Introduction

Syphilis is a sexually transmitted infection (STI) that occurs when the gram-negative bacterium *Treponema pallidum* penetrates the epidermis or mucous membranes of an individual [1, 2]. People that engage in unprotected vaginal, anal, or oral sex, live in urban areas, or belong to minority groups are at higher risk for syphilis [1, 3]. Although the incidence of primary and secondary syphilis has increased in most ethnic groups, Caucasians are still 7.0 times less likely than African Americans and 2.0 times less likely than Hispanics to contract syphilis. This disparity may be due to differences in income, education, drug/alcohol use, health-care access, and prevalence of other diseases, such as HIV infection [4]. Congenital syphilis is also more commonly passed from mothers with no antenatal care or a history of substance abuse [5].

The virulence of *T. pallidum* stems from the pathogen's affinity for many different extra cellular matrix (ECM) molecules in mammalian tissue and the paucity of outer membrane proteins recognized by the human immune system. Langerhans cells (LCs) in the skin and dendritic cells (DCs) in the mucosa may phagocytize *T. pallidum* and produce inflammatory cytokines through signaling of toll-like receptors (TLR2s) in response to degraded lipid portions of TpN17 and TpN47. DCs can also present the pathogen to T cells [2].

K. Kinser, BS • A.R. Dominguez, MD, BS (✉)
Department of Dermatology,
University of Texas Southwestern Medical School,
5323 Harry Hines Blvd, Dallas, TX 75390, USA
e-mail: arturo.dominguez@utsouthwestern.edu

D. Jackson-Richards, A.G. Pandya (eds.), *Dermatology Atlas for Skin of Color*,
DOI 10.1007/978-3-642-54446-0_36, © Springer-Verlag Berlin Heidelberg 2014

36.2 Clinical Features

Primary syphilis is marked by a singular, indolent ulcer known as a chancre at the site of inoculation, usually on the penis or vulva (Fig. 36.1). This stage is usually asymptomatic but can be associated with localized tender lymphadenopathy [6]. Symptoms of secondary syphilis include fever, headache, sore throat, malaise, or generalized lymphadenopathy. The cutaneous manifestations differ based on the pathogen's virulence and the patient's individual reaction to the treponeme [6]. Secondary syphilis lesions commonly occur in a palmoplantar distribution but can also involve the face, trunk, and extremities [1]. Since the lesions of secondary syphilis have such a wide variety of morphologic presentations, this disease has often been called "the great imitator" (Figs. 36.2, 36.3, 36.4, 36.5, 36.6, and 36.7). Diffuse, discrete, and pale macular lesions tend to spare the face and are not contagious [2, 6]. These lesions may fade, disappear, or change shape over time [6, 7]. Papular lesions can be brownish in color with a collarette of scale [7]. When a papular lesion involves warm, moist intertriginous areas, condyloma lata can develop [1, 2]. These verrucous, gray plaques are very contagious and occur more commonly in African American women or

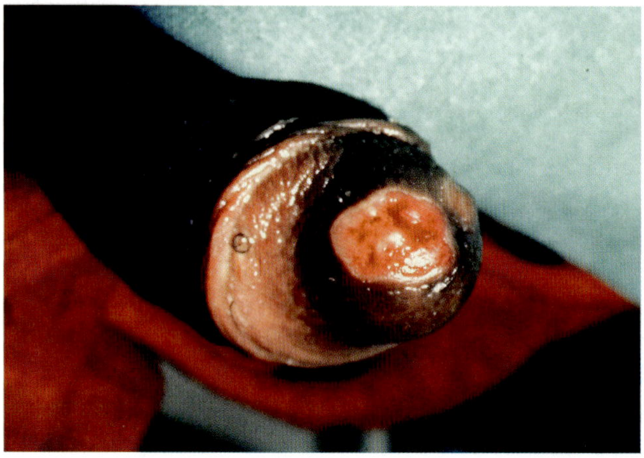

Fig. 36.1 Chancre due to syphilis in an African American male

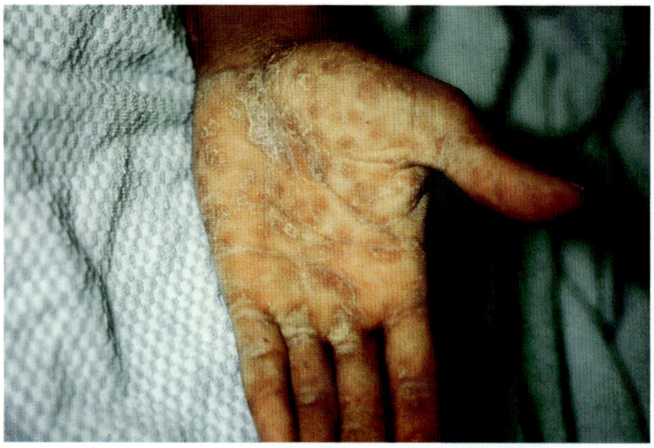

Fig. 36.2 Scaly pigmented plaques on the palms due to secondary syphilis in an African American male

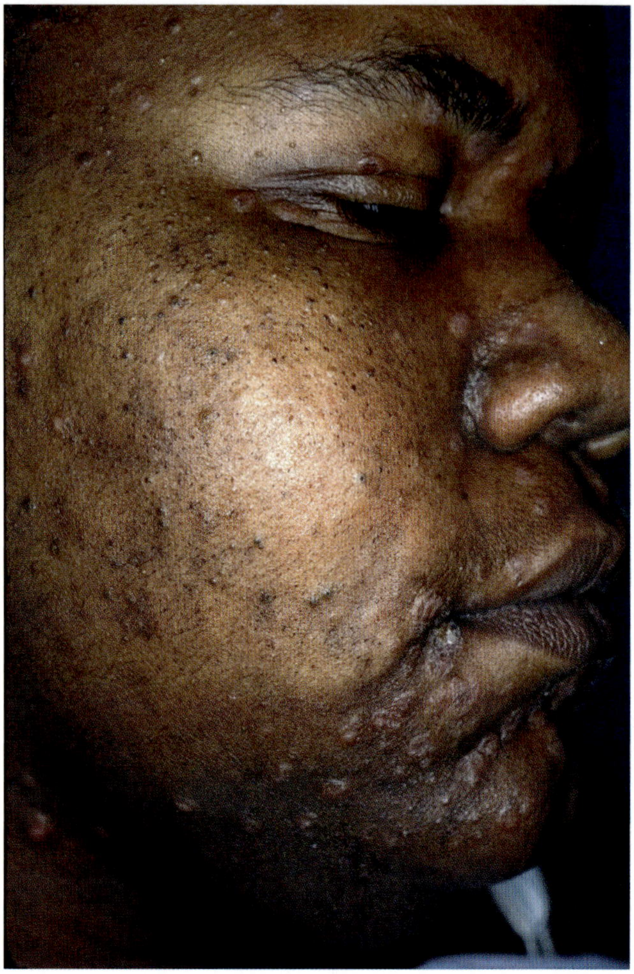

Fig. 36.3 Papules on the face and neck due to secondary syphilis in an African American female (Courtesy of Dr. Chauncey McHargue)

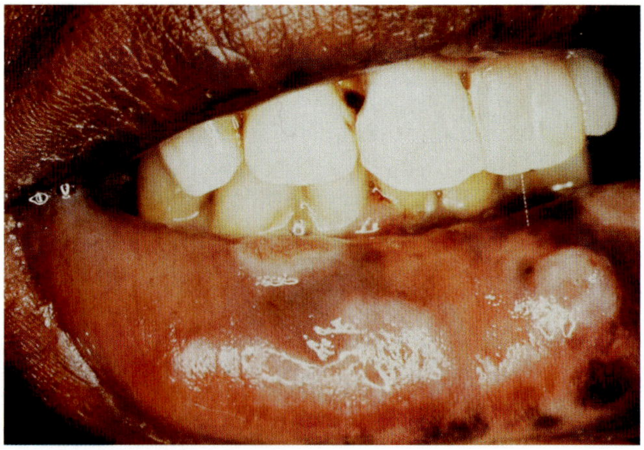

Fig. 36.4 Mucous patches on the lower lip due to secondary syphilis in an African American male

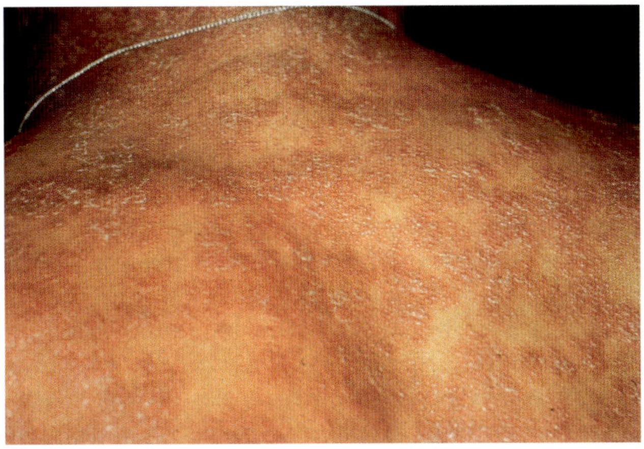

Fig. 36.5 Thin scaly plaques on the back due to secondary syphilis in a Hispanic male

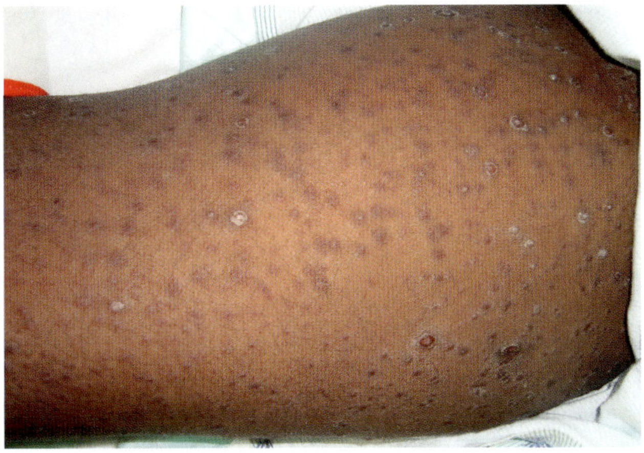

Fig. 36.7 Multiple scaly papules on the leg due to secondary syphilis in an African American male

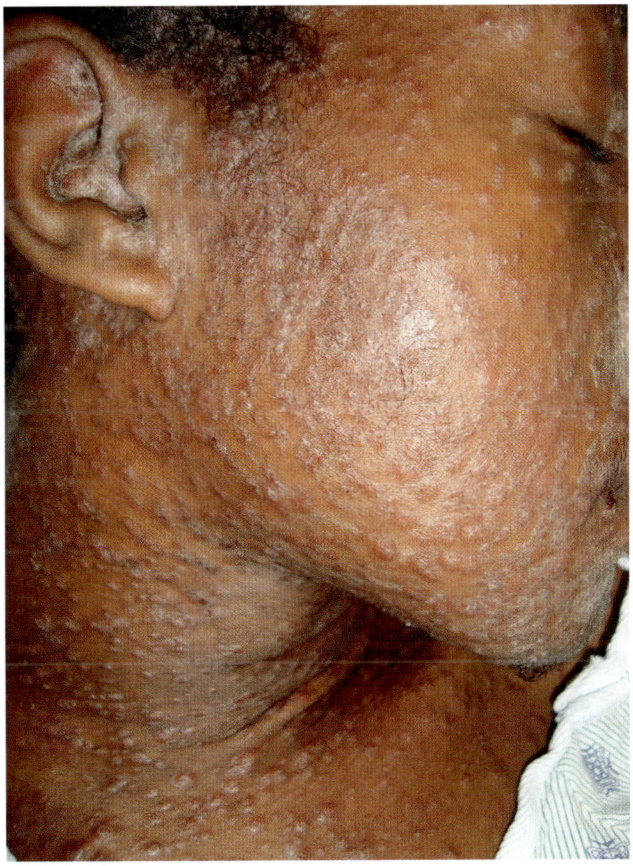

Fig. 36.6 Multiple scaly papules due to secondary syphilis in an African American male

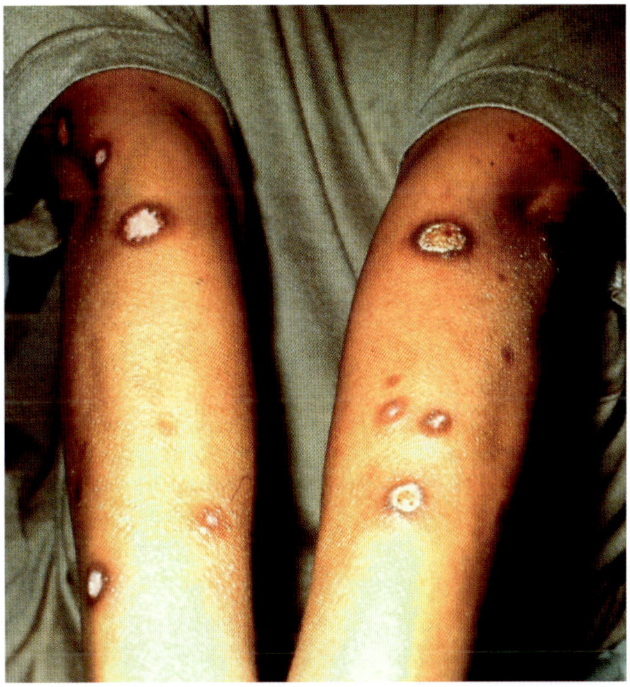

Fig. 36.8 Ulcerative lesions on the arms due to lues maligna in an African American female

patients with recurrent syphilis [1, 7]. Cutaneous lesions can be pustular, nodular, lichenoid, follicular, psoriasiform, and hyper- or hypopigmented. Annular, reddish-brown lesions close to the angles of the mouth and vesicular lesions are more commonly seen in African Americans. Although rare, lesions can also be corymbose, frambosiform, or kerato-pustular [7]. If hair follicles are infected, "moth-eaten" alopecia can occur [2]. Eroded, pink to gray mucous patches can occur in or around the mouth of some individuals with secondary syphilis. Transitory, indolent nonerosive plaques can appear on the tongue or anogenital region. These mucosal ulcers are most commonly seen in African American women [7].

Individuals infected with HIV are more likely to have concurrent primary and secondary syphilis [6]. Patients with HIV can also present with lues maligna, a form of secondary syphilis with necrotic, ulcerating, pustular lesions and early presentation of neurosyphilis (Figs. 36.8 and 36.9) [2, 6, 8].

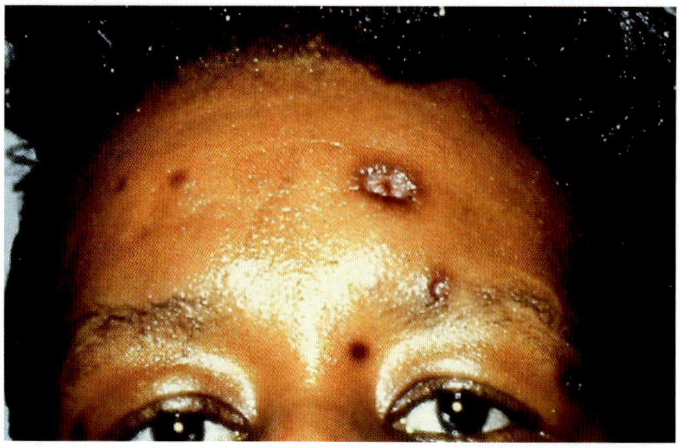

Fig. 36.9 Ulcerative lesions on the upper face due to lues maligna in an African American female

Tertiary syphilis can occur 10–30 years after a primary infection. Granulomatous, painless, necrotic lesions known as gummas arise from subcutaneous tissue and are found on the head, calf, or sternum [2, 9]. During this stage, neurological and systemic organ damage can occur, resulting in dementia, paralysis, blindness, hepatitis, or aortitis [2].

36.3 Natural History and Prognosis

Primary syphilis occurs roughly 14–21 days after initial contact. Within 8 weeks, the resulting chancre will resolve even without treatment. Four to ten weeks later, secondary syphilis may develop, which marks the systemic spread of treponemes through the lymphatics into the bloodstream. Macular lesions are transitory and last 2–3 days. Other lesion types can last for weeks [6]. Secondary syphilis will spontaneously resolve in 3–12 weeks, but healed lesions may result in depigmentation [6, 9]. The term "collar of Venus" has been used to describe hypopigmented macules that can be seen around the neck [7, 9]. Tertiary syphilis can appear years later and result in a progressive decline in health unless treated. Healed gummas can result in permanent, retractile scarring [9]. If syphilis is treated early on, the disease is easily curable. However, if the disease progresses to the tertiary stage or if significant organ or brain damage occurs, full treatment and recovery can be more difficult, if not impossible [1]. Patients who have had syphilis once are not immune from becoming reinfected [6].

36.4 Histopathologic Features

A biopsy of syphilitic lesions reveals hyperkeratosis and elongated interpapillary ridges [6, 8]. Cellular infiltrates consist of lymphocytes, macrophages, and plasma cells in the superficial and deep dermis [6, 8, 10]. Treponemes can be found in all but secondary macular lesions [6]. The degree of tissue reaction and inflammation depends on the type of lesion [10].

36.5 Diagnosis and Differential Diagnosis

Diagnosis of syphilis depends on a detailed clinical exam combined with serological testing. Non-treponemal tests (VDRL and RPR) are used more frequently than treponemal tests (FTA-ABS, TP-PA, MHA-TP), which are mainly used to confirm test results [1, 5, 6]. Non-treponemal tests are based on an antigen-antibody reaction, so other viral infections can cause false positives [5, 6]. A false negative RPR may be seen in acutely infected patients due to a prodromal effect. Dark-field microscopy can provide definitive results, but this form of testing is not used very often anymore [6].

The differential diagnosis of syphilis depends on the stage of the disease, but high clinical suspicion is necessary in patients with multiple risk factors, as syphilis has often been described as "the great mimicker" [6–8].

36.6 Treatment

Primary and secondary syphilis are treatable with a single injection of IM benzathine penicillin G at a dose of 2.4×10^6 units [1]. If the patient is allergic to penicillin, oral macrolide or tetracycline antibiotics can be used, but these are not as effective as penicillin [6]. In latent syphilis of unknown duration, Benzathine penicillin G 7.2 million units total, administered as 3 doses of 2.4 million units IM each at 1-week intervals is recommended. Pregnant mothers with a penicillin allergy must be desensitized and treated with penicillin because macrolides and tetracyclines are contraindicated during pregnancy [5]. During treatment of secondary syphilis, a patient may experience the Jarisch-Herxheimer reaction, which involves fever, a morbilliform rash, and worsening of cutaneous symptoms [8]. This reaction to cytokines and treponemal endotoxins resolves in 24 h [7, 8].

References

1. Ramoni S, Cusini M, Crosti C. An atlas of syphilis in a single case. Arch Dermatol. 2011;147:869–70.
2. LaFond R, Lukehart S. Biological basis for syphilis. Clin Microbiol Rev. 2006;19:29–49.
3. Owsu-Edusel Jr K, et al. The association between racial disparity in income and reported sexually transmitted infections. Am J Public Health. 2012;103:910–6.
4. Centers for Disease Control and Prevention. 2011. Sexually Transmitted Diseases Surveillance: STDs in racial and ethnic minorities. http://www.cdc.gov/std/stats11/min orities.htm. Accessed 27 July 2013.
5. Walker J, Walker G. Congenital syphilis: a continuing but neglected problem. Semin Fetal Neonatal Med. 2007;12:198–206.
6. Baughn R, Musher D. Secondary syphilitic lesions. Clin Microbiol Rev. 2005;18:205–16.
7. Mullooly C, Higgins S. Secondary syphilis: the classical triad of skin rash, mucosal ulceration, and lymphadenopathy. Int J STD AIDS. 2010;21:537–45.
8. Shimizu S, et al. Unusual cutaneous features of syphilis in patients positive for human immunodeficiency virus. Clin Exp Dermatol. 2009;35:169–72.
9. Varma R, Estcourt C, Mindel A. Syphilis, sexually transmitted diseases. 2nd ed. San Diego: Academic Press; 2013.
10. McMillan A, McQueen A, McLaren C. A histopathological study of secondary syphilis. J Eur Acad Dermatol Venereol. 1996;7:235–9.

Hansen's Disease

37

Amy Thorne and Jack B. Cohen

Contents

A. Thorne, MFA, DO
Department of Dermatology, University of New Mexico,
1021 Medical Arts Ave. NE, Albuquerque, NM 87131-5231, USA

J.B. Cohen, DO (✉)
Department of Dermatology,
University of Texas Southwestern Medical Center,
5323 Harry Hines Blvd., Dallas, TX 75390-9190, USA

Department of Dermatology,
Dallas County Health & Human Services,
2377 N. Stemmons Freeway, Suite 522, Dallas, TX 75207-2710, USA
e-mail: jbcohendo@aol.com; jack.cohen@utsouthwestern.edu

37.1 Epidemiology

Leprosy, usually referred to as Hansen's disease to decrease stigmatization of the diagnosis, is a chronic infectious granulomatous disease with an affinity for skin and nerves. An estimated two million people are infected worldwide with the highest incidence in equatorial Asia, Africa, Central and South America, and the Caribbean [1]. However, calculation of incidence has been hindered in recent years by a low number of reports submitted to the World Health Organization by member states which previously had a high number of annual new cases [2]. Endemic areas in the USA are Texas and Louisiana. In the USA, the average number of new annual cases over the last 10 years has been 130 [3].

37.2 Etiology

Mycobacterium leprae, a slow-growing, acid-fast bacillus and the only obligate intracellular mycobacteria, causes leprosy. These unique mycobacteria survive in macrophages in the skin and Schwann cells [1]. *M. leprae* has yet to be grown in cell-free culture and can be grown in limited viable quantities on the foot pad of the athymic nude mouse and armadillo models for study. Spread of these mycobacteria is poorly understood, but thought to occur through airborne droplets from nasal mucosa of the upper airways of an untreated infected person, or through prolonged skin contact [3]. Incubation of Hansen's disease ranges widely from 2 to even 20 years [3]. Hansen's disease has a low communicability with about 95 % of the world's population having a natural immunity to the bacteria [3]. A newly identified organism, *M. lepromatosis,* with identical clinical features has been described [4].

Highly complex interactions between *M. leprae* and the human host will determine if the host is even susceptible to leprosy, as well as the subsequent clinical form of the infection. Genome research indicates that evidence of specific genes and polymorphisms on chromosomes 6, 9, 11, 12, 13,

D. Jackson-Richards, A.G. Pandya (eds.), *Dermatology Atlas for Skin of Color*,
DOI 10.1007/978-3-642-54446-0_37, © Springer-Verlag Berlin Heidelberg 2014

15, 16, 17, and 20 influences activation of the toll-like receptors (TLRs) induction of antimicrobial pathways of innate defense [5]. Activation of TLRs 1 and 2 influences the adaptive immune response by upregulating antigen presentation molecules and cytokine secretion that define the Th1 or Th2 response of the T lymphocyte [6]. Finally, the natural diverse response of the T lymphocyte (cell-mediated immunity) will determine the clinical form of the presentation.

37.3 Clinical Features

Ridley and Jopling classified the spectrum seen in Hansen's disease based on the number of lesions on clinical presentation, the histopathology, and number of organisms seen on the skin biopsy [7]. Tuberculoid (paucibacillary) and lepromatous (multibacillary) leprosy are opposing polar forms of the disease. The middle of the leprosy spectrum is borderline tuberculoid, borderline, and borderline lepromatous types of leprosy. Tuberculoid leprosy (TT) is characterized by one or very few sharply bordered, asymmetrically distributed indurated plaques that are often annular, slightly dry in texture, with central clearing and hypopigmentation. Central anesthesia usually occurs and these lesions are less commonly accompanied by peripheral motor neuropathy (Figs. 37.1, 37.2, 37.3, and 37.4). This host response represents strong immunity with very few or no organisms seen on biopsy.

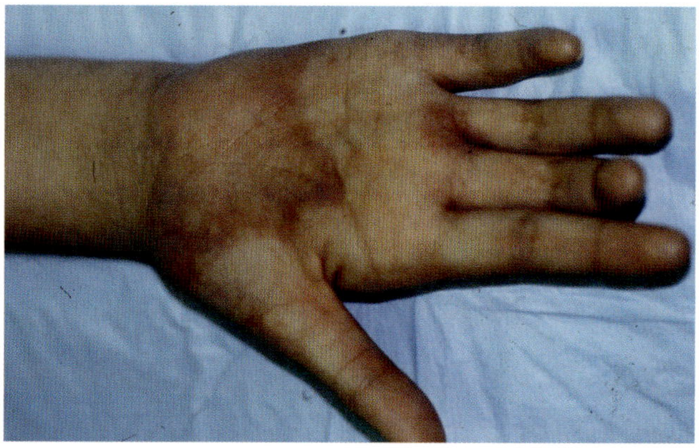

Fig. 37.1 TT leprosy – Annular plaque on right hand with weakness in an ulnar distribution in an Indian woman

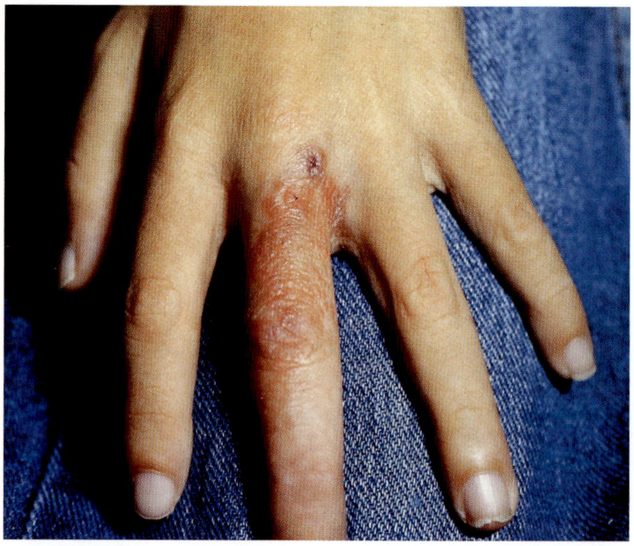

Fig. 37.2 TT leprosy – Erythematous plaque on dorsal aspect of the middle finger in an Asian male

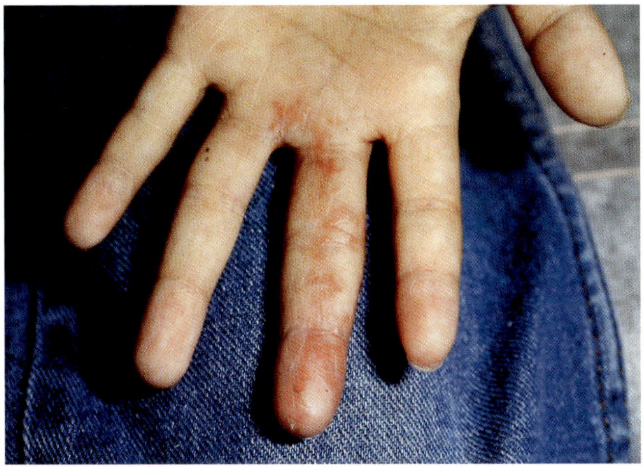

Fig. 37.3 TT leprosy – Erythematous plaque on volar aspect of the middle finger in an Asian male

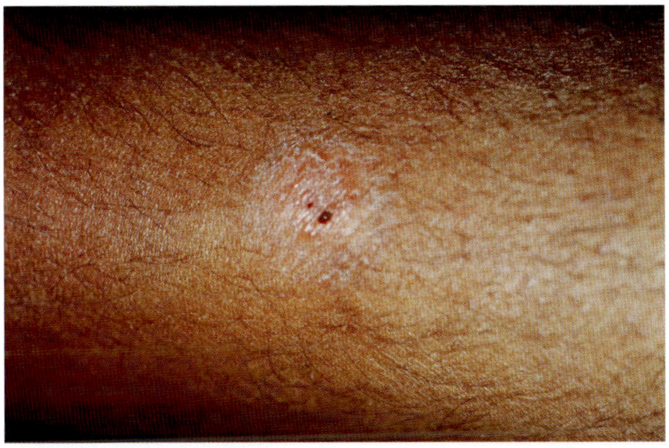

Fig. 37.4 TT leprosy – Hypopigmented scaly macule which is anesthetic to pinprick testing in an Indian male

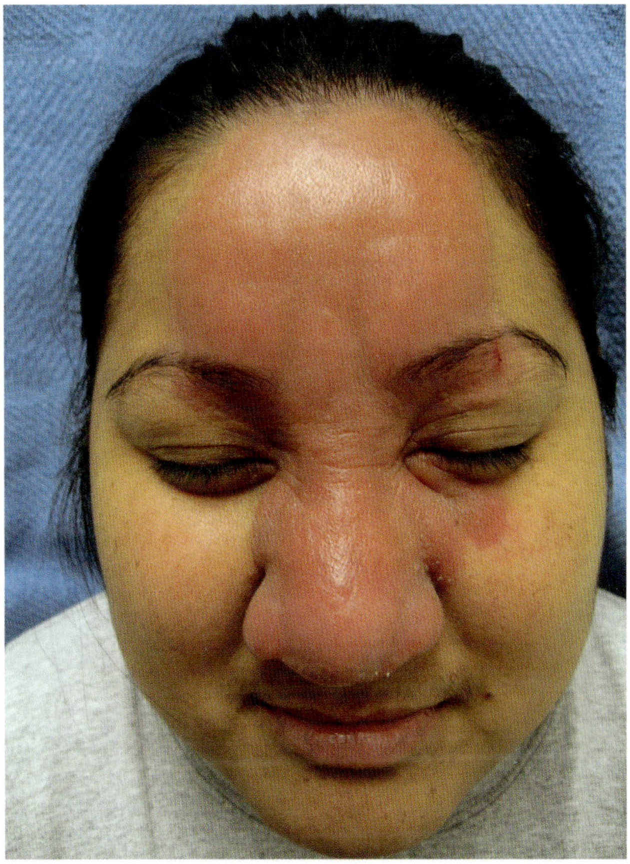

Fig. 37.5 BT leprosy – Raised bordered plaque on the midface of a Pacific Island female

Self-cure is possible with over half of these cases resolving without treatment [1].

In borderline tuberculoid leprosy (BT), the immune system is able to partially inhibit bacillary growth, but not enough to self-cure. Large annular, anesthetic, hypopigmented plaques greater than 10-cm in diameter or multiple asymmetric well-demarcated plaques can develop (Fig. 37.5). Borderline leprosy (BB) is a rarely seen immunologic midpoint of the granulomatous spectrum, with features of both the tuberculoid and lepromatous types of Hansen's disease [1] (Fig. 37.6). BB is an unstable form of leprosy that quickly changes to a more stable tuberculoid or progresses to the lepromatous zone. Annular lesions with a sharp interior and less distinct exterior border are characteristics of BB leprosy. Moderate numbers of bacilli are also seen upon biopsy.

Borderline lepromatous leprosy (BL), also called dimorphic leprosy, has a highly varied presentation with asymmetric annular plaques with sharp interior and less distinct exterior borders along with nodules and papules symmetrically distributed [1] (Fig. 37.7). Hypo- or hyperpigmented lesions can be anesthetic, can be hyperesthetic, or can have intact sensation. Moderate to large numbers of organisms are seen. A high incidence of symmetric nerve palsies occurs, and, if severe, acral stocking-glove anesthesia will be present. Untreated borderline lepromatous leprosy progresses slowly, along with increasing skin and nerve damage.

Lepromatous leprosy (LL) is characterized by a lack of cellular immunity, which allows unrestricted bacillary growth with widespread, multiorgan disease possible. Symmetric, usually poorly defined nodules, with occasional dermatofibroma-like papules occur (Figs. 37.8 and 37.9). Diffuse subclinical infiltration of the skin with widening nasal bridge and loss of the eyebrows can occur giving the so-called leonine facies (Fig. 37.10). Fusiform swelling of the fingers can occur along with symmetrical stocking-glove anesthesia.

Rare forms of leprosy include as follows: (1) indeterminate leprosy which is a term assigned to an early hypopigmented macule with or without sensory deficit and occasionally with a few acid-fast bacilli on biopsy. This rare form of leprosy occurs before the host makes a definitive immunologic commitment to cure or to react with an overt

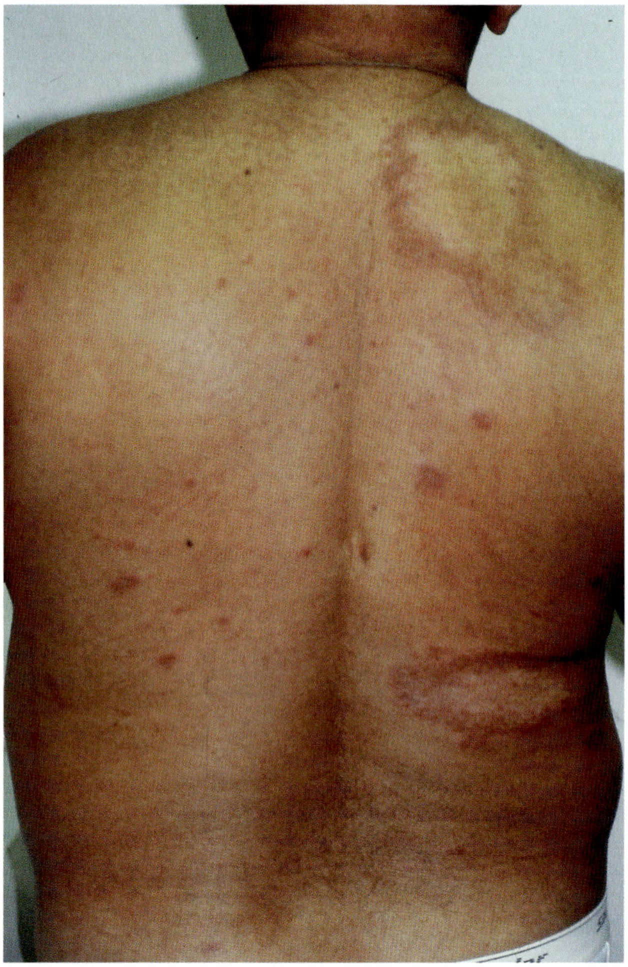

Fig. 37.6 BB leprosy – Asymmetric annular plaques with central hypopigmentation and nodules in a Brazilian male

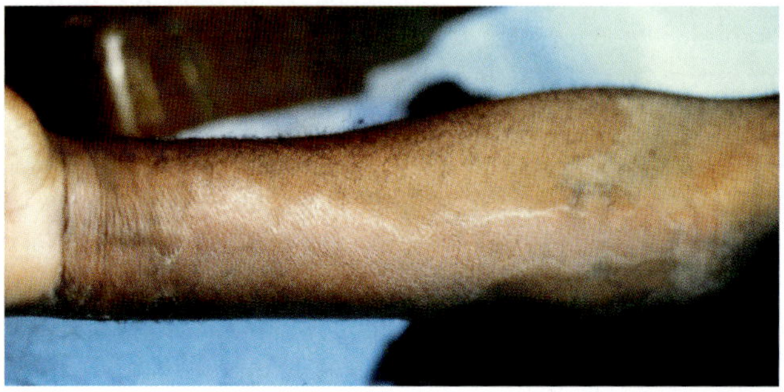

Fig. 37.7 BL leprosy – Symmetrical plaques and nodules with sensory and motor neuropathy in a Central African male

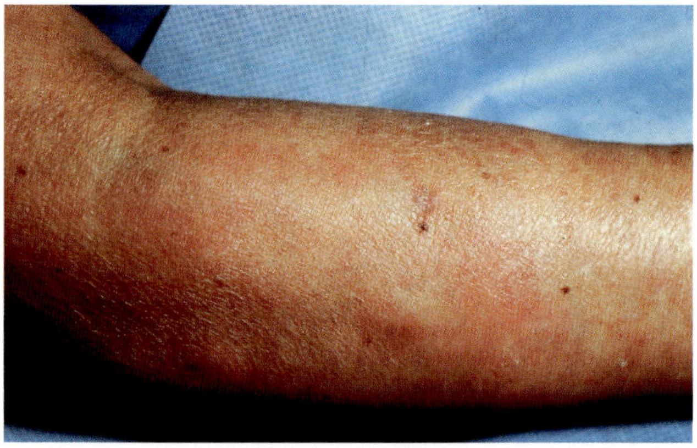

Fig. 37.8 LL leprosy – Diffuse edema, plaques, and erythema on the arm of an Asian female

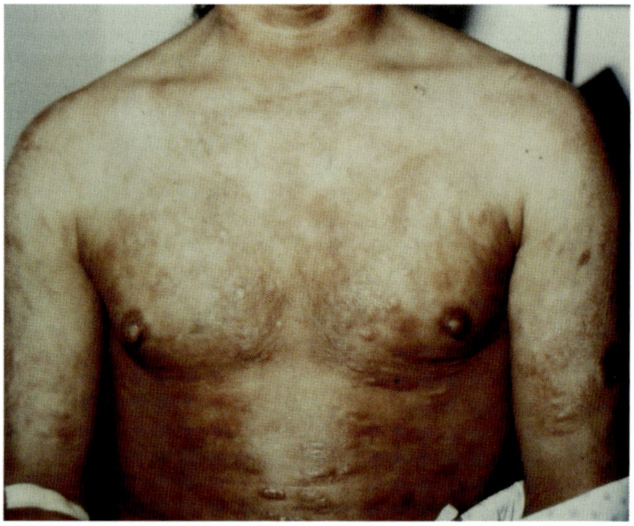

Fig. 37.9 LL leprosy – Diffuse ill-defined nodules and plaques on the trunk and arms in a Central American male

granulomatous response. (2) Diffuse leprosy of Lucio and Latapí (Latapí's lepromatosis) is considered the most anergic form of leprosy, characterized by generalized infiltration of the skin which never transforms into nodules. Diffuse alopecia of the eyebrows and eyelashes, a widened nasal root, symmetrical acral anesthesia, purple discoloration of the hands and feet, and telangiectasias can occur. (3) Pure neuritic leprosy (PNL) presents with numbness and paresthesias in the absence of skin lesions. This diagnosis of PNL is made on nerve biopsy.

Peripheral nerve abnormalities include (1) enlargement of nerves close to skin surface such as the great auricular, ulnar, median, superficial peroneal, sural, and posterior tibial nerves; (2) sensory loss in skin lesions; (3) nerve palsies secondary to granulomatous inflammation within nerves causing sensory and motor loss; and (4) acral distal symmetric anesthesia. A common complaint is pain in the extremities and a burning sensation in the soles of the feet [3].

In addition to sensory or motor loss, denervation causes anhydrosis and decreased oil production in the skin. Thus, the skin becomes dry, inelastic, and difficult to heal when trauma occurs. Most of the deformity and disability associated with Hansen's disease is secondary due to repetitive trauma and infection of areas which have become insensitive [3].

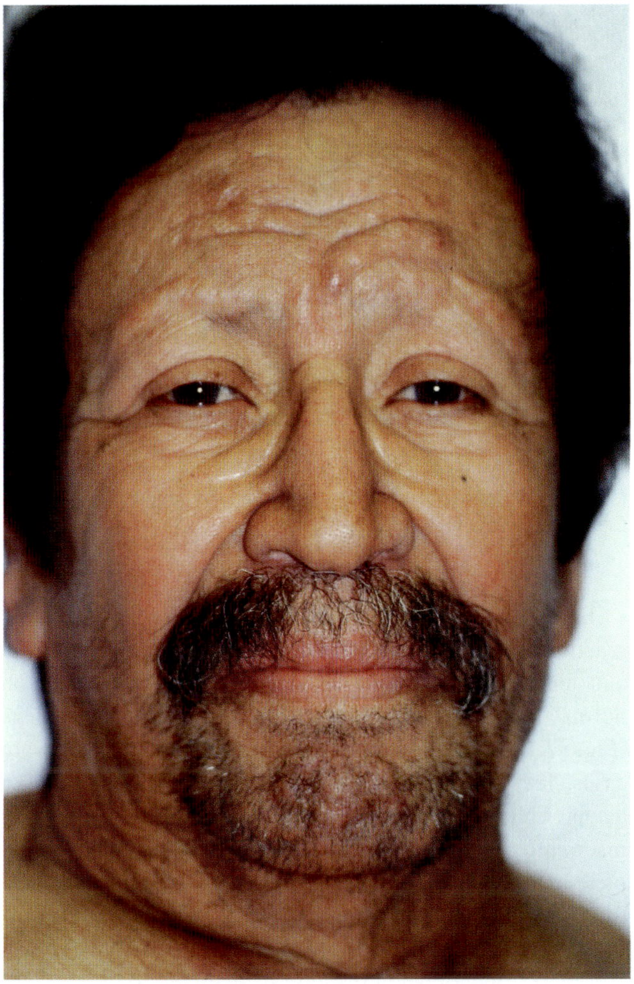

Fig. 37.10 LL leprosy – Leonine face with infiltrated skin and loss of eyebrows in a Central American male

37.4 Histopathologic Features

Histology is very helpful in the diagnosis of leprosy, especially for multibacillary forms, where the Fite stain identifies multiple acid-fast bacilli. In the tuberculoid or paucibacillary forms, the diagnosis is often suggestive, but not diagnostic, except when the granulomas are within nerves. Bacilli in the perineurium, influx of inflammatory cells, bulky bacillary material in Schwann cells and invading macrophages, and fibrosis of the inflamed nerve can all contribute to the permanent nerve damage seen in Hansen's disease. Globi, which are amphophilic collections of mycobacterium, may form in lepromatous leprosy [9].

37.5 Diagnosis and Differential Diagnosis

Differential diagnosis includes other granulomatous infections, including atypical mycobacteria infections, cutaneous tuberculosis, and deep fungal infections. Noninfectious conditions are also in the differential diagnoses, including sarcoidosis, vitiligo, and pityriasis alba.

The diagnosis of leprosy should be entertained in anyone who was born or resided in an endemic area, has a blood relative with the disease (transmission, common genetic factors, and common exposures), and who simultaneously presents with skin lesions and peripheral nerve abnormalities. A confirmed diagnosis of leprosy requires the presence of a consistent peripheral nerve abnormality or the demonstration of mycobacterium in tissues [1]. Molecular and immunological tests for tissue specimens have been developed for leprosy diagnosis and prognostics, including polymerase chain reactions (PCR) and enzyme-linked immunosorbent assay (ELISA) [8].

37.6 Treatment

Paucibacillary disease (TT or BT), defined as less than five lesions by the WHO, is treated according to the WHO recommendations with two-drug therapy for 6 months, usually dapsone 100 mg daily and rifampin 600 mg daily (or q monthly supervised). Alternative medications in case of allergies or nonresponse include clofazimine 50 mg daily, minocycline 100 mg daily, or ofloxacin 400 mg daily. Multibacillary disease defined as greater than five lesions (BB, BL, and LL) requires three-drug therapy for 1 year, usually dapsone 100 mg daily, rifampin 600 mg daily (or q monthly supervised), and clofazimine 50 mg daily or one of the alternative medications [3].

37.7 Leprosy Host Reactions

Leprosy host reaction states can occur and have significant morbidity and mortality if not treated promptly. Jopling's type 1 reaction ("reversal reaction") and Jopling's type 2 reaction (erythema nodosum leprosum, "ENL") are common with 25–50 % of patients experiencing a reaction state sometime during the course of the disease and even years after treatment has been discontinued. Lucio reactions associated with the diffuse leprosy of Lucio and Latapí are rarely seen. In untreated leprosy, nerve damage is insidious, but in a reaction state, the nerve damage can occur quite rapidly and become the major cause of disability.

Reversal reaction (Jopling's type 1 reaction, delayed-type hypersensitivity reaction) represents an "upgrade" in the immune response with an abrupt worsening of clinical nodules and plaques associated with tenderness, fever, and malaise (Fig. 37.11). Neurologic deficits can worsen with the inflammation of the involved nerve roots to cause palsies. Reversal reactions almost always occur after initiation of therapy, rarely before or after treatment. This most commonly occurs with multibacillary forms of leprosy. Treatment is with prednisone slowly tapered over at least 2–3 months, but this painful type of reaction state may need to be treated for years.

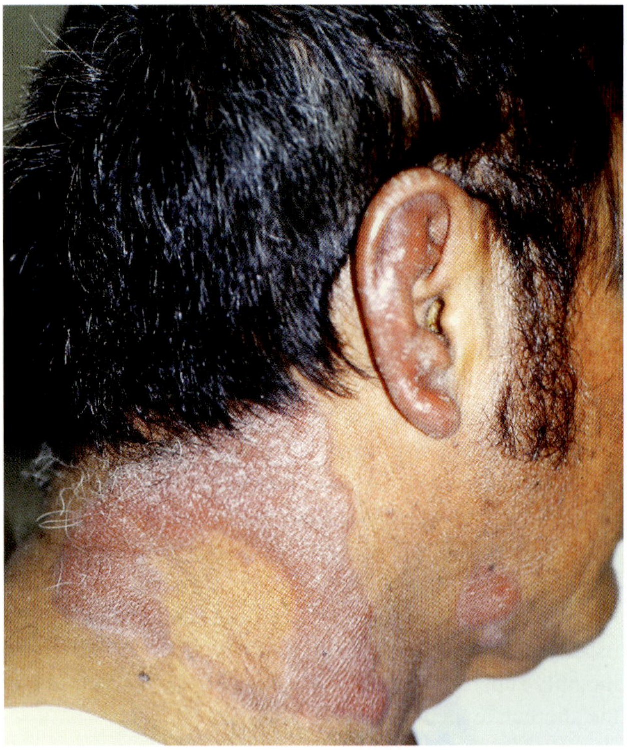

Fig. 37.11 Reversal reaction – Warm, edematous inflamed well-defined plaques on the neck and ears of a Central American male

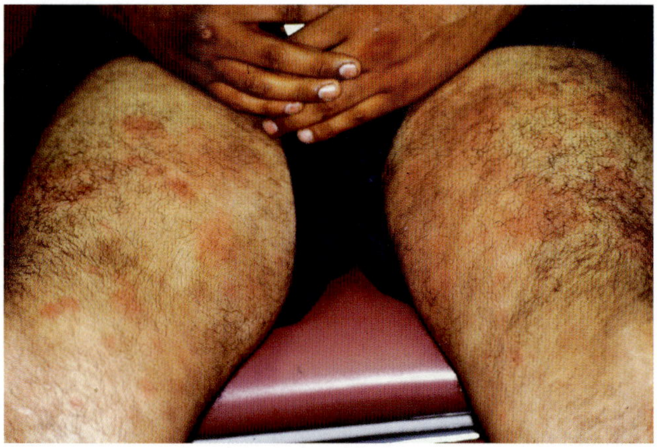

Fig. 37.12 Erythema nodosum leprosum – Crops of erythematous, tender, ill-defined subcutaneous nodules on the thighs and legs in a Central American male

Erythema nodosum leprosum (ENL, Jopling's type 2 reaction) is a leprosy-specific response with crops of painful and tender ill-defined subcutaneous nodules that arise on normal skin usually symmetrically on the arms and legs (Fig. 37.12). Facial nodules occur in 50 % of cases. In severe cases, fever, malaise, epididymitis, orchitis, and iritis can occur. ENL can occur before the diagnosis of leprosy is made, after treatment is initiated, or after treatment is complete and may last for years. Treatment is with prednisone, thalidomide (its only indication), or less commonly clofazimine or pentoxifylline.

Lucio's phenomenon reaction is restricted to diffuse leprosy of Lucio and Latapí. Painful, but nontender, hemorrhagic infarcts resembling septic infarcts develop on the arms and lower extremities. Bullae and ulcers may occur. This reaction is common in Mexico and the Caribbean. New lesions cease within 1 week after treatment with rifampin but may worsen if treated with dapsone alone.

37.8 Case Management

Management of leprosy starts by correctly making the diagnosis, then classifying the type of leprosy on clinical and histological criteria before initiating appropriate therapy. Skin lesion development and resolution, as well as sensory and motor function, should be periodically documented. Monitoring the patient while on medication and obtaining appropriate laboratory tests to avoid toxicity are important. Evaluating and treating other skin infections and injuries, particularly in areas with anesthesia, helps to prevent further tissue damage. One may need to obtain consultations with neurology, ophthalmology, ENT, orthopedic surgery, podiatry, and occupational or physical therapy depending on the situation. Above all, education of the patient and family members helps to alleviate fears, overcome stigmas, improve compliance, and reduce anxiety associated with Hansen's disease.

References

1. Rea TH, Modlin RL. Fitzpatrick's dermatology in general medicine. 7th ed. New York: McGraw-Hill; 2008. Chapter 186, p. 1786–96.
2. World Health Organization. Weekly epidemiological record. http://www.who.int/wer. 24 Aug 2012.
3. National Hansen's Disease Programs. Manual from the National Hansen's Disease Program booklet from Baton Rouge, LA published in 2012.
4. Han XY, Seo YH, Sizer KC, et al. A new mycobacterium species causes diffuse lepromatous leprosy. Am J Clin Pathol. 2008;130:856–64.
5. Goulart LR, Bernardes-Goulart IM. Leprosy pathogenetic background: a review and lessons from other mycobacterial diseases. Arch Dermatol Res. 2009;301:123–37.
6. Krutzik SR, Ochoa MT, Seiling PA, et al. Activation and regulation of Toll-like receptors 1 and 2 in human leprosy. Nat Med. 2003;9:525–32.
7. Ridley DS, Jopling WH. Classification of leprosy according to immunity: a five-group system. Int J Lepr Other Mycobact Dis. 1966;34:255–73.
8. Goulart LR, Bernardes-Goulart IM. Leprosy: diagnostic and control challenges for a worldwide disease. Arch Dermatol Res. 2008;300:269–90.
9. Elston D, Ferringer T. Dermatopathology. Requisites in dermatology. Philadelphia: Elsevier; 2009. Chapter 17, p. 245.

Skin Signs of HIV Infection

38

Thao Duong and Arturo Ricardo Dominguez

Contents

T. Duong, MD
Department of Internal Medicine, University of Texas at Southwestern, 5323 Harry Hines Blvd., Dallas, TX 75392, USA
e-mail: thao.duong@phhs.org

A.R. Dominguez, MD (✉)
Department of Dermatology, University of Texas Southwestern Medical Center, 5323 Harry Hines Blvd., Dallas, TX 75390, USA

Abbreviations

AIDS	Acquired immunodeficiency syndrome
CMV	Cytomegalovirus
HAART	Highly active antiretroviral therapy
HHV-8	Human herpesvirus-8
HIV	Human immunodeficiency virus
HPV	Human papillomavirus
HSV	Herpes simplex virus
MC	Molluscum contagiosum
OHL	Oral hairy leukoplakia
PUVA	Psoralen + ultraviolet A
TNF	Tumor necrosis factor
UVB	Ultraviolet B
VZV	Varicella-zoster virus

38.1 Etiology

The human immunodeficiency virus (HIV) is a blood-borne retrovirus that attacks white blood cells, primarily CD4+ T cells, which may ultimately lead to acquired immunodeficiency syndrome (AIDS). Sexual intercourse is the most common mode of transmission, but the virus can also be transmitted during childbirth, breastfeeding, or via shared contaminated needles in intravenous drug users.

38.2 Epidemiology

Although HIV infection affects people of all races, it disproportionately affects ethnic minorities, notably African Americans and Hispanics in the United States [1]. Ethnic minorities have also been observed to have a greater incidence of cutaneous diseases [2]. African American race is an independent risk factor for developing dermatologic disorders in HIV + patients [2].

In 2006, African Americans made up only 12 % of the US population but represented 46 % of all people with HIV,

D. Jackson-Richards, A.G. Pandya (eds.), *Dermatology Atlas for Skin of Color*,
DOI 10.1007/978-3-642-54446-0_38, © Springer-Verlag Berlin Heidelberg 2014

compared with Caucasians, who only represented 35 % of cases [3]. Prevalence was almost eight times greater among blacks than whites [1]. Hispanics accounted for 15 % of the US population and 18 % of people with HIV with the prevalence rate almost three times greater than whites [3]. Of all HIV-positive patients, it has been estimated that greater than 90 % of patients have mucocutaneous complaints, some causing significant morbidity [2].

38.3 Clinical Features

HIV infection usually undergoes three clinical stages: acute infection, latency period, and progression to AIDS (Table 38.1). Primary HIV infection is often asymptomatic, but 25–75 % of patients will develop a mononucleosis-like illness, including fever, malaise, myalgia, lymphadenopathy, and a morbilliform rash [4]. After this stage, the body mounts a strong immune response to decrease the absolute level of viremia but active virus replication persists in lymphoid tissues. During this latency period, the immune system is still functional and can keep infections under control. However, it has been found that seropositive patients have an increased risk of developing psoriasis, seborrheic dermatitis, atopic dermatitis, xerosis, eosinophilic folliculitis, and papular pruritic eruption compared to the general population [5].

Table 38.1 Cutaneous manifestations by HIV disease stage

Acute	Generalized morbilliform rash
Latent	Seborrheic dermatitis, psoriasis, xerosis/atopic dermatitis, HPV infections, varicella zoster, candidiasis, oral hairy leukoplakia
Progression to AIDS	Kaposi's sarcoma, opportunistic fungal infections, extensive molluscum contagiosum, disseminated CMV and HSV, eosinophilic folliculitis, papular pruritic eruption of HIV

38.4 Seborrheic Dermatitis

Seborrheic dermatitis is more common in HIV-positive patients than seronegative patients and affects up to 85 % of all seropositive patients at some point during the course of their disease [5]. As the name suggests, seborrheic dermatitis involves areas with an abundance of sebaceous glands, particularly the face and scalp (Figs. 38.1 and 38.2). Similarly to immunocompetent patients, the disease presents as greasy, scaly thin papules and plaques over an erythematous base that may itch or burn and is often more severe and recalcitrant to treatment. Treatment consists of topical corticosteroids, antifungals, sulfacetamide, or antimicrobial shampoos.

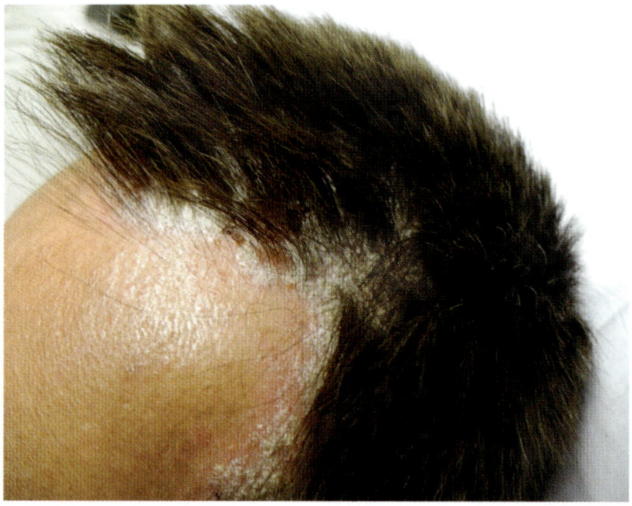

Fig. 38.1 Seborrheic dermatitis of the scalp in a Hispanic male with HIV infection

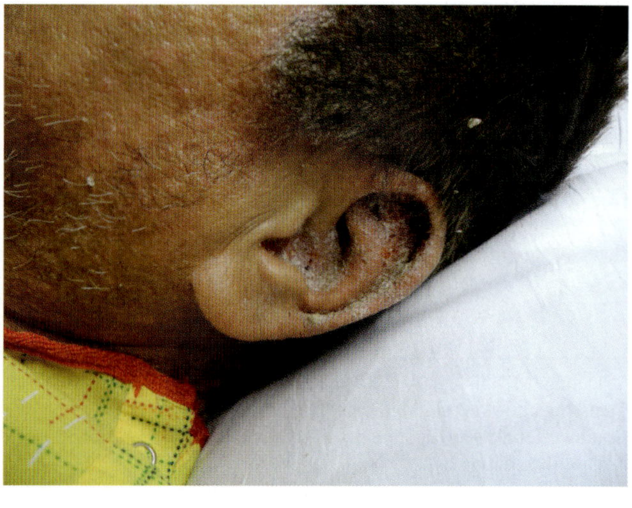

Fig. 38.2 Seborrheic dermatitis of the ear in a Hispanic male with HIV infection

38.5 Psoriasis

The rate of psoriasis in HIV + patients is similar to the general population but it is often more severe and resistant to treatment [5]. The disease manifests as well-demarcated, silvery scale overlying an erythematous plaque on extensor surfaces that can be pruritic and painful. Lesions may be numerous and even present as erythroderma (Fig. 38.3). Nail pitting, onycholysis, and subungual hyperkeratosis can also be present. Although the rate of psoriasis is similar between seropositive and seronegative patients, psoriatic arthritis is much more common in HIV + patients [5]. Treatment consists of emollients, corticosteroids, fluocinonide, vitamin D derivatives, and retinoids for mild disease, phototherapy with UVB or PUVA for moderate disease, and systemic agents such as methotrexate or cyclosporine for severe disease resistant to other forms of treatment. TNF inhibitor therapy may also be safe and effective in HIV-infected patients [6].

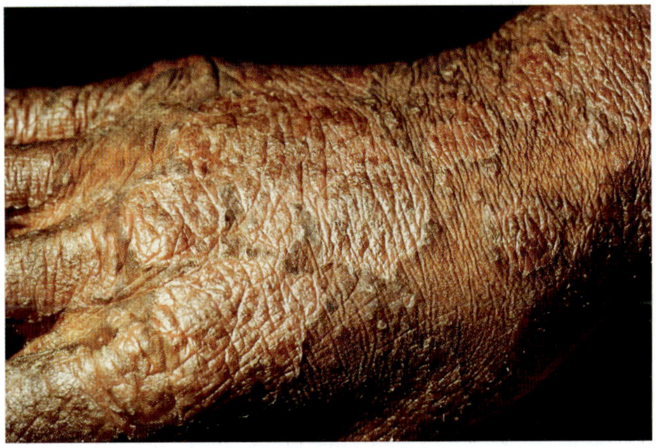

Fig. 38.3 Psoriasis of the hand in an African American male with HIV infection

38.6 Xerosis/Atopic Dermatitis

Xerosis and atopic dermatitis are the most common skin conditions of patients infected with HIV [5]. Xerosis occurs in greater than 20 % of patients even when the CD4 count is >400×10^6/L and can transform to ichthyosis once it drops below 50×10^6/L [5, 6]. Atopic dermatitis is seen in approximately 30–50 % of patients [5]. Xerosis in AIDS patients can present with atopic dermatitis-like lesions, with erythema, oozing, crusting, and lichenified plaques. Xerosis is usually generalized, whereas atopic dermatitis is more common in flexural areas, eyelids, neck, flanks, hands, and lower legs. Both conditions are managed with improved skin hygiene, including short lukewarm showers, mild soaps, and emollients, but a topical corticosteroid is often added for those with significant itching and inflammation. Antihistamines such as hydroxyzine are also recommended for patients complaining of pruritus, which is common in both diseases.

38.7 Eosinophilic Folliculitis/Papular Pruritic Eruption of HIV

Eosinophilic folliculitis and papular pruritic eruption of HIV are both extremely pruritic eruptions that are relatively unique to HIV infection. Both conditions present as multiple erythematous small papules but the distribution is different in the two conditions. Eosinophilic folliculitis centers around follicles and favors the face, neck, scalp, and upper trunk (Fig. 38.4), whereas papular pruritic eruptions of HIV favor the extremities [7]. Treatment of choice for both conditions is immune reconstitution with HAART, but emollients, topical steroids, antifungals, metronidazole, isotretinoin, and UVB therapy have been used with varying success [8].

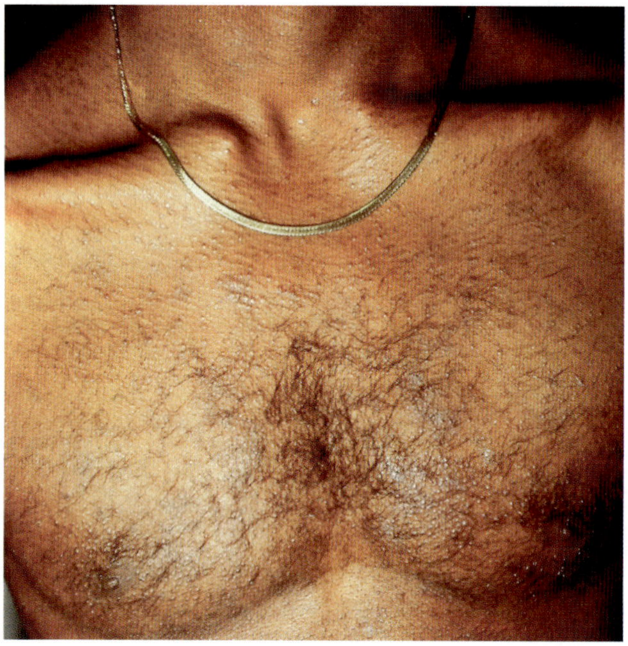

Fig. 38.4 Eosinophilic folliculitis of the chest in an African American male with HIV infection

38.8 Kaposi's Sarcoma

Kaposi's sarcoma, an AIDS-defining illness caused by the human herpesvirus-8 (HHV-8), is a vascular neoplastic disorder that affects the skin, oral mucosa, lymph nodes, and visceral organs with skin being the most common site. Rarely, a patient can have visceral organ involvement without cutaneous disease [9]. Early lesions are often pink or yellowish green, simulating bruises, purpura, or dermatofibromas before developing into typical dark red, brown, or violaceous macules, papules, plaques, nodules, or tumors that are distributed singly, grouped, or coalesced together (Figs. 38.5, 38.6, 38.7, 38.9, 38.10, and 38.11). Initially, lesions are commonly found on the face and trunk and arranged parallel to skin tension lines, but one-third to half of patients develop lesions on their lower extremities which can ulcerate and cause severe pain [9]. Extracutaneous lesions are frequently seen in the lymph nodes, respiratory tract, and gastrointestinal tract with the general rule of one internal lesion for every

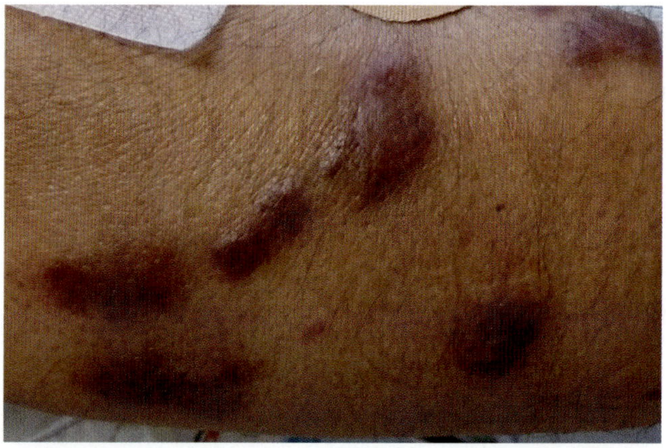

Fig. 38.5 Kaposi's sarcoma of the forearm in a Hispanic male with HIV infection

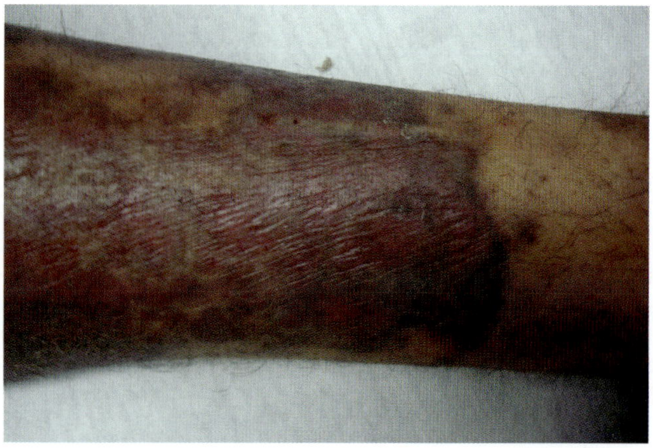

Fig. 38.6 Kaposi's sarcoma of the calf in a Hispanic male with HIV infection

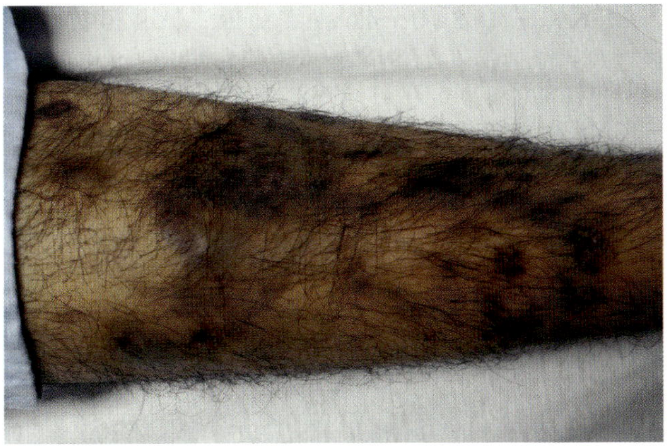

Fig. 38.7 Gray-brown Kaposi's sarcoma of the calf in a Hispanic male with HIV infection

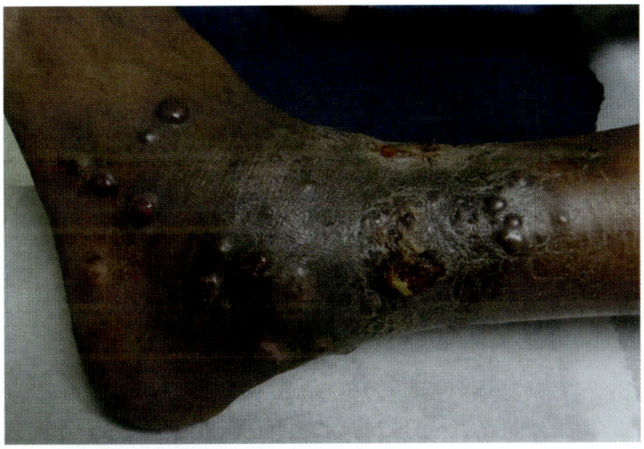

Fig. 38.8 Nodular Kaposi's sarcoma of the foot and lower leg in an African American male with HIV infection

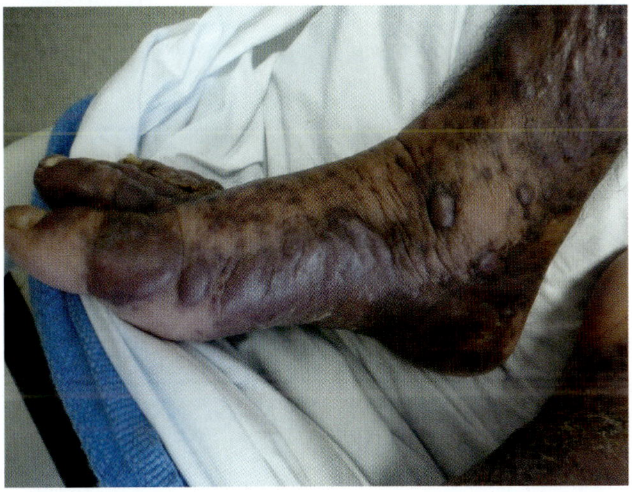

Fig. 38.9 Hypertrophic Kaposi's sarcoma of the foot and ankle in an African American male with HIV infection

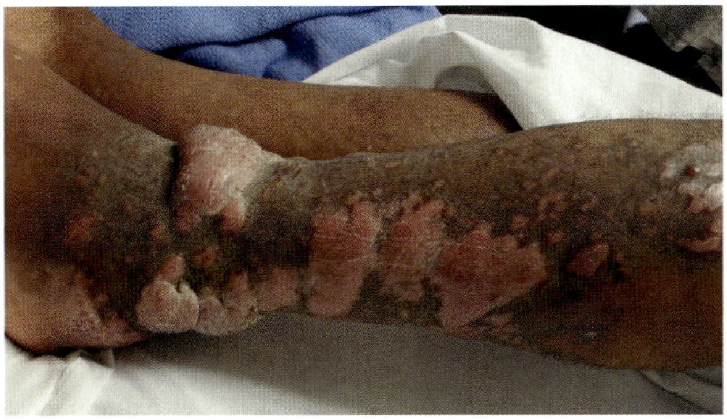

Fig. 38.10 Hypertrophic Kaposi's sarcoma of the calf and ankle in an African American male with HIV infection

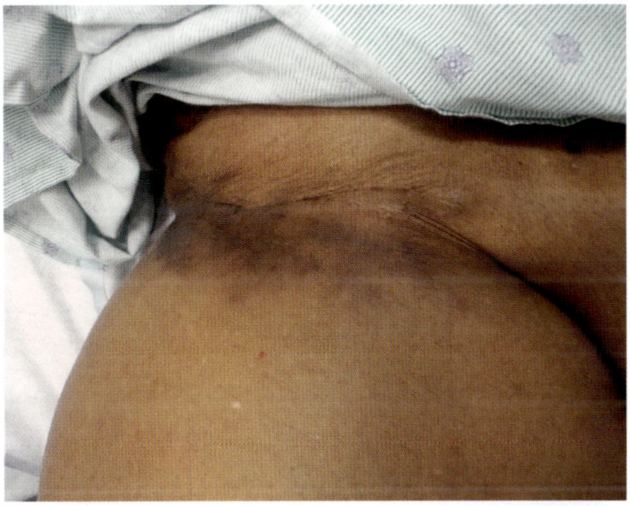

Fig. 38.11 Kaposi's sarcoma of the inguinal fold in an African American male with HIV infection

five skin lesions [9]. Lymph node involvement can cause lymphedema due to the obstruction of lymphatic channels. Gastrointestinal involvement can cause nausea, abdominal pain, ulceration, bleeding, and bowel obstruction, and pulmonary involvement can present with cough, dyspnea, chest pain, and respiratory distress, which can mimic an opportunistic infection.

The introduction of HAART (highly active antiretroviral therapy) has significantly decreased the incidence and altered the clinical course of Kaposi's sarcoma and is the first line of treatment [9]. Immune reconstitution can sometimes cause resolution of lesions. However, patients with visceral disease may need chemotherapy in addition to HAART. Locally symptomatic lesions can be treated with radiation, cryosurgery, laser surgery, excisional surgery, electrocauterization, or intralesional injections of vinblastine, vincristine, and interferon-alpha [9].

38.9 HPV Infections

Condyloma acuminata, also known as anogenital warts, are caused by the human papillomavirus (HPV), particularly by HPV serotypes 6 and 11. In men, the disease commonly affects the penis, urethra, scrotum, perianal, anal, and rectal areas as well as oral mucosa and in women, the labia, introitus, and perineum [8]. Condyloma can present with a variety of different morphologies ranging from smooth verrucous papules to rough exophytic fungating masses with color ranging from skin colored to brown (Fig. 38.12). Although most lesions are asymptomatic, some can cause pain and pruritus and extensive perianal condylomata, as often seen in HIV-positive patients, and can cause secondary constipation and urinary obstruction [8]. Infections with HPV serotypes 16 and 18 are less prevalent but are the types most commonly associated with cervical and anal cancer. HIV-positive patients have an increased risk of acquisition and persistence of HPV infection, and invasive cervical cancer is the third most common AIDS-defining malignancy, after non-Hodgkin's lymphoma and Kaposi's sarcoma. HPV serotypes 7 and 32 affect oral surfaces and can occur on all oral mucosal surfaces [10]. Patients with HIV infection may also develop large or numerous common or flat warts on normal skin (Fig. 38.13).

No treatment is 100 % effective in eradicating HPV, but multiple options are available to treat lesions, including antiproliferative agents (e.g., podophyllotoxin), destructive therapies (e.g., cryotherapy, topical trichloroacetic acid, electrocautery, CO_2 laser treatment, and surgical excision), and antiviral agents (e.g., cidofovir and interferons). Immunomodulators (e.g., imiquimod) are less effective than in immunocompetent patients. Similar to Kaposi's sarcoma, HAART can cause regression of disease with improvement of the immune system.

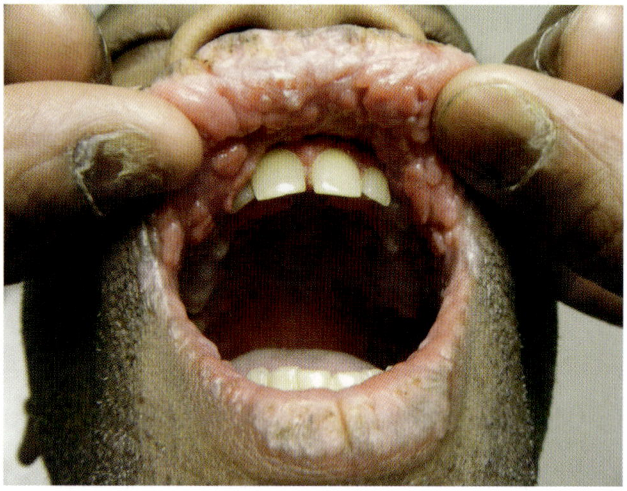

Fig. 38.12 Multiple mucosal warts in an African American male with HIV infection

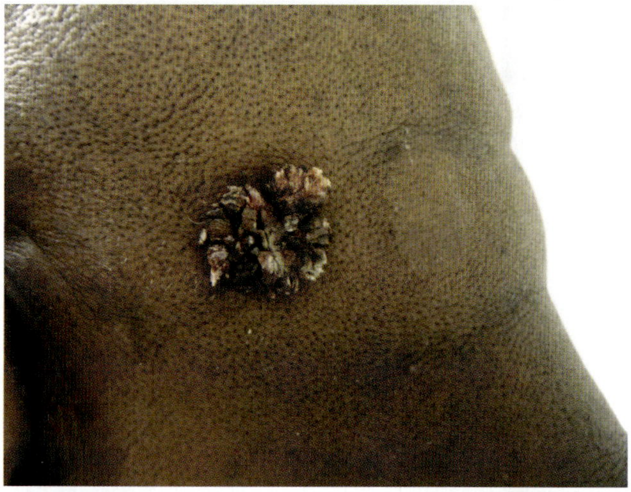

Fig. 38.13 Filiform verruca of the scalp in an African American male with HIV infection

38.10 HSV/VZV/CMV

Herpes simplex virus-2 (HSV-2), varicella-zoster virus (VZV), and cytomegalovirus (CMV) all belong to the viral family *Herpesviridae*. The viruses share a common structure but cause significantly different clinical diseases. HSV-2 is transmitted through direct contact with active lesions or exchange of bodily fluids during sexual intercourse and generally causes anogenital disease. Initially, clinical presentation is similar to immunocompetent hosts with grouped vesicles on erythematous bases in peri-genital areas, but with deterioration of immune status, lesions become more numerous, verrucous, ulcerative, and recalcitrant (Figs. 38.14, 38.15, and 38.16).

Primary infection with VZV causes chickenpox but the virus remains latent in dorsal root ganglia indefinitely after the infection and reactivation causes herpes zoster or "shingles." Initial occurrence manifests as painful grouped or confluent papules, vesicles, or crusted erosions distributed in a dermatomal pattern without crossing the midline and spontaneously resolves in 2–3 weeks, similarly to immunocompetent hosts [4]. However, with depressed immunity, disease becomes more severe, persistent, and recurrent. Disseminated VZV, defined as greater than 20 vesicles outside of contiguous dermatomes, can spread systemically, causing hepatitis, pneumonitis, and encepahlitis.

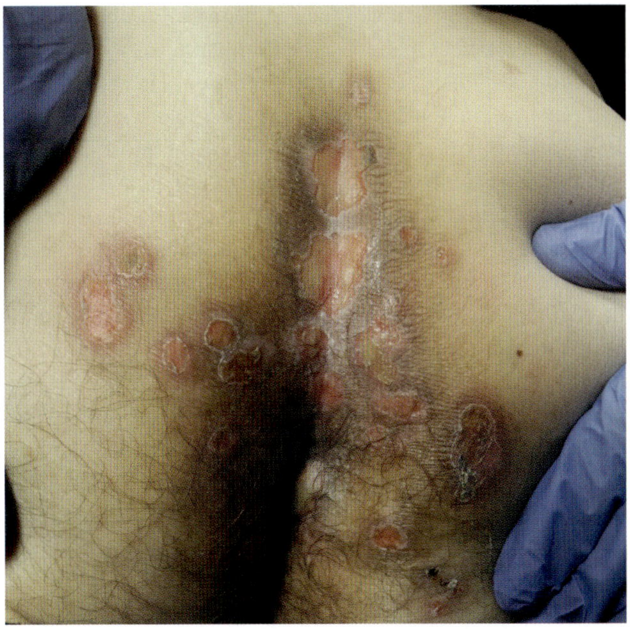

Fig. 38.15 Severe ulcerative herpes simplex virus infection of the buttocks in a Hispanic male with HIV infection

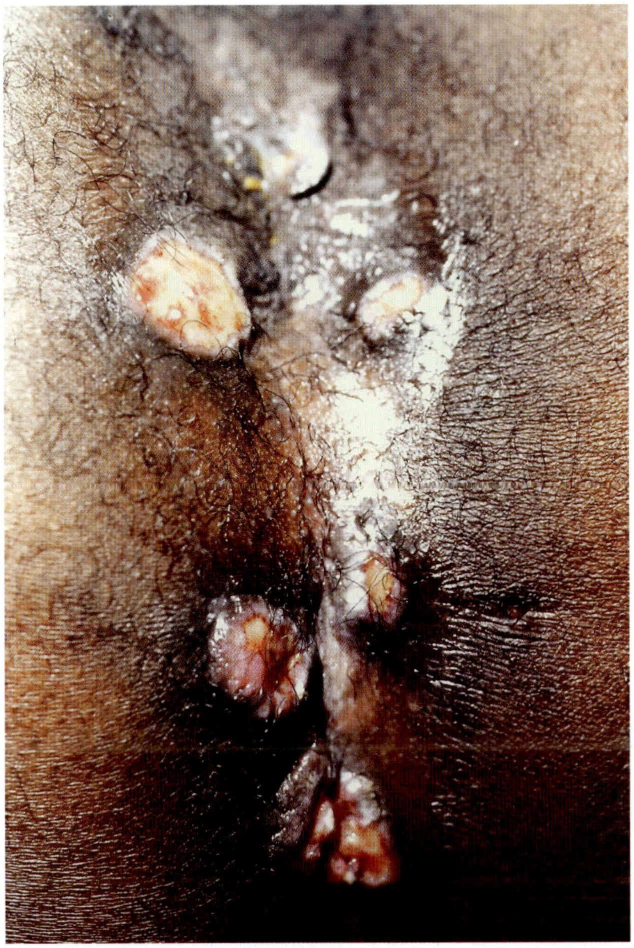

Fig. 38.14 Ulcerative herpes simplex virus infection of the buttocks in an African American male with HIV infection

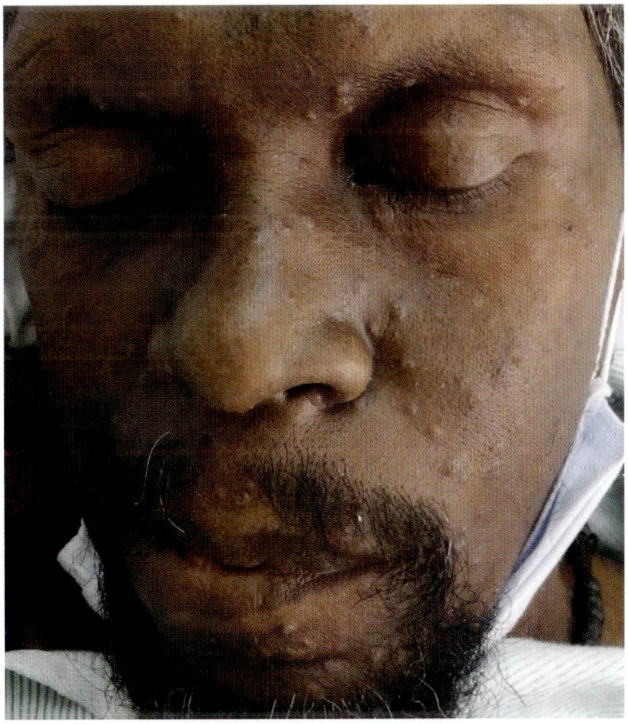

Fig. 38.16 Vesicles of the face due to disseminated herpes simplex virus infection in an African American male with HIV infection

CMV infection is ubiquitous and generally subclinical in immunocompetent patients [4]. Similarly to VZV, CMV infection is divided into primary infection, latent infection, and reactivation. It affects almost every organ system and, in HIV-positive patients, represents one of the most common opportunistic infections. Cutaneous disease is rare but more prevalent in immunocompromised than immunocompetent patients [8]. Cutaneous CMV infection can present as ulcers, verrucous lesions, and palpable purpuric papules in the genital region, chest, and oral mucosa. Vesicles, bullae, generalized morbilliform, and vesiculobullous and perifollicular papulopustular eruptions have also been reported [8]. Acyclovir is the drug of choice for both HSV and VZV infections, while foscarnet is used for acyclovir-resistant strains. Ganciclovir is the drug of choice for CMV infection, with foscarnet being a second-line drug.

38.11 Opportunistic Fungal Infections

Histoplasmosis, blastomycosis, and coccidioidomycosis are all opportunistic fungal infections transmitted via inhalation of spores found in the soil. *Histoplasma capsulatum*, *Blastomyces dermatitidis*, and *Coccidioides immitis* are endemic to certain regions, and individuals living in or having traveled to these regions harbor latent pulmonary infection. However, in immunocompromised hosts, the infection can become reactivated and disseminate hematogenously, causing significant morbidity and mortality.

Cryptococcus neoformans is a ubiquitous encapsulated yeast found in the soil that commonly presents as subacute meningitis or meningoencephalitis in HIV-positive patients. 5–10 % of patients with disseminated disease may also develop cutaneous lesions [11]. The most common presentation is umbilicated skin-colored papules or nodules, similar to molluscum contagiosum (MC), distributed in the head and neck area (Fig. 38.17) [11]. Less commonly, it can present as pustules, ulcers, abscesses, cellulitis, panniculitis, and plaques.

Both histoplasmosis, endemic to the Ohio and Mississippi River Valleys, and coccidioidomycosis, endemic to the southwestern United States, Mexico, and Central and South America, can produce lesions identical to cutaneous cryptococcosis in patients with disseminated disease (Figs. 38.18 and 38.19) [11]. In addition, lesions caused by coccidioidomycosis can coalesce and become confluent, forming abscesses with draining sinus tracts that heal with

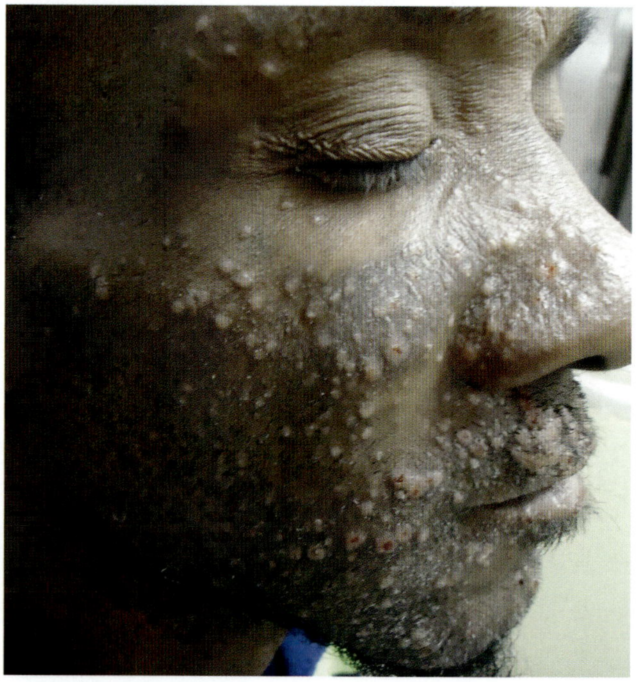

Fig. 38.17 Multiple lesions of cutaneous cryptococcosis of the face in an African American male with HIV infection

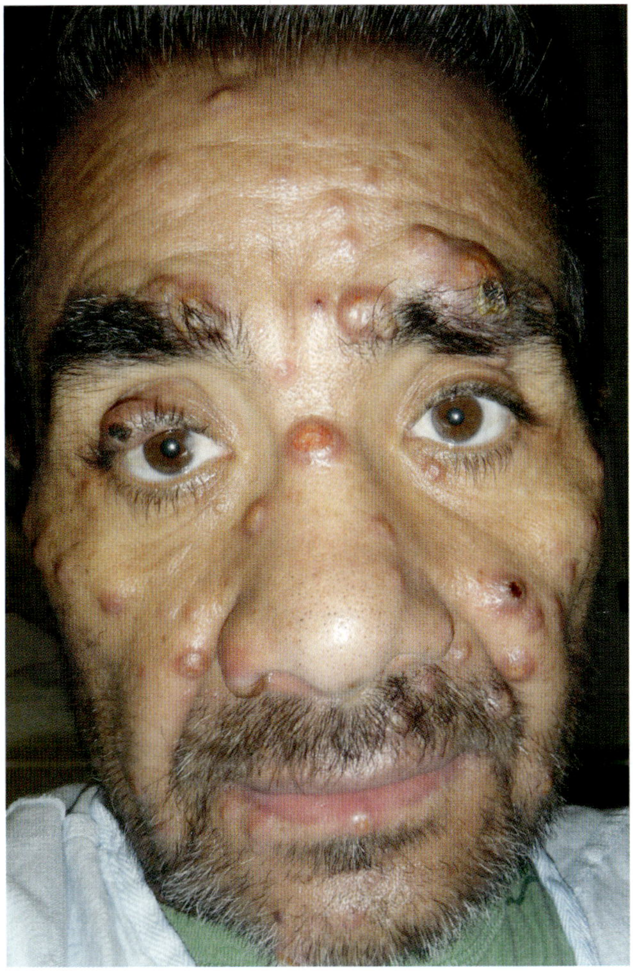

Fig. 38.18 Cutaneous lesions of histoplasmosis of the face in a Hispanic male with HIV infection

scarring [11]. Blastomycosis initially presents as papules or pustules but if left untreated can progress to large ulcerated plaques with violaceous verrucous borders that heal with scarring.

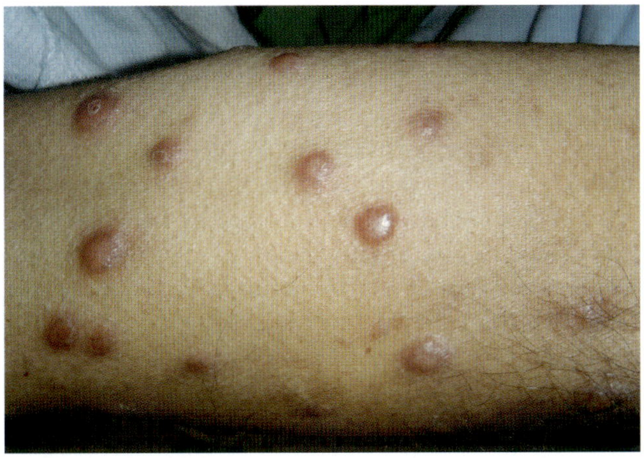

Fig. 38.19 Cutaneous lesions of histoplasmosis of the upper arm in a Hispanic male with HIV infection

Clinically, the three dimorphic fungi may present very similarly and diagnosis requires isolation of organisms from a clinical specimen. In addition to these opportunistic infections, molluscum contagiosum should also be in the differential, since MC lesions in patients with immune suppression often are larger, more diffuse, and can progress to nodular, tumor-like lesions that become necrotic, resembling cryptococcosis.

Treatment for all four infections consists of induction with intravenous amphotericin B until clinical improvement is observed and then maintenance with fluconazole or itraconazole for several weeks to months. Treatment for disseminated *Cryptococcus* may also include flucytosine. Afterward, patients with disseminated histoplasmosis, blastomycosis, or cryptococcosis are maintained on oral azoles for 1 year or longer. Treatment can be discontinued in patients who show an immune response to HAART. In contrast, patients with disseminated coccidioidomycosis are maintained on azoles indefinitely [11].

38.12 Oral Candidiasis/Oral Hairy Leukoplakia

Oral candidiasis and oral hairy leukoplakia (OHL) are both common oral manifestations of HIV infection. Oral candidiasis is most often caused by *Candida albicans*, part of normal flora, and OHL is caused by the Epstein-Barr virus [12]. Oral candidiasis presents in a variety of ways with pseudomembranous (thrush) and erythematous candidiasis being the most common. Thrush characteristically presents as white/creamy curd-like plaques on an erythematous base on the oral mucosa which can easily be removed. Erythematous candidiasis appears as red macules of varying sizes on the palate and dorsal surface of the tongue. Symptoms for both include pain, dysphagia, and changes in taste [12].

OHL can resemble thrush but, in contrast to thrush, it does not rub off. Lesions are asymptomatic and most commonly present as whitish corrugated "hairy" plaques on the lateral tongue but can occur anywhere in the mouth (Fig. 38.20) [12].

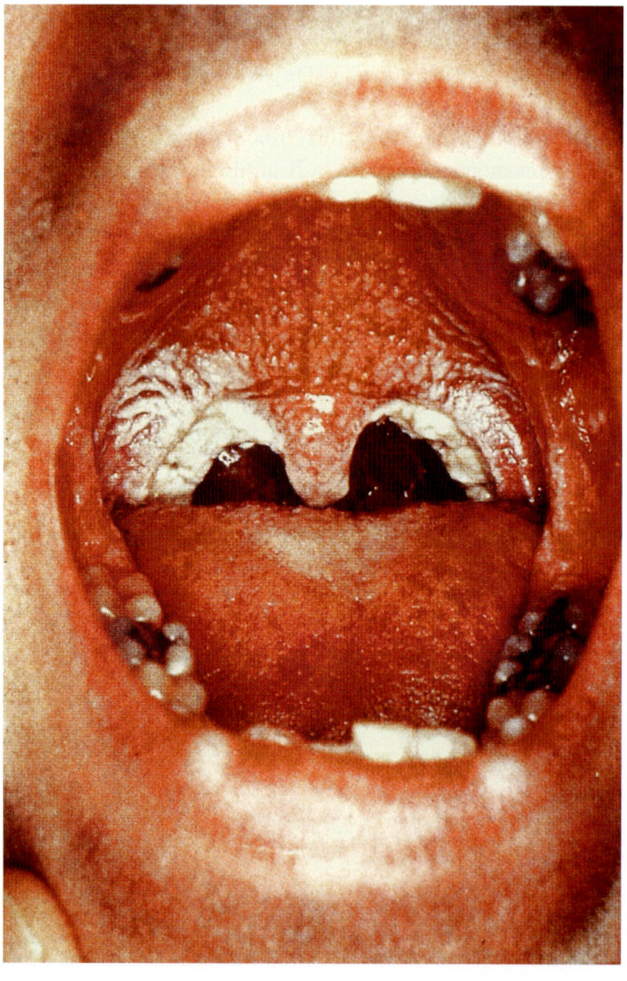

Fig. 38.20 Oral hairy leukoplakia of the oral mucosa in a Hispanic male with HIV infection

Oral candidiasis can be treated either topically or systematically. Topical medications are preferred over systemic treatments because they limit systemic absorption and include clotrimazole, nystatin, and amphotericin B. Systemic therapies include fluconazole, ketoconazole, itraconazole, and amphotericin B. Treatment for OHL is often not necessary but if desired, acyclovir, topical podophyllin resin, or topical isotretinoin can be used [8]. However, lesions typically recur once therapy is discontinued.

38.13 Lipodystrophy

HAART has transformed HIV infection from a once fatal disease into a chronic condition for patients that have access to these medications. However, one of the most common adverse effects of HAART is lipodystrophy, a syndrome characterized by a constellation of body composition and metabolic changes. Body composition changes include fat redistribution due to lipoatrophy or lipohypertrophy, and metabolic changes consist of insulin resistance and dyslipidemia, resembling metabolic syndrome. There is a wide variation regarding the prevalence of HIV lipodystrophy reported in the literature ranging anywhere from 2 to 80 % [13]. Lipodystrophy commonly presents as a loss of subcutaneous fat in the extremities or face with a gain in truncal and upper body fat content. The stigma associated with these changes, particularly temporal wasting and loss of subcutaneous fat from the buccal and dorsocervical fat pads, can cause patients to become less compliant or even refuse therapy [14]. The disorder is often progressive, and treatment options include (1) avoidance of antiviral agents that are more commonly associated with lipodystrophy, such as thymidine analog nucleoside reverse-transcriptase inhibitors and protease inhibitors such as stavudine or zidovudine, and (2) discontinuation of causative medications in favor of an alternative that includes medications such as tenofovir or possibly abacavir, which tend to have less of an association with lipodystrophy. The presence of preexisting HIV drug resistance and the patient's treatment history must be considered prior to changing antiretrovirals and is best left to the patient's primary HIV provider [14]. Discontinuation of the causative agents can partially reverse these changes; however, some may be nonreversible. Diet, exercise, weight loss, plastic surgery, and dermal fillers are alternative options for patients who are on effective antiviral regimens. Currently, there are two dermal fillers that are FDA approved for treating facial lipoatrophy in HIV patients: poly-L-lactic acid (PLLA or Sculptra™) and calcium hydroxylapatite (Radiesse™). Thiazolidinediones have also been studied for the treatment of HIV lipoatrophy but studies have demonstrated conflicting outcomes [15].

References

1. Moore RD. Epidemiology of HIV infection in the United States: implications for linkage to care. Clin Infect Dis. 2011;52 Suppl 2:S208–13.
2. Strachan DD. The dermatological manifestations of HIV infection in ethnic skin. New York: Springer; 2009.
3. HIV/AIDS Surveillance Report. 2007. Accessed 2013, at http://cdc.gov/hiv/topics/surveillance/resources/reports/2007report/pdf/2007SurveillanceReport.pdf.
4. Su W, Berthelot C, Cockerell CJ. Viral infections in HIV disease. In: Cockerell C, Calame A (eds.) Cutaneous manifestations of HIV disease. London: Manson Publishing; 2012; pp 11–37.
5. Cedeno-Laurent F, Gomez-Flores M, Mendez N, et al. New insights into HIV-1-primary skin disorders. J Int AIDS Soc. 2011;14:1–11.
6. Morrell P, Calame A, Cockerell CJ. Papulosquamous skin disorders in HIV infection. London: Manson Publishing; 2012.
7. Amerson EH, Maurer TA. Dermatologic manifestations of HIV in Africa. Top HIV Med. 2010;18:16–22.
8. Aftergut K, Cockerell CJ. Update on the cutaneous manifestations of HIV infection. Clinical and pathologic features. Dermatol Clin. 1999;17:445–71, vii.
9. Berthelot C, Cockerell CJ. Cutaneous neoplastic manifestations of HIV disease. London: Manson Publishing; 2012.
10. Hagensee ME, Cameron JE, Leigh JE, Clark RA. Human papillomavirus infection and disease in HIV-infected individuals. Am J Med Sci. 2004;328:57–63.
11. Kamalpour J, Calame A, Cockerell CJ. Cutaneous manifestations of deep fungal infections in HIV disease. London: Manson Publishing; 2012.
12. Cook-Norris RH, Calame A, Cockerell CJ. Oral and ocular manifestations of HIV infection. London: Manson Publishing; 2012.
13. Safrin S, Grunfeld C. Fat distribution and metabolic changes in patients with HIV infection. AIDS. 1999;13:2493–505.
14. Singhania R, Kotler DP. Lipodystrophy in HIV patients: its challenges and management approaches. HIV AIDS (Auckl). 2011;3:135–43.
15. Cofrancesco Jr J, Freedland E, McComsey G. Treatment options for HIV-associated central fat accumulation. AIDS Patient Care STDS. 2009;23:5–18.

Part VII

Neoplasms

Seborrheic Keratoses, Dermatosis Papulosa Nigra, and Dermatofibromas

39

Diane Jackson-Richards

Contents

39.1 Epidemiology and Etiology

Seborrheic keratoses (SKs) are among the most common benign skin lesions seen in the general population. SKs are such a common incidental skin finding that epidemiological studies are lacking. SKs typically may present as early as the 30's but become more common with advancing age. SKs occur worldwide and in all races and equally between the sexes. In general SKs are felt to be more common in Caucasians. Dermatosis papulosa nigra (DPN) is felt to be a subset of seborrheic keratoses as they share common histopathologic features. DPNs are seen primarily in persons of African descent but are also common in other darker-skinned races such as Hispanics and Asians. Similar to SKs, DPNs have a familial tendency and become more frequent with age. The etiology of SKs and DPNs is unknown. SKs occur in covered and sun-exposed areas of the body; however, because of the high frequency of both these lesions on the face, sun exposure has been hypothesized as a possible etiologic factor. A study by Yeatman et al. [1] examined SKs in Australians and found a higher prevalence of lesions in sun-exposed areas. A study by Kwon et al. evaluated SKs in 303 Korean males. They found that 88.1 % of Korean males, aged 40–70, had at least one SK. This is similar to the incidence seen in Caucasians. They examined the number and location of lesions and history of sun exposure. SKs on exposed skin (face and hands) involved a greater surface area and lesions steadily grew in size [2]. DPNs were the focus of a study done by Niang et al. in Dakar, Senegal. Thirty patients were examined and treated for DPNs over a 6-month period. They found a genetic predisposition in 93.3 % as well as a female predominance and presentation mainly in sun-exposed areas [3].

Dermatofibromas are very common, benign dermal tumors composed of fibrohistiocytes. The exact etiology is unknown. There is debate as to whether they are neoplasms or rather reactive hyperplasia to minor cutaneous trauma or insect bites. Initial minor insult to the skin may incite a reactive hyperplasia with eventual autonomous growth that yields a benign neoplasm [4]. Dermatofibromas usually are seen in middle-aged adults and more frequently in females [4].

D. Jackson-Richards, MD
Department of Dermatology, Multicultural Dermatology Center, Henry Ford Hospital, 3031 West Grand Blvd., Detroit, MI 48202, USA
e-mail: djackso1@hfhs.org

D. Jackson-Richards, A.G. Pandya (eds.), *Dermatology Atlas for Skin of Color*,
DOI 10.1007/978-3-642-54446-0_39,© Springer-Verlag Berlin Heidelberg 2014

39.2 Clinical Features

SKs can occur on any skin area other than the palms, soles, or mucous membranes. The face and trunk are the most common areas involved, followed by the upper and lower extremities (Figs. 39.1, 39.2, 39.3, 39.4, and 39.5). SKs are well-demarcated papules and plaques with an average size of 0.4–1.5 cm. Lesions as large as 5 cm occasionally occur. The color varies from yellow or flesh-colored to dark brown or black with brown being most common. Keratotic plugging can be seen within lesions and is helpful in making the diagnosis. SKs are asymptomatic unless external irritation occurs. Pruritus, and more rarely tenderness, may occur. DPNs are dark brown to black, flat-topped, or pedunculated 1–5 mm papules (Figs. 39.6, 39.7, and 39.8). The most common location is the malar area of the face or periorbital region but the neck and upper trunk are also involved. Both SKs and DPNs have a strong familial tendency and become more numerous with age; however, DPNs may have onset as early as the mid 20's. The cosmetic appearance is a predominant concern for most patients.

Dermatofibromas present as firm, smooth papules or nodules that are 2–10 mm in size. Lesions can be up to 2 cm but these are much less common. Dermatofibromas are usually hyperpigmented especially in darker skin but color can vary from flesh-colored to pink to dark brown. Most commonly they present on the lower extremities followed by the upper extremities and proximal trunk (Figs. 39.9, 39.10, 39.11, and 39.12). Rarely are lesions found on the face, fingers, or toes. When lesions are gently palpated or pinched, there is a downward movement producing what is referred to as the "dimple sign." Dermatofibromas are usually asymptomatic and remain stable for many years. Multiple eruptive dermatofibromas have been described in the setting of lupus erythematosus profundus, immunosuppression, and HIV infection.

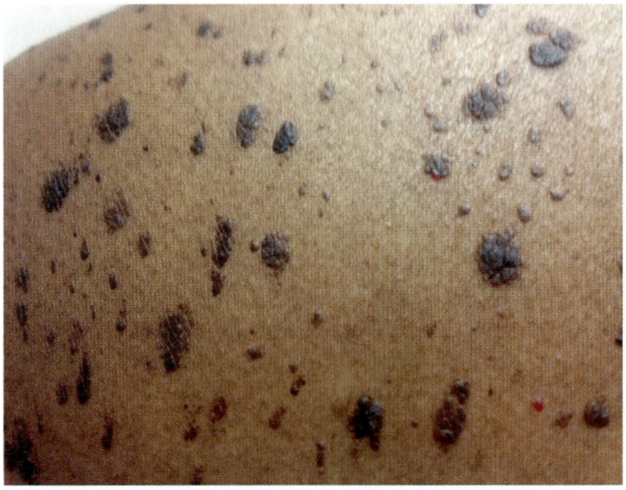

Fig. 39.1 Seborrheic keratoses on the back of an African-American female

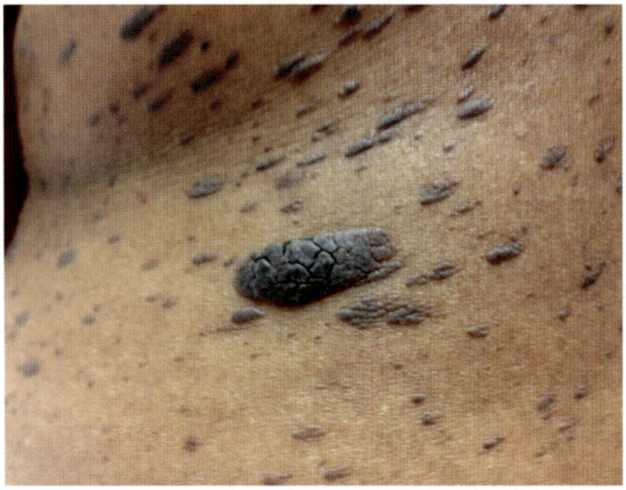

Fig. 39.2 Seborrheic keratoses on the trunk of an African-American female

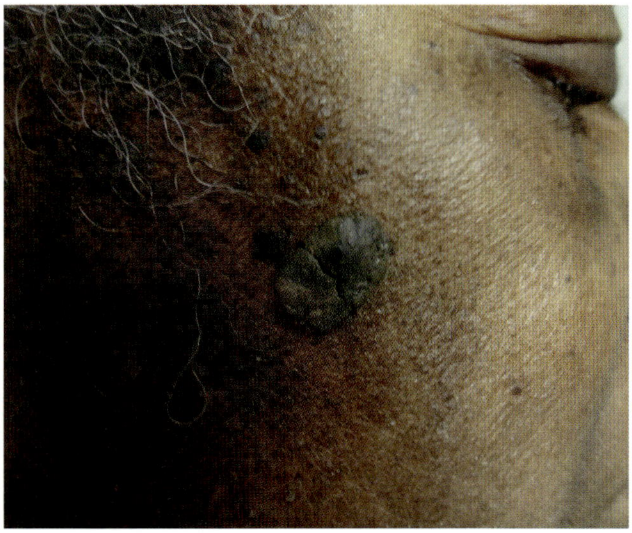

Fig. 39.3 Large seborrheic keratosis on the face of an African-American female

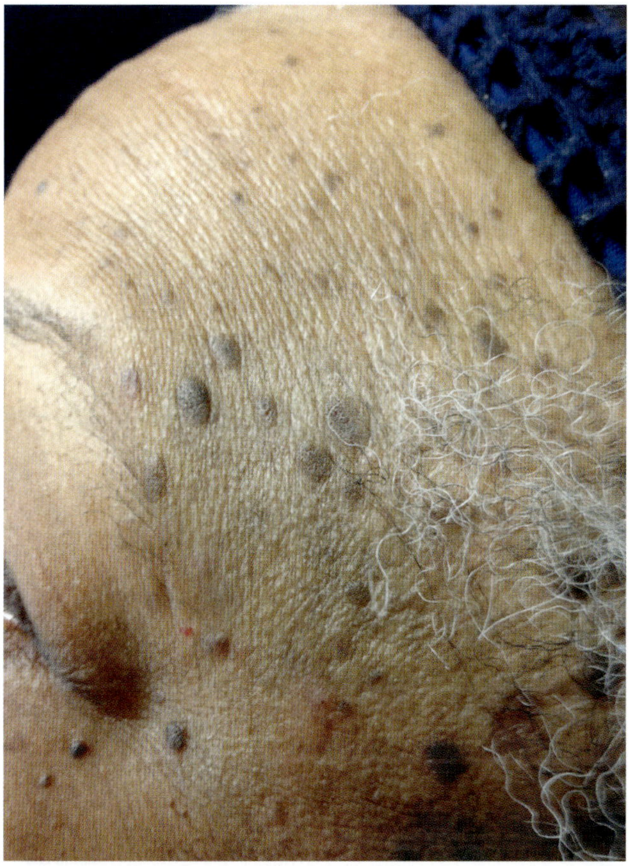

Fig. 39.4 Seborrheic keratoses on the temple and forehead of an African-American female

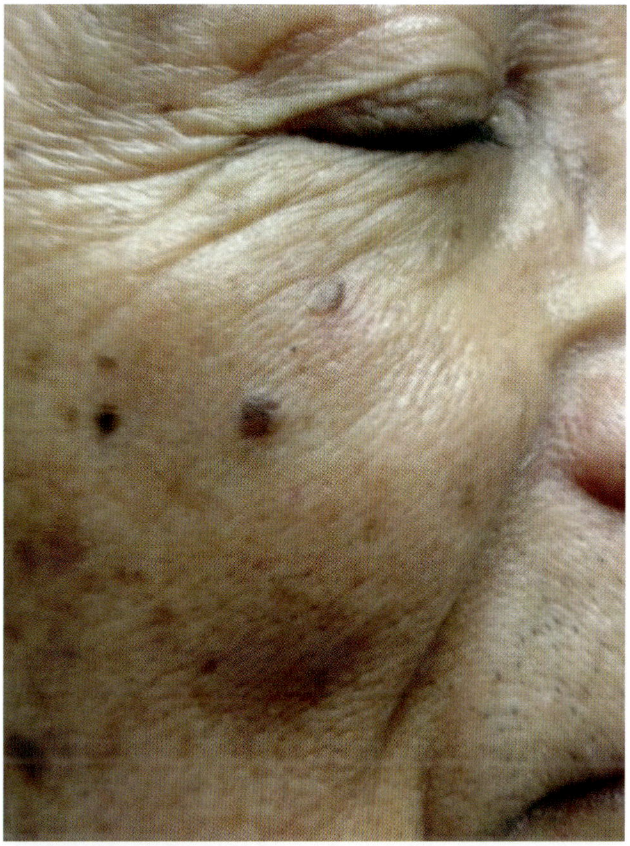

Fig. 39.5 Seborrheic keratoses on the cheek of an Asian male

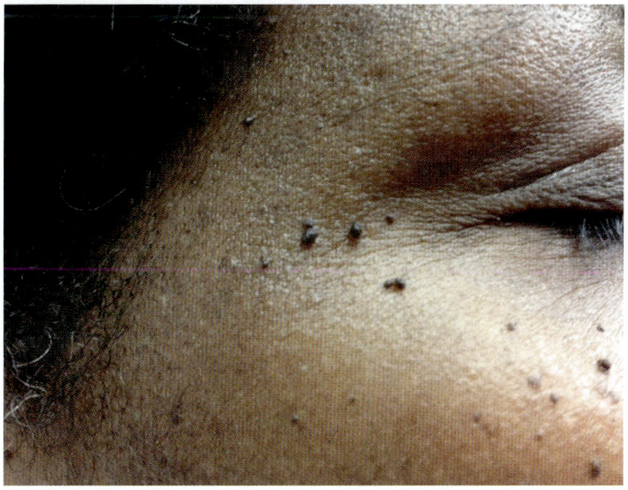

Fig. 39.6 Dermatosis papulosa nigra on the cheek of an African-American female

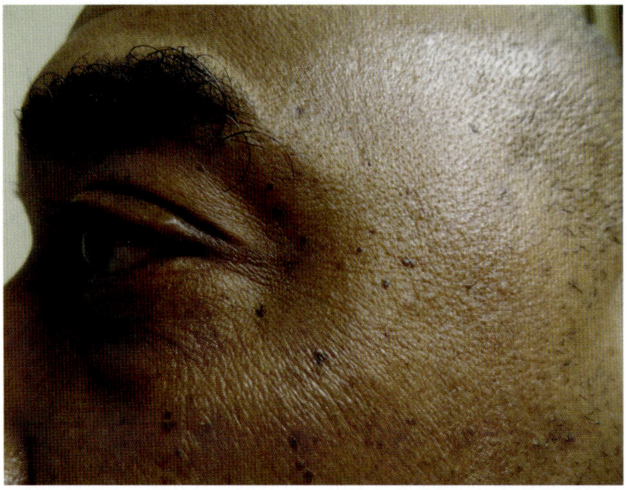

Fig. 39.7 Dermatosis papulosa nigra on the temple and cheek of an African-American male

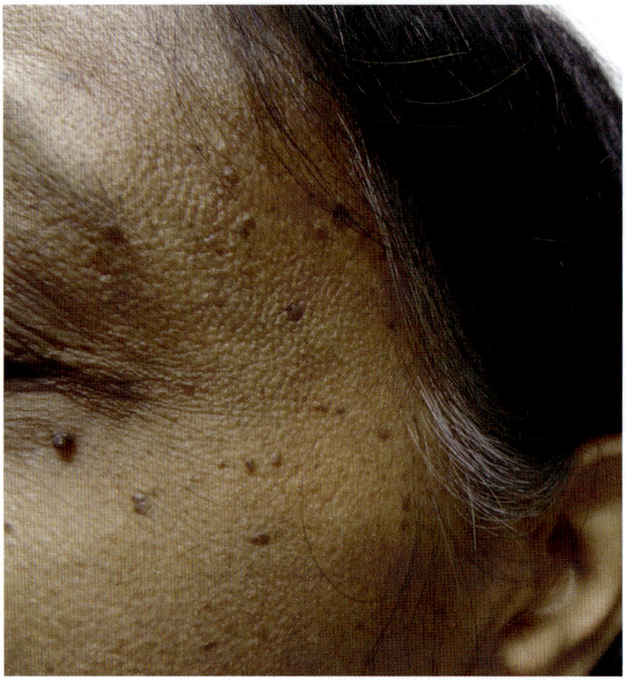

Fig. 39.8 Dermatosis papulosa nigra on the temple of a South Asian female

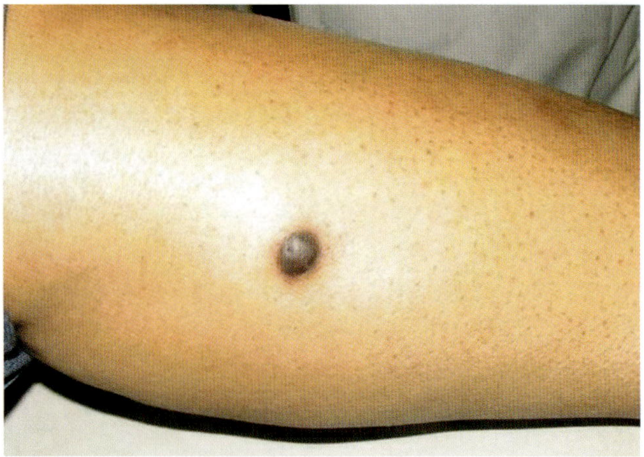

Fig. 39.9 Dermatofibroma on the leg of an AA female

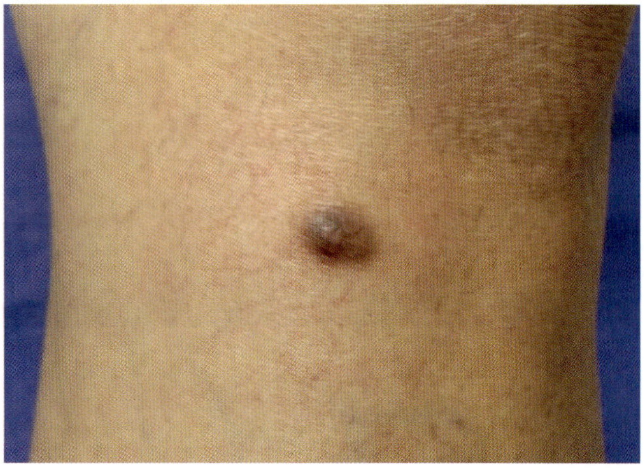

Fig. 39.10 Dermatofibroma below the knee of an AA female

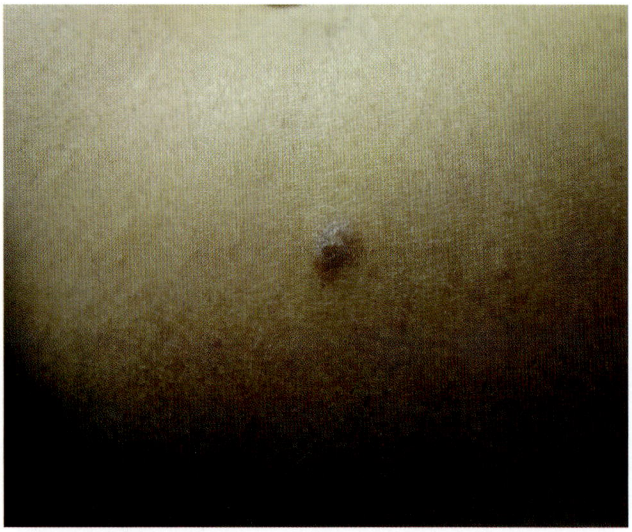

Fig. 39.11 Dermatofibroma on the leg of a Hispanic female

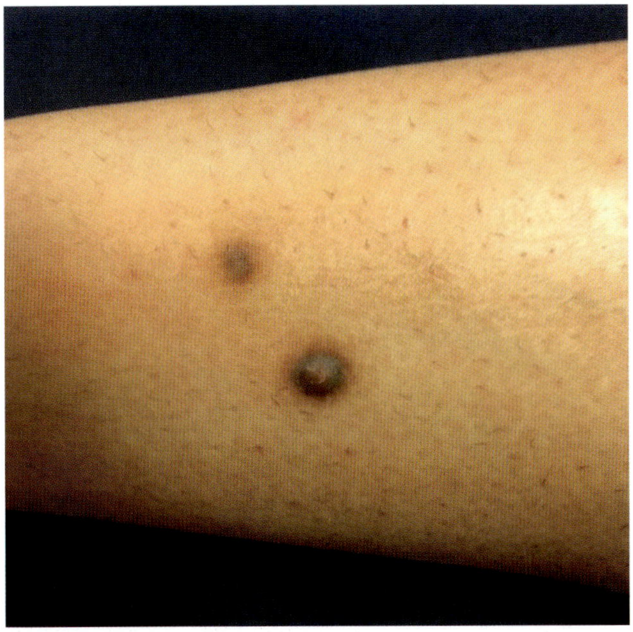

Fig. 39.12 Dermatofibromas on the lower leg of an AA female

39.3 Histopathologic Features

Six different histologic types of seborrheic keratosis have been reported, including acanthotic, hyperkeratotic, reticulated, clonal, irritated, and melanoacanthoma. The acanthotic type is most common. All seborrheic keratoses show hyperkeratosis, acanthosis, and papillomatosis. The acanthosis is due to the upward growth of the SK and the lesions are often described as having a straight line forming the lower border of the lesion. Acanthotic SKs show a thickened epidermis with mild hyperkeratosis and papillomatosis. The thickened epidermis is primarily composed of basaloid cells as opposed to squamous cells. A characteristic feature is pseudo-horn cysts that are completely keratinized horny invaginations. Melanin is increased in the keratinocytes. If lesions are inflamed, there may be a lichenoid infiltrate. DPNs have the same histology as acanthotic SKs, however, the epidermis shows more squamous cells rather than basaloid cells [5].

DFs show a hyperplastic epidermis with hyperpigmentation of the basal layer. The dermal tumor component consists of spindle-shaped fibroblasts along with histiocytes. Histiocytes may be mono- or multinucleated with a vacuolated or foamy cytoplasm. Hyalinized collagen bundles are seen at the periphery of the tumor. Adnexal structures are rare at the center of the lesion, however, hyperplastic sebaceous glands and aggregates of basaloid cells emanating from the epidermis can be seen. Hemorrhage into a dermatofibroma or hemosiderin in macrophages can be seen. Positive immunohistochemical staining with smooth muscle actin and factor XIIIa along with negative CD34 supports the diagnosis. Dermatofibromasarcoma protuberans shows a net-like permeation of the subcutis and positive CD34 staining [6].

39.4 Differential Diagnosis

The dark brown or black color of SKs often brings about concern for atypical melanocytic nevi or melanoma to the inexperienced observer. The differential diagnosis also includes acrochordon, verruca vulgaris, or Bowen's disease. Early SKs with minimal elevation may be mistaken for solar lentigines. SKs in the genital area are difficult to distinguish from condyloma acuminata. DPNs may present like acrochordons and vice versa.

39.5 Treatment

Since SKs and DPNs are benign lesions, treatment is usually for cosmetic reasons. Cryotherapy, shave or snip excision, curettage, electrodessication, or destruction with lasers have all been used successfully. The method of destruction has to be considered carefully in darker skin because of the risk of hypo- or hyperpigmentation. Cryotherapy is particularly destructive to melanocytes and often leaves hypopigmentation. There are reports of 532-diode laser [7], potassium-titanyl-phosphate laser [8], and 1,064 nm Nd:YAG laser being used to treat DPNs with good cosmetic outcome.

Treatment of dermatofibromas is usually unnecessary, as the resultant scar is usually worse than the original lesion. Excision can be performed if the diagnosis is uncertain or for cosmetic reasons.

References

1. Yeatman J, Kilkenny M, Marks R. The prevalence of seborrheic keratosis in an Australian population: does exposure to sunlight play a part in their frequency? Br J Dermatol. 1997;137:411–4.
2. Kwon OS, Hwang EJ, Bae JH, Park HE, Lee JC, Youn JI, Chung JH. Seborrheic keratosis in the Korean males: causative role of sunlight. Photodermatol Photoimmunol Photomed. 2003;19:73–80.
3. Niang SO, Kane A, Diallo M, Choutah F, Dieng MT, Ndiaye B. Dermatosis papulosa nigra in Dakar, Senegal. Int J Dermatol. 2007; 46 Suppl 1:45–7.
4. Hugel H. Fibrohistiocytic skin tumors. J Dtsch Dermatol Ges. 2006; 4(7):544–55.
5. Lever WF, Schaumburg-Lever G. Histopathology of the skin. 7th ed. Philadelphia: JB Lippincott; 1990.
6. Kamino H, Salcedo E. Histopathologic and immunohistochemical diagnosis of benign and malignant fibrous and fibrohistiocytic tumors of the skin. Dermatol Clin. 1999;17(3):487–505.
7. Lupo M. Dermatosis papulosis nigra: treatment options. J Drugs Dermatol. 2007;6:29–30.
8. Kundu RV, Joshi SS, Suh K, Boone SL, Huggins RH, Alam M, White L, Rademaker AW, West DP, Yoo S. Comparison of electrodesiccation and potassium-titanyl-phosphate laser for treatment of dermatosis papulosa nigra. Dermatol Surg. 2009;35:1079–83.

Keloids

40

Tiffany T. Mayo and Donald A. Glass II

Contents

40.1 Introduction

Keloids are exuberant cutaneous scars that form due to the abnormal growth of fibrous tissue following an injury. They were first described in the Smith papyrus around 1700 BC and have been depicted in West Nigerian sculptures as early as the thirteenth century [1]. The word *keloid* is a derivative of *chele*, a Greek term meaning "crab claw," proposed by Alibert in the early nineteenth century to describe their lateral extension into normal skin [2].

Though keloids are seen in all races, they are 15 times more common in patients of African, Hispanic, or Asian lineage than in Caucasians [2]. The prevalence of keloids is estimated to be between 4 and 6 % in those of African descent, though it has been reported as high as 16 % [3]. They occur equally in males and females [2]. The highest incidence of keloids occurs in the second and third decades of life; they rarely occur in childhood or in the elderly [2, 4]. Most keloids occur sporadically, but there are families with multiple generations affected. Familial keloids most commonly occur in an autosomal dominant inheritance pattern with incomplete penetrance and variable expressivity [5]. Keloids often occur in patients with Rubinstein-Taybi syndrome (mutations in CREBBP and EP300), whereas there are no known reports of keloids in albinos [2].

The most frequent precipitating event causing keloid formation is trauma, including surgery, abrasions, lacerations, and piercings (Fig. 40.1). Acne is another relatively common cause of keloids (Fig. 40.2). Minor burns and vaccinations have also been associated with keloids. Spontaneous keloid formation has been reported, particularly on presternal skin [3, 6].

T.T. Mayo, BS, MS, MD
Department of Dermatology,
University of Alabama at Birmingham,
EFH 414, 1530 3rd Avenue South,
Birmingham, AL 35294-0009, USA
e-mail: tmayo@uabmc.edu

D.A. Glass II, MD, PhD (✉)
Department of Dermatology,
University of Texas Southwestern Medical Center,
5323 Harry Hines Blvd., 9069,
Dallas, TX 75390-9069, USA
e-mail: donald.glass@utsouthwestern.edu

D. Jackson-Richards, A.G. Pandya (eds.), *Dermatology Atlas for Skin of Color*,
DOI 10.1007/978-3-642-54446-0_40, © Springer-Verlag Berlin Heidelberg 2014

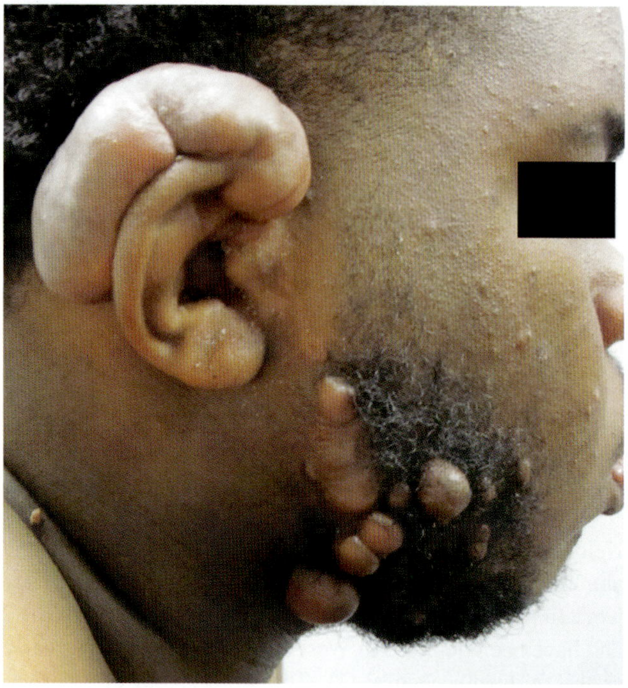

Fig. 40.1 African-American male with keloids on the ear and beard area due to dog bites

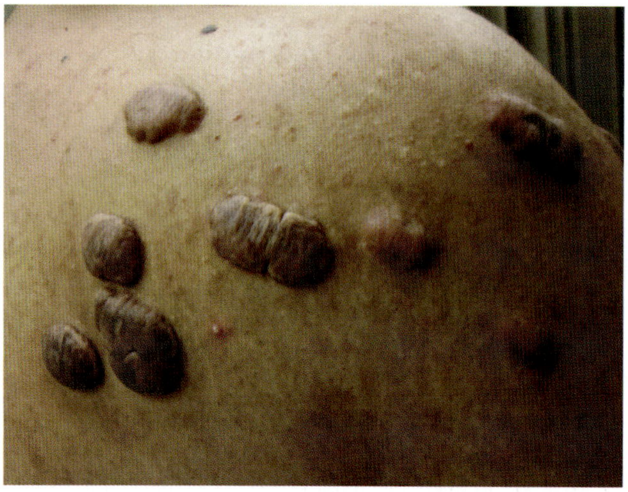

Fig. 40.2 Hispanic male with acne-induced keloids. Note the pustules on the patient's back

40.2 Clinical Features

Keloids appear as firm, well-demarcated nodules or tumors with shiny surfaces and irregular borders (Fig. 40.3). They are usually pink, skin colored, or hyperpigmented (Fig. 40.4). Telangiectasias may also be present. The morphological appearance can vary depending on the anatomic location. Keloids are most commonly located on the presternal area, back, shoulders, earlobes, and posterior neck (Figs. 40.5 and 40.6) [4]. The beard area of the face and the upper extremities are more often affected than the lower extremities. Keloids rarely occur on the genitalia, palms, or soles. Pain, pruritus, and paresthesias are frequently reported symptoms [2, 4, 6]. Infection and ulceration may also occur [3].

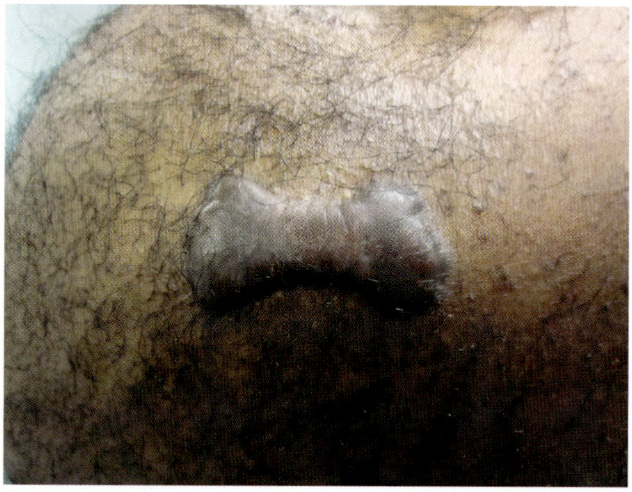

Fig. 40.3 African-American male with hyperpigmented dumbbell-shaped keloid scar on the shoulder

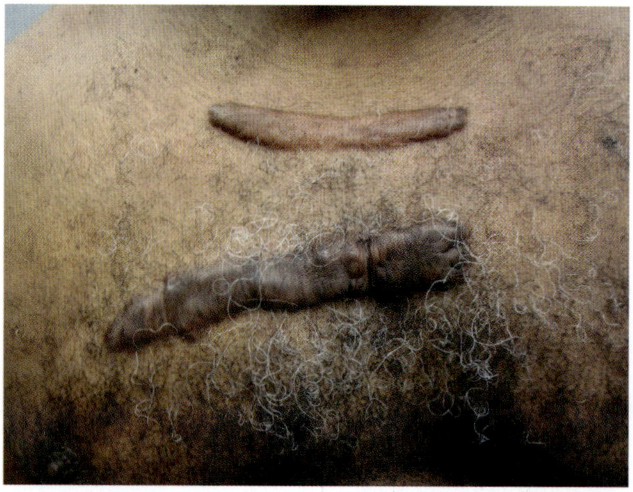

Fig. 40.4 A skin-colored and a hyperpigmented linear keloid on the chest of an African male

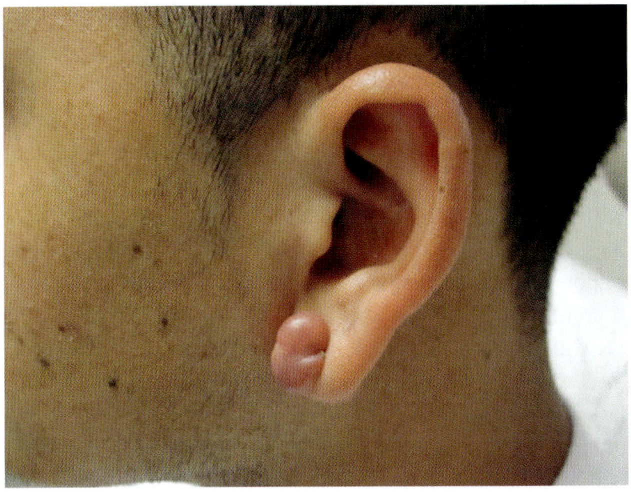

Fig. 40.5 Erythematous small keloid on the left earlobe of a Hispanic male

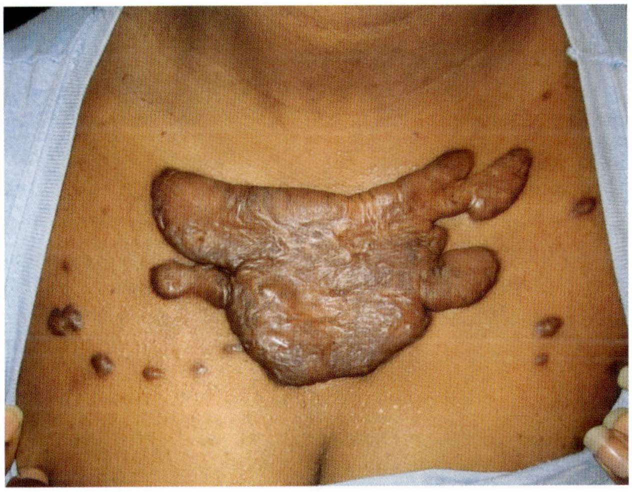

Fig. 40.6 Large keloid with smaller surrounding lesions on the chest of an African-American female

40.3 Natural History and Prognosis

Keloids usually appear within 3 months of a precipitating trauma but their emergence may be delayed by several years. They have a gradual onset and can remain actively growing for many years. The characteristic feature distinguishing keloids from hypertrophic scars is the tendency of the former to grow past the boundaries of the original injury and invade into the surrounding normal skin. Hypertrophic scars, in contrast, remain confined to the margins of the original cutaneous injury. Keloids do not undergo spontaneous regression and tend to recur after surgical excision [2–4].

40.4 Histopathologic Features

Keloids are histologically characterized by a nodular proliferation of fibroblasts with haphazardly arranged, thick eosinophilic hyalinized collagen fibers in the dermis. Hypertrophic scars differ from keloids in that they tend to have epidermal atrophy, are often more cellular, and have less hyalinized collagen fibers than keloids [7].

40.5 Diagnosis and Differential Diagnosis

The diagnosis of keloids is often a clinical diagnosis because biopsy may induce further growth. Differential diagnoses include other benign conditions (e.g., dermatofibroma and adult onset juvenile xanthogranuloma), systemic fibrotic/sclerotic conditions (e.g., nodular scleroderma), and malignant tumors (e.g., dermatofibrosarcoma protuberans) [8]. Lobomycosis should be considered for keloid-like lesions occurring on the ears.

40.6 Treatment

Preventing unnecessary trauma is the most effective way to manage keloid formation in those who are predisposed. There are a number of modalities available to treat formed keloids but none are 100 % effective in preventing regrowth or recurrence (Fig. 40.7). If acne is the cause of keloids, it must be treated aggressively to prevent lesions long-term.

Surgical excision is a commonly used therapeutic technique. When surgery is indicated, suturing techniques that reduce skin tension should be attempted in those with a history of keloids or those at risk for keloid formation. When used alone, surgical excision has a rate of recurrence ranging from 45 to 100 %; therefore, it is usually used in combination with other therapies [9].

Intralesional corticosteroids remain a first-line therapeutic option in the treatment of keloids. They are often effective in producing softer, flatter, and smaller lesions. Aside from pain associated with the injection, over 60 % of patients are reported to experience side effects such as atrophy, dyspigmentation, and telangiectasias (Fig. 40.8) [9].

Pressure therapy is a common intervention used to prevent hypertrophic scars and is also used to prevent keloid recurrence after surgical excision, especially on the earlobes. Mechanical pressure devices are applied maintaining pressures between 24 and 30 mmHg for up to 12 months [9].

Silicone gel is an effective and painless option for treating keloids. The sheets are placed over the keloid or site of trauma and are thought to work due to the direct effects of occlusion, including increased hydration and possibly increased oxygen tension [9]. They are much more effective in preventing keloid occurrence after trauma than in reducing the size of an already formed keloid.

Radiation therapy is used in keloids refractory to other therapeutic modalities and is most often used in combination with surgery. When used as a monotherapy, recurrence rates have been reported between 50 and 100 %. Due to concerns of potential carcinogenic side effects, this therapy is reserved for adults with refractory keloids [9, 10].

Multiple lasers have been used to treat keloids in the past three decades. More recently the Nd:YAG and pulsed-dye lasers have been used and are thought to be effective in reducing pain and pruritus, hyperpigmentation, and the height of keloids [10].

Cryotherapy has been found to be useful in flattening small keloids. It can cause hypopigmentation and is therefore not used frequently in patients with darker skin [10]. Intralesional cryotherapy, rather than external application, is an emerging new treatment modality.

Interferon, 5-fluorouracil (5-FU), and bleomycin are relatively new promising therapies to treat keloids. Intralesional interferon injections have been shown to increase the breakdown of collagen. 5-FU injections have also demonstrated promise and work by inhibiting fibroblast proliferation. Bleomycin has demonstrated a flattening effect but also has hyperpigmentation as a reported side effect [9, 10]. Though new techniques are promising, more research is needed in the genetics, prevention, and treatment of keloids.

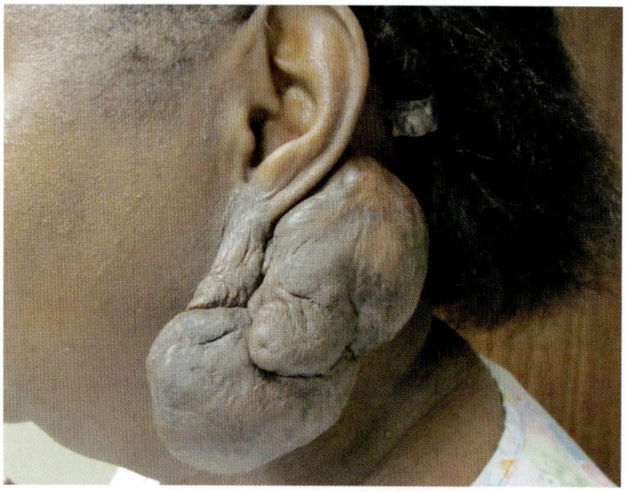

Fig. 40.7 African-American female with a recurrent earlobe keloid despite several excisions, intralesional triamcinolone, and radiation therapy

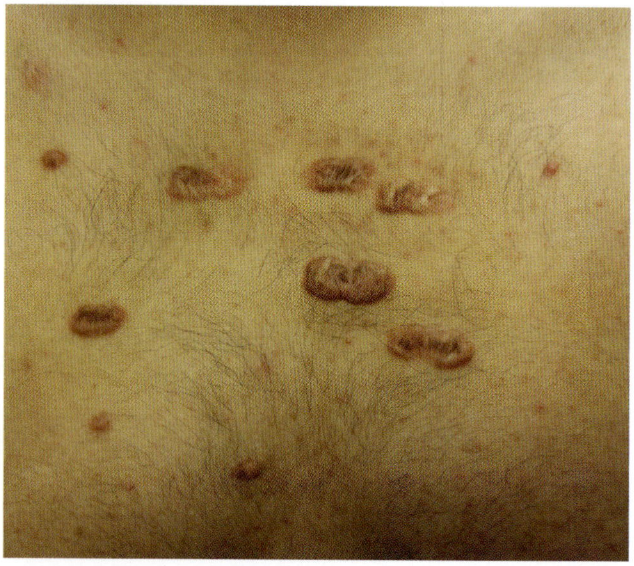

Fig. 40.8 Softer, less-raised keloids with dyspigmentation after intralesional steroids on a Hispanic male (same patient as Fig. 40.2)

References

1. Berman B, Bieley HC. Keloids. J Am Acad Dermatol. 1995; 33:117–23.
2. Niessen FB, Spauwen PH, Schalkwijk J, Kon M. On the nature of hypertrophic scars and keloids: a review. Plast Reconstr Surg. 1999; 104:1435–58.
3. Cosman B, Crikelair GF, Ju DMC, Gaulin JC, Lattes R. The surgical treatment of keloids. Plast Reconstr Surg. 1961;27:335–58.
4. Datubo-Brown DD. Keloids: a review of the literature. Br J Plast Surg. 1990;43:70–7.
5. Marneros AG, Norris JE, Olsen BR, Reichenberger E. Clinical genetics of familial keloids. Arch Dermatol. 2001;137:1429–34.
6. Alhady SM, Sivanantharajah K. Keloids in various races. A review of 175 cases. Plast Reconstr Surg. 1969;44:564–6.
7. Calonje E, McKee P, Fletcher C. Tumors of the dermis and subcutaneous fat. In: McKee P, editor. Pathology of the skin. London: Mosby-Wolfe; 1996.
8. Ogawa R, Akaishi S, Hyakusoku H. Differential and exclusive diagnosis of diseases that resemble keloids and hypertrophic scars. Ann Plast Surg. 2009;62:660–4.
9. Mustoe TA, Cooter RD, Gold MH, Hobbs FD, Ramelet AA, Shakespeare PG, et al. International clinical recommendations on scar management. Plast Reconstr Surg. 2002;110:560–71.
10. Shaffer JJ, Taylor SC, Cook-Bolden F. Keloidal scars: a review with a critical look at therapeutic options. J Am Acad Dermatol. 2002;46:S63–97.

Acne Keloidalis Nuchae

41

Richard H. Huggins

Contents

41.1 Introduction

The condition that would later come to be known as acne keloidalis nuchae (AKN) was first described by Kaposi as dermatitis papillaris capillitii in 1879. Bazin renamed it acne keloidalis in 1882 [1]. AKN is a chronic inflammatory follicular disorder, primarily affecting black men, which presents with persistent papules and, in some cases, keloidal plaques on the occipital scalp and posterior neck.

41.2 Epidemiology

AKN overwhelmingly affects men of African descent. The prevalence in this population is estimated to be 1.3–16.3 % [2]. The condition tends to develop after puberty, with AKN being observed rarely in young children. Black women may infrequently be affected, with a male to female ratio of 20:1 reported [2]. There are only a few case reports of AKN in Caucasians.

R.H. Huggins, MD
Department of Dermatology, Henry Ford Hospital,
3031 West Grand Blvd., Suit 800 Dermatology,
Detroit, MI 48202, USA
e-mail: rhuggin1@hfhs.org

D. Jackson-Richards, A.G. Pandya (eds.), *Dermatology Atlas for Skin of Color*,
DOI 10.1007/978-3-642-54446-0_41, © Springer-Verlag Berlin Heidelberg 2014

41.3 Clinical Features

The typical initial presentation of AKN is the presence of small, firm, and persistent papules on the occiput and posterior neck (see Figs. 41.1, 41.2, and 41.3). In some cases these lesions coalesce to form fibrotic, alopecic, and keloid-like plaques (see Figs. 41.4, 41.5, 41.6, and 41.7). At any point, secondary infection may develop, manifested as pustules or purulent drainage in early lesions (see Fig. 41.8) and abscesses in more advanced lesions. Early disease may be asymptomatic or associated with varying degrees of pruritus. Plaque-stage disease is often associated with severe pruritus and significant pain.

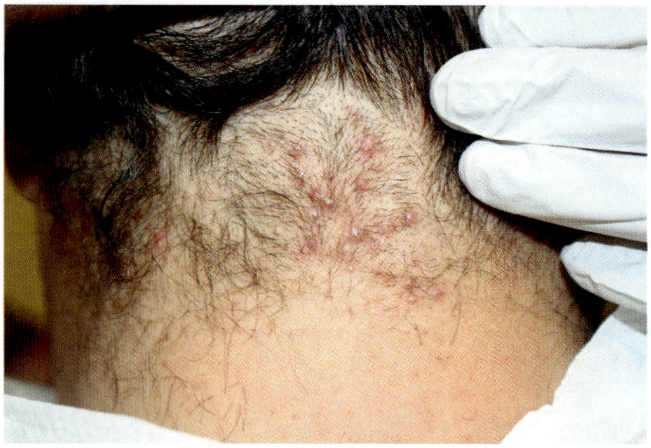

Fig. 41.3 Erythematous follicular papules in a Hispanic male

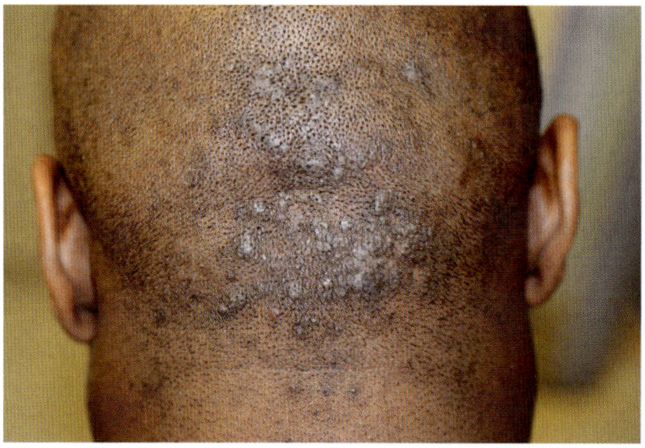

Fig. 41.1 Hyperpigmented, follicular papules in an African-American male

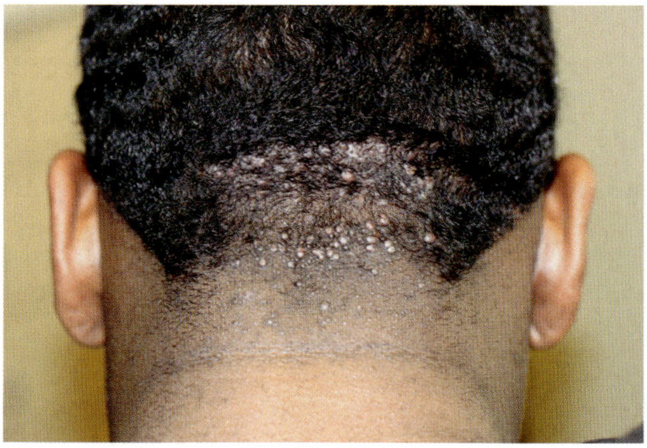

Fig. 41.4 Several hyperpigmented and erythematous follicular papules in an African-American male

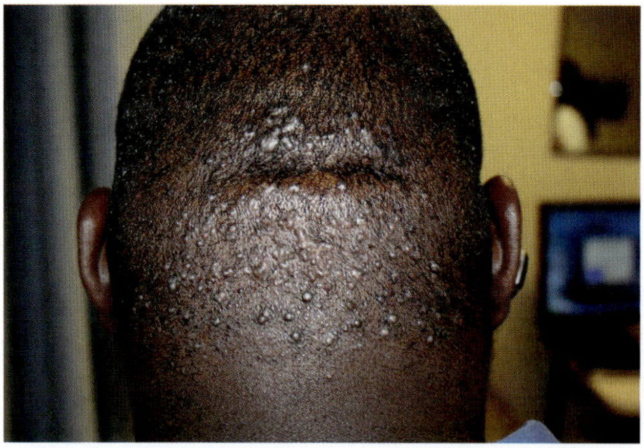

Fig. 41.2 Numerous hyperpigmented follicular papules and early plaques in an African-American male

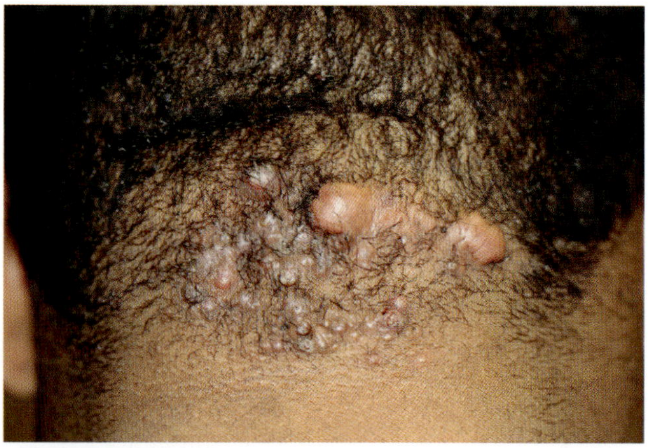

Fig. 41.5 Erythematous and flesh-colored follicular papules and keloidal plaques in an African-American male

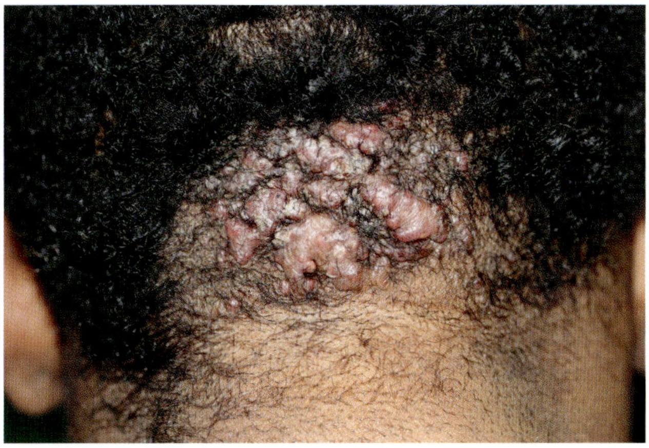

Fig. 41.6 Several erythematous keloidal plaques in an African-American male

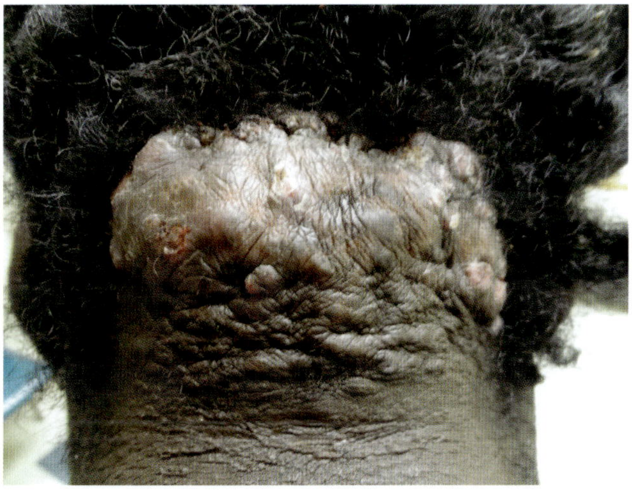

Fig. 41.7 Large coalescent keloidal plaque in an African-American male (Courtesy of Diane Jackson-Richards, MD)

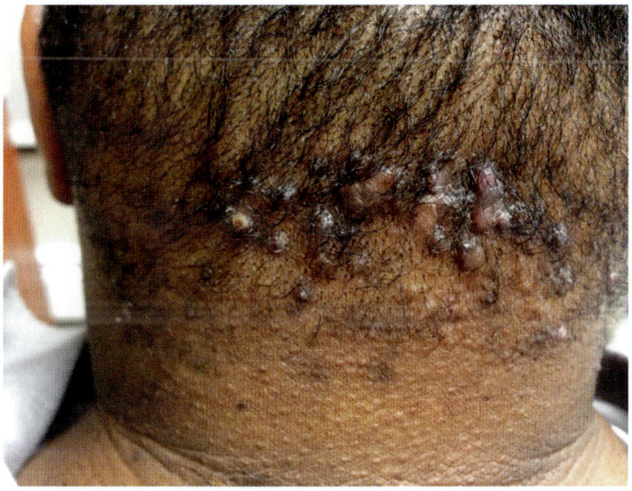

Fig. 41.8 Erythematous follicular papules and plaques and a single follicular pustule in an African-American male (Courtesy of Diane Jackson-Richards, MD)

41.4 Etiology

The complete pathogenesis of AKN has not yet been fully elucidated, but in all likelihood the etiology is multifactorial. Chronic trauma to the occipital scalp and posterior neck appears to be important in AKN development. Nearly 90 % of AKN cases are observed in individuals who have their hair cut closely with clipper. A significant proportion of AKN patients report crusting, new papule development, and even bleeding temporally associated with their haircuts, further supporting the traumatic nature of close haircuts [2]. Additionally, such individuals commonly have their hair cut every 1–2 weeks, hence the chronicity of this trauma. The highest prevalence of AKN is reported in African-American professional football players, individuals in whom helmets are sources of regular vigorous friction [2]. Constant neck irritation by collared shirts is another potential source of chronic trauma in affected patients.

There is evidence for a role of androgen excess in the development of AKN. Higher levels of testosterone have been found in men with the condition [3]. The predominant development of AKN after puberty further supports the possibility that androgens may be involved in AKN development. AKN has also been associated with seborrhea, certain medications (i.e., anticonvulsants and immunosuppressants), microorganisms, and a family history of AKN [3].

Of note, ingrown hairs are not seen on biopsies of AKN, making this an unlikely contributor to AKN development [4].

A histopathologic study of AKN suggests the following cascade in the pathogenesis of AKN. The trigger of the initial perifollicular inflammation is unclear, but potential agents include microbes, other extrinsic substances (i.e., cosmetics), sebum, or desquamated keratinocytes. Subsequently, the epithelium of the follicular wall is thought to be weakened by the acute inflammation caused by the trigger, leading to rupture of the hair follicle and release of the hair shaft into the dermis. It is believed this is followed by a granulomatous foreign-body reaction initiated by the presence of the naked hair shaft within the dermis, resulting in the appearance of papules on exam. As the condition progresses, the granulomatous inflammatory response predominates, resulting in fibrosis at the cellular level and keloid-like plaque development [4].

41.5 Histopathological Features

Because AKN has such a typical presentation, the diagnosis is usually based solely on clinical observation of characteristic lesions. When lesions are biopsied, the findings vary with the stage of development of the condition. Early lesions typically show a dense inflammatory infiltrate of neutrophils and lymphocytes both within and around the hair follicles, destruction of the follicular wall, and localized granulomatous inflammation. In more advanced lesions, scar formation, naked hair shafts within the dermis, and more widespread granulomatous inflammation are observed [4].

41.6 Treatment

AKN treatment should be tailored to the stage of development in each affected patient. Early lesions, primarily consisting of papules, may be amenable to medical and laser treatments. Topically, mid-strength to super-potent corticosteroids, retinoids, and imiquimod have been used with varying degrees of success. Intralesional corticosteroids may also be beneficial with papular disease. Topical and, in severe cases, systemic antibiotics are indicated when pustules or other signs of infection are present. Oral antibiotics with anti-inflammatory activity, such as tetracycline derivatives, may be useful even in the absence of obvious infection. Serial treatments with both the diode and long-pulsed neodymium-doped yttrium aluminum garnet (Nd: YAG) lasers have been used successfully to treat AKN. The Nd: YAG is thought to be safer to use in dark skin due to a lower incidence of complications, such as post-inflammatory hyperpigmentation [5–7].

For advanced disease, in which keloidal plaques are present, surgical excision should be considered. This has been performed successfully with the wounds being left to heal by secondary intention following excision with either a CO_2 laser or an electrosurgical unit. Healing time ranges between 6 and 8 weeks and the resulting cosmetic appearance is operator and patient dependent [8, 9].

References

1. Cosman B, Wolff M. Acne keloidalis. Plast Reconstr Surg. 1972;50:25–30.
2. Khumalo NP, Gumedze F, Lehloenya R. Folliculitis keloidalis nuchae is associated with the risk for bleeding from haircuts. Int J Dermatol. 2011;50:1212–6.
3. George AO, Akanji AO, Nduka EU, et al. Clinical, biochemical and morphologic features of acne keloidalis in a black population. Int J Dermatol. 1993;32:714–6.
4. Sperling LC, Homoky C, Pratt L, et al. Acne keloidalis is a form of primary scarring alopecia. Arch Dermatol. 2000;136:479–84.
5. Shah GK. Efficacy of diode laser for treating acne keloidalis nuchae. Indian J Dermatol Venereol Leprol. 2005;71:31–4.
6. Esmat SM, Abdel Hay RM, Abu Zeid OM. The efficacy of laser-assisted hair removal in the treatment of acne keloidalis nuchae; a pilot study. Eur J Dermatol. 2012;22:645–50.
7. Abergel RP, Dwyer RM, Meeker CA, et al. Laser treatment of keloids: a clinical trial and an in vitro study with Nd: YAG laser. Lasers Surg Med. 1984;4:291–5.
8. Kantor GR, Ratz JL, Wheeland RG. Treatment of acne keloidalis nuchae with carbon dioxide laser. J Am Acad Dermatol. 1986;14(2 Pt 1):263–7.
9. Beckett N, Lawson C, Cohen G. Electrosurgical excision of acne keloidalis nuchae with secondary intention healing. J Clin Aesthet Dermatol. 2011;4:36–9.

Basal Cell Carcinoma

42

Thao Duong and Divya Srivastava

Contents

T. Duong, MD (✉)
Department of Internal Medicine,
University of Texas at Southwestern, 5323 Harry Hines Blvd.,
Dallas, TX 75392, USA
e-mail: thao.duong@phhs.org

D. Srivastava, MD
Department of Dermatology,
University of Texas Southwestern Medical Center,
5939 Harry Hines Blvd., Suit 100, Dallas, TX 75390-9191, USA
e-mail: divya.srivastava@utsouthwestern.edu

42.1 Introduction

Basal cell carcinoma is a slow-growing skin cancer typically found on the head and neck that is induced by ultraviolet radiation. Individuals with darker skin types have inherent protection from ultraviolet light due to an increase in epidermal melanin causing sun-induced skin cancer to be less prevalent [1]. Although diagnosis and management are similar across different skin types, delays in diagnosis and treatment exist in darker skin types as there are false perceptions regarding inherent photoprotection and the ability to develop skin cancer.

42.2 Epidemiology

BCC is the most common skin cancer in Caucasians, Hispanics, Chinese, and Japanese and the second most common skin cancer in Blacks and Asian Indians. However, because melanin is photoprotective, BCC is 19 times more common in Caucasians than in Blacks [2]. BCC comprises 65–75 % of skin cancer in Caucasians, compared to 30 % in Indians, 12–35 % in American Blacks, and 2–8 % in African Blacks. Considering the diversity of skin color with different concentrations of melanin in the epidermis, inherent sun protection varies widely in skin color leading to variable prevalence rates [3].

42.3 Etiology

Basal cell carcinoma is associated with long-term cumulative ultraviolet radiation (UVR) exposure, particularly UVB. UVB directly damages DNA and RNA causing a transition mutation in the nucleic acid sequence [2]. Although UVR plays a significant role in the development of BCC, it is not the only risk factor, as BCC can also occur in non-sun-exposed skin. Other factors predisposing to BCC are ingestion of arsenic, radiation, scars, ulcers, albinism, nevus sebaceous, immunosuppression, and genetic conditions such as Gorlin's syndrome and xeroderma pigmentosum.

D. Jackson-Richards, A.G. Pandya (eds.), *Dermatology Atlas for Skin of Color*,
DOI 10.1007/978-3-642-54446-0_42,

42.4 Clinical Features

In skin of color patients, similar to Caucasians, BCC most commonly occurs in patients over age 50. Seventy to ninety percent of BCCs develop on the head and neck region, followed by the trunk, then extremities. The clinical presentation and histologic features of BCC are somewhat different in people of color than Caucasians [1, 4]. The most common clinical presentation across skin types is nodular BCC, which typically presents as a solitary asymptomatic papule or nodule with telangiectasias and a rolled border. As lesions progress, they may develop ulceration (Figs. 42.1, 42.2, and 42.3). The classic findings of telangiectasias and a pearly rolled border may be challenging to appreciate in darker skin types [5]. BCCs in Asians often appear brown to glossy black and are described as having a "pearly black" appearance. Pigmented BCC, a variant of nodular BCC, is much more common in darker-skinned patients and represents more than 50 % of BCCs in Blacks, Hispanics, and Asians, compared to 6 % in Caucasians (Figs. 42.4 and 42.5) [1, 5]. Superficial BCC presents as an erythematous scaly plaque most commonly on the trunk or extremity (Fig. 42.6). Morpheaform BCC is less common in Blacks than Caucasians and presents with a porcelain-colored plaque with smooth indistinct borders that may be atrophic or indurated (Fig. 42.7).

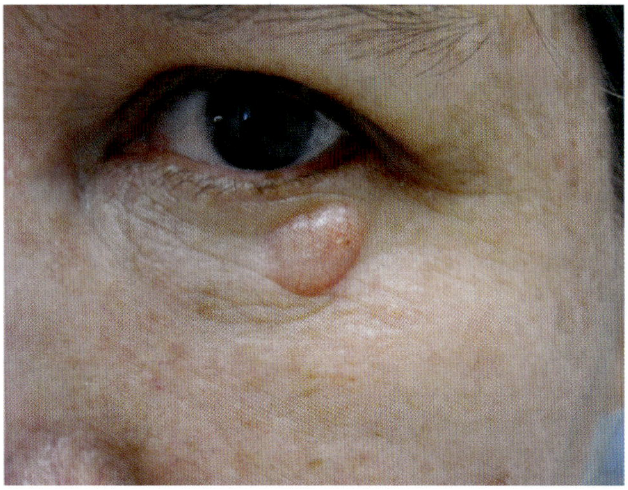

Fig. 42.1 Nodular BCC presenting as a pearly papule with telangiectasias on the lower eyelid of a Hispanic female

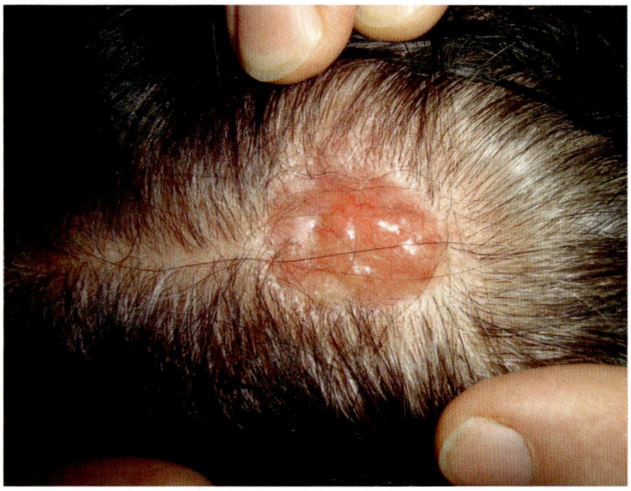

Fig. 42.3 Large nodular BCC on the scalp of an elderly Hispanic female

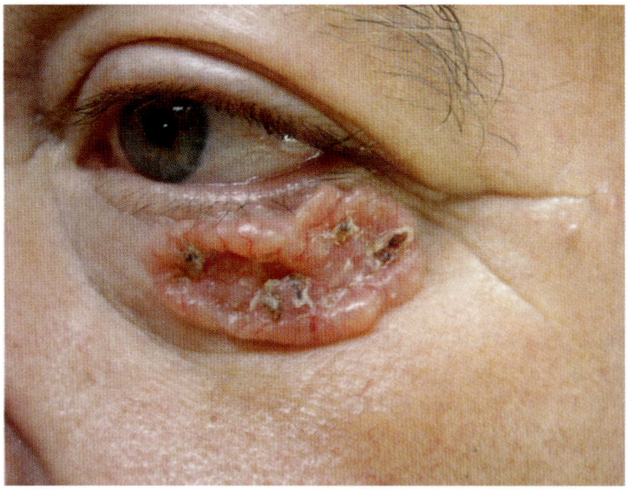

Fig. 42.2 Large nodular BCC with prominent telangiectasias, a translucent rolled border, and early central ulceration on the lower eyelid of a Hispanic female

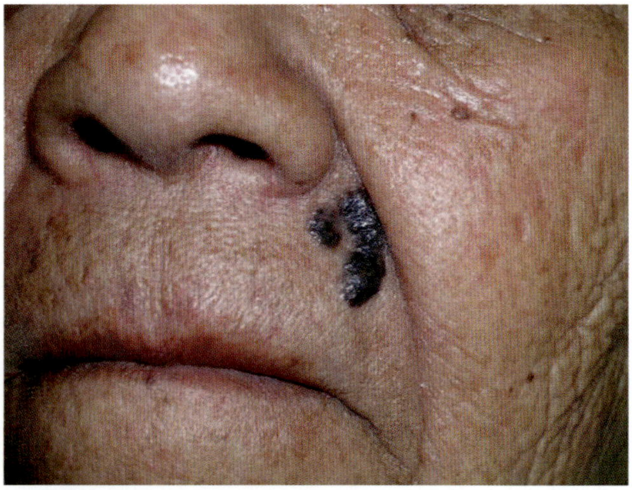

Fig. 42.4 Pigmented BCC with glossy black or pearly black appearance on the upper cutaneous lip of a Hispanic male

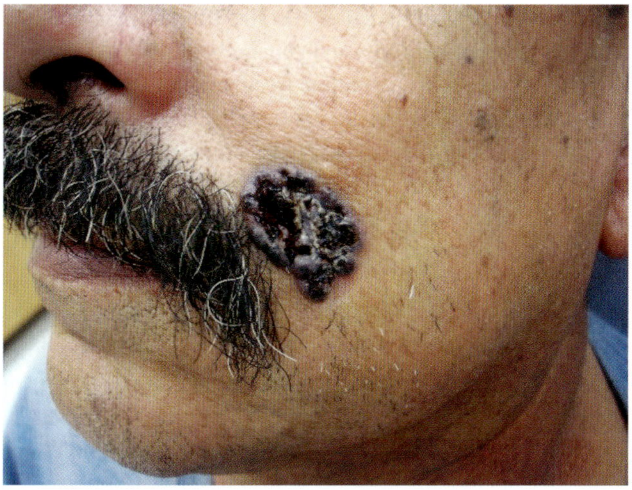

Fig. 42.5 Pigmented BCC with rolled border and central ulceration on the cheek of a Hispanic male

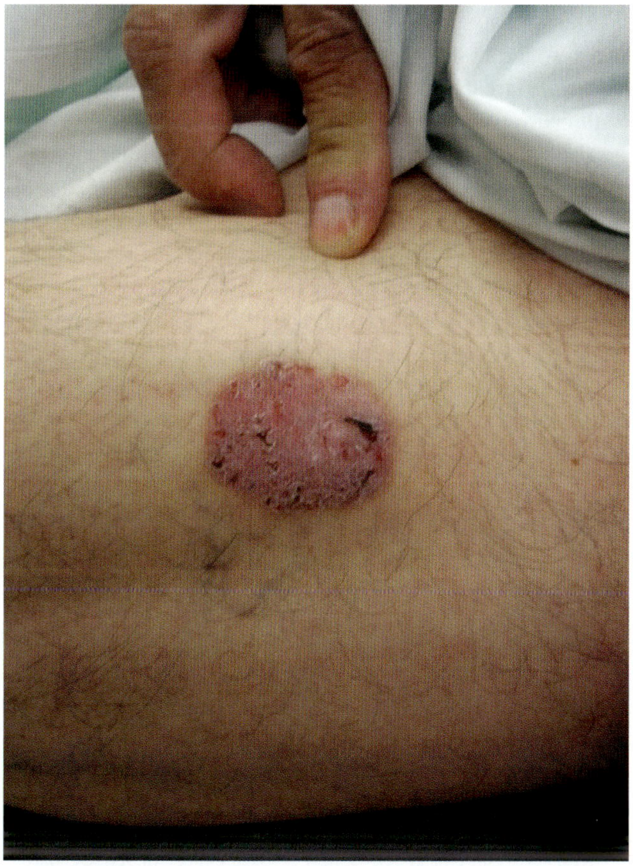

Fig. 42.6 Superficial BCC presenting as erythematous scaly plaque on the arm of a Hispanic male

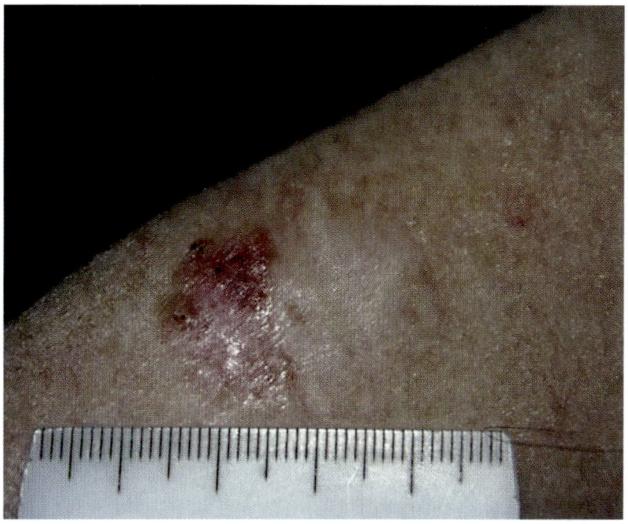

Fig. 42.7 Morpheaform BCC with features of pearliness and porcelain-white areas on the arm of a Hispanic female

42.5 Natural History and Prognosis

Although BCCs are slow-growing neoplasms that rarely metastasize, they can be locally invasive and can cause significant morbidity and cosmetic disfigurement. Metastatic rates range from 0.0028 to 0.1 % and do not vary based on skin type.

42.6 Histopathology

BCC is classified into five main histologic and clinical subtypes. The most common subtype, nodular BCC, is characterized by basophilic aggregates with peripheral palisading and retraction artifact in the papillary and reticular dermis. Pigmented BCC also has melanin and melanocytes within the tumor. Superficial BCC has similar basophilic aggregates with peripheral palisading and clefting arising from the epidermis. Micronodular BCC is similar to nodular BCC, with smaller tumor islands that are widely dispersed. Infiltrative BCC presents with cords and strands of neoplastic cells infiltrating through collagen fibers often deep in the dermis. A fibrotic stroma and frequent mitoses are observed. Morpheaform BCC is marked by strands of basaloid neoplastic cells embedded in a characteristic heavily fibrotic stroma.

42.7 Diagnosis and Differential Diagnosis

The diagnosis of BCC is made on clinical examination and histology. Physical examination should focus on identifying tumor size, palpating clinical margins, and lymph node exam. Diagnosis is confirmed with a skin biopsy of a suspicious lesion. The differential diagnosis for a BCC includes squamous cell carcinoma, actinic keratosis, seborrheic keratosis, melanoma, nevi, angiofibroma, and sebaceous hyperplasia. Pigmented BCC can be particularly challenging to differentiate from seborrheic keratoses, blue nevi, lentigines, or melanoma.

42.8 Treatment

A variety of treatment options exist for BCC. Clinical and histologic traits such as tumor size, location, and histology determine whether the tumor is low risk or high risk. The goal is complete removal of the tumor with maximal preservation of function and cosmetic appearance. The treatment modality should be tailored to the individual patient with consideration for the location and size of the cancer and the patient's preferences, age, and general health.

Surgery is the most common treatment modality for basal cell carcinoma. The three modalities used are electrodessication and curettage, wide local excision, and Mohs micrographic surgery. In electrodessication and curettage, the tumor is removed by curettage followed by electrodessication of the lesion with a 2–3 mm margin. This method is indicated for smaller superficial or nodular BCCs on the trunk and extremity. A wide local excision with 4–6 mm is considered for well-defined larger skin cancers on the trunk and extremity. Mohs micrographic surgery can offer superior histologic margin control and maximum tissue conservation. Indications for Mohs micrographic surgery in individuals with BCC include location on central face, ear or lip, tumors >2 cm on the trunk, recurrent lesions, incompletely excised lesions, tumors with morpheaform or infiltrative histology, poorly defined lesions, lesions with perineural invasion, lesions arising in scar/radiation sites, immunosuppression, and history of genetic conditions such as Gorlin's syndrome and xeroderma pigmentosum.

Topical treatments can be employed for low-risk patients with primary superficial BCC who cannot undergo surgery or radiation or in patients with multiple primary tumors even though the cure rate is lower than surgical excision. Both imiquimod and topical 5-fluorouracil are approved by the US Food and Drug Administration for the treatment of superficial BCC <2 cm on the trunk and extremity.

Vismodegib is a novel therapeutic agent that targets the Hedgehog signaling pathway and was recently approved by the FDA in 2012 for the treatment of metastatic BCC.

References

1. Gloster Jr HM, Neal K. Skin cancer in skin of color. J Am Acad Dermatol. 2006;55(5):741–60; quiz 61–4. PubMed PMID: 17052479. Epub 2006/10/21. eng.
2. Roewert-Huber J, Lange-Asschenfeldt B, Stockfleth E, Kerl H. Epidemiology and aetiology of basal cell carcinoma. Br J Dermatol. 2007;157 Suppl 2:47–51. PubMed PMID: 18067632. Epub 2007/12/11. eng.
3. Battie C, Gohara M, Verschoore M, Roberts W. Skin cancer in skin of color: an update on current facts, trends, and misconceptions. J Drugs Dermatol. 2013;12(2):194–8. PubMed PMID: 23377393. Epub 2013/02/05. eng.
4. Kim GK, Del Rosso JQ, Bellew S. Skin cancer in Asians: part 1: nonmelanoma skin cancer. J Clin Aesthet Dermatol. 2009;2(8):39–42. PubMed PMID: 20729955. Pubmed Central PMCID: 2923966. Epub 2010/08/24. eng.
5. Ahluwalia J, Hadjicharalambous E, Mehregan D. Basal cell carcinoma in skin of color. J Drugs Dermatol. 2012;11(4):484–6. PubMed PMID: 22453586. Epub 2012/03/29. eng.

Squamous Cell Carcinoma

43

Ryan Thorpe and Divya Srivastava

Contents

R. Thorpe, BS (✉)
Department of Dermatology, University of Texas Southwestern Medical School, 100 Kings Row Drive, Mansfield, TX 76063, USA
e-mail: ryan.thorpe@utsouthwestern.edu

D. Srivastava, MD
Department of Dermatology, University of Texas Southwestern Medical Center, 5939 Harry Hines Blvd., Suite 100, Dallas, TX 75390-9191, USA
e-mail: divya.srivastava@utsouthwestern.edu

43.1 Introduction

Squamous cell carcinoma (SCC) of the skin, like other nonmelanoma skin cancers (NMSC), is more common in fair-skinned individuals but is seen in all races [1]. Although SCC is diagnosed and treated similarly across ethnicities, significant discrepancies mark the etiology, presentation, and prognosis of SCC in skin of color. Knowledge of SCC in these patients is important for clinicians, as patients with skin of color comprise the majority of the world's population, and it is predicted that by 2050, Hispanics, Asians, and Blacks will comprise 50 % of the US population [2].

43.1.1 Epidemiology

In patients with skin of color, NMSC occurs at a rate of 3.4/100,000 compared with 230/100,000 in lightly pigmented individuals. SCC is the most common cutaneous malignancy diagnosed in Blacks and Asian Indians, comprising 30 and 65 % of skin cancers, respectively, and is the second most common skin cancer in Chinese and Japanese populations [2, 3]. The ratio of BCC to SCC is reversed in Blacks, with darker-skinned patients having a ratio of 1.1:1 compared to 4:1 in Caucasians [2]. The incidence of SCC in Chinese, Malays, and Indians is reported to be 3.2/100,000 in men and 5.8/100,000 in women [3]. The lower incidence of SCC in skin of color is likely a consequence of inherent photoprotection provided by increased epidermal melanin and more dispersed melanosomes [1, 2].

D. Jackson-Richards, A.G. Pandya (eds.), *Dermatology Atlas for Skin of Color*, DOI 10.1007/978-3-642-54446-0_43,

43.1.2 Etiology

Ultraviolet radiation (UVR) is the most significant risk factor for SCC in Caucasians and Asians in whom lesions are found in sun-exposed areas. However, the etiopathogenesis of SCC in darkly pigmented individuals, in whom lesions are diagnosed in non-sun-exposed areas, is less clear. Significant risk factors in this patient population include a history of chronic inflammation, unremitting ulcers, and scarring, with 20–40 % of SCCs diagnosed in these clinical scenarios [1–3]. Other risk factors for SCC include albinism, lupus erythematosus, hidradenitis suppurativa, vitiligo, HPV, exposure to chemical carcinogens, and certain genetic disorders (Fig. 43.1) [1–5].

Squamous cell carcinoma evolves under a classic cancer model with precursors, tumor progression, and potential for metastasis [1]. Mutations in p53 are implicated in the development of SCC in this model. Precursor lesions, including actinic keratosis and Bowen's disease or squamous cell carcinoma in situ, are uncommon in dark skin but can be seen in Asians and Hispanics [1–3].

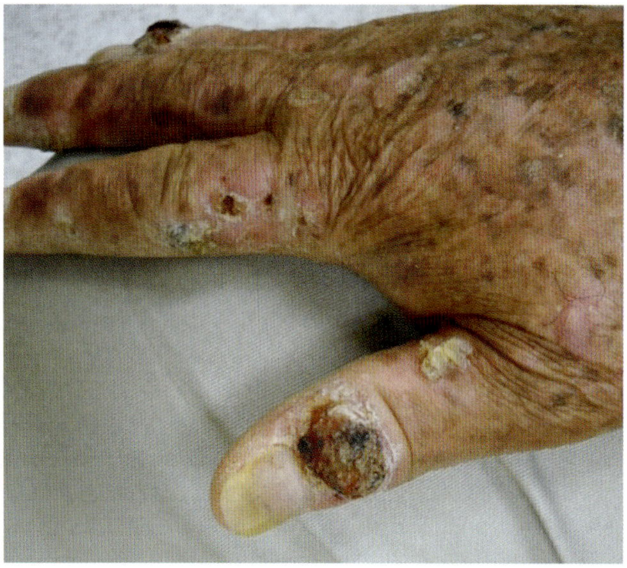

Fig. 43.1 Squamous cell carcinoma on the dorsal thumb in a Hispanic male with xeroderma pigmentosum

43.2 Clinical Features

The clinical features of SCC depend on the location, background pigmentation of the patient, and clinical setting. While 65 % of SCC in Caucasians are found on the head and neck region, only 35 % of SCC in skin of color are found on sun-exposed areas of the head and neck (Fig. 43.2) [1]. In one report, SCC was 8.5 times more frequently found in non-sun-exposed areas in Blacks compared with Caucasians [2]. In all, 30–40 % of SCC in people of color develop in scars or chronic, nonhealing ulcers, compared to less than 2 % in Whites; therefore, it is particularly important to look for suspicious lesions in patients with such lesions [1, 3]. In African-Americans, SCC presents in the anogenital region in 10–23 % of cases (Fig. 43.3) [2].

SCC is typically described as a slowly or rapidly growing erythematous hyperkeratotic papule or nodule (Fig. 43.4) [1]. Lesions can vary in color from erythematous to skin-colored [1, 3]. Advanced lesions can present with ulceration, friability, and induration (Fig. 43.5). Based on a review of cases in African-Americans in Atlanta, Georgia, one study concluded that the combination of hyperkeratotic lesions with mottled pigmentation should alert the physician to the possibility of SCC [2]. SCC in situ is uncommon in persons of color, but when seen, it is often found as an erythematous, hyperkeratotic patch on the lower extremeties [1, 2, 4]. Rare pigmented variants of SCC in situ are described in Caucasians and are relatively more common in skin of color (Fig. 43.6) [3]. Keratoacanthoma, a well-defined crateriform nodule, is a rapidly growing variant of SCC that can be associated with a history of trauma (Fig. 43.7).

In rapidly growing SCC, lesions may be tender. In advanced SCC, paresthesia, anesthesia, and pain may be signs of perineural invasion [1]. Systemic findings are infrequently related to the primary lesion but are a result of metastasis to lymph nodes and distant organs. Consequently, a full history and physical should be performed on any patient suspicious for invasive carcinoma [3].

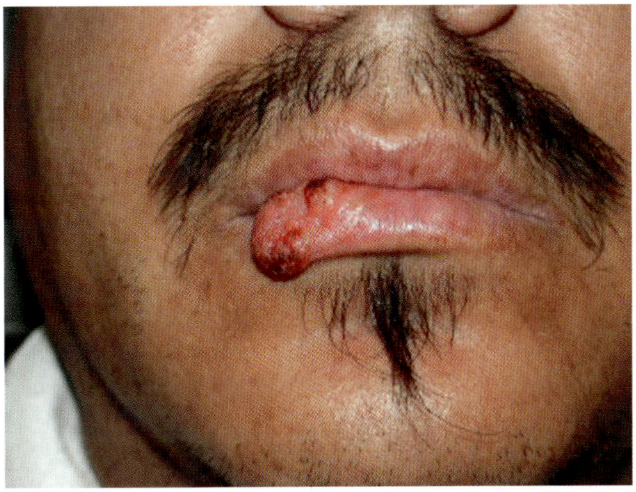

Fig. 43.2 Squamous cell carcinoma on the lip of a Hispanic male

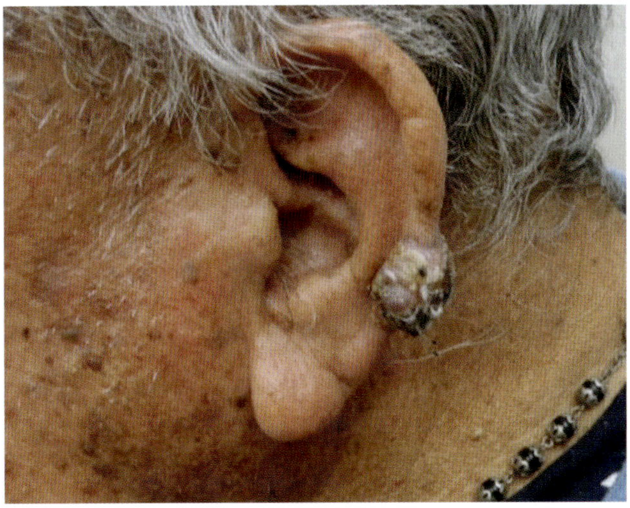

Fig. 43.4 Squamous cell carcinoma presenting as a hyperkeratotic nodule on the ear of a Hispanic male

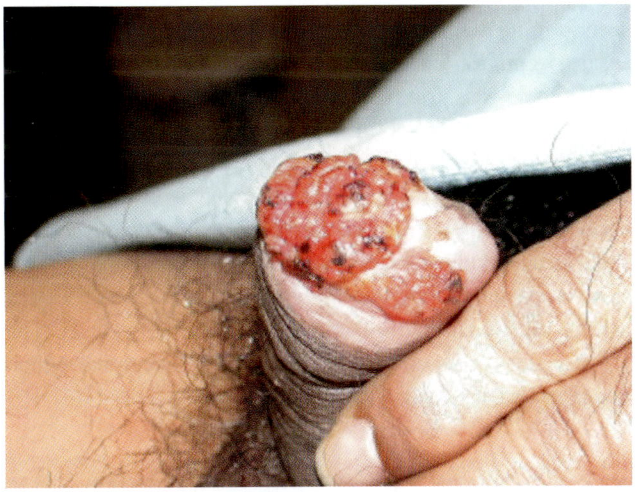

Fig. 43.3 Penile squamous cell carcinoma associated with human papillomavirus infection in an African-American male

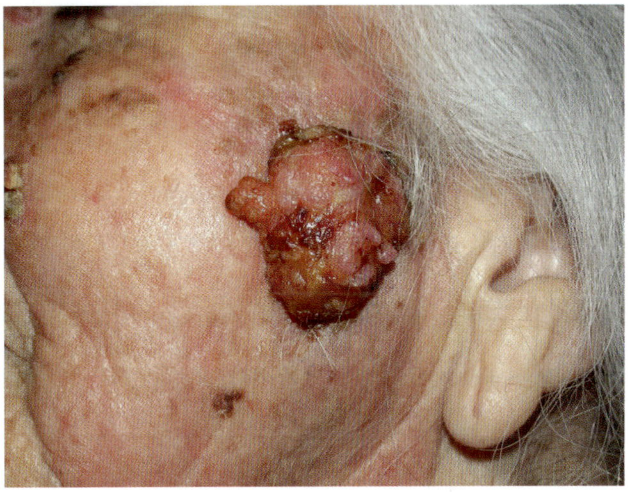

Fig. 43.5 Advanced squamous cell carcinoma presenting as a large friable ulcerated tumor on the cheek in a Hispanic female

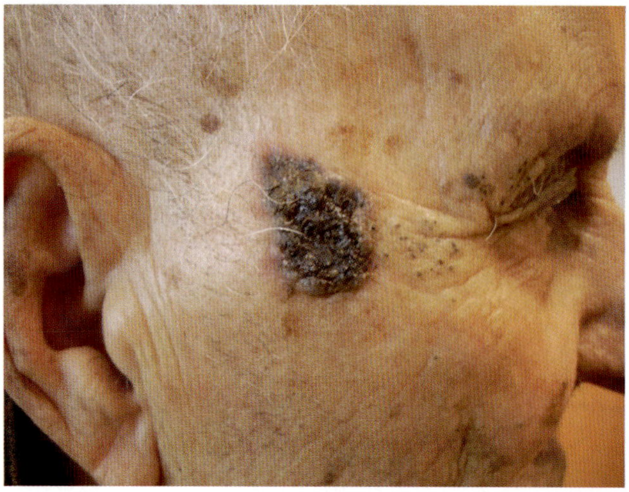

Fig. 43.6 Pigmented Bowen's disease on the zygoma in a Hispanic male

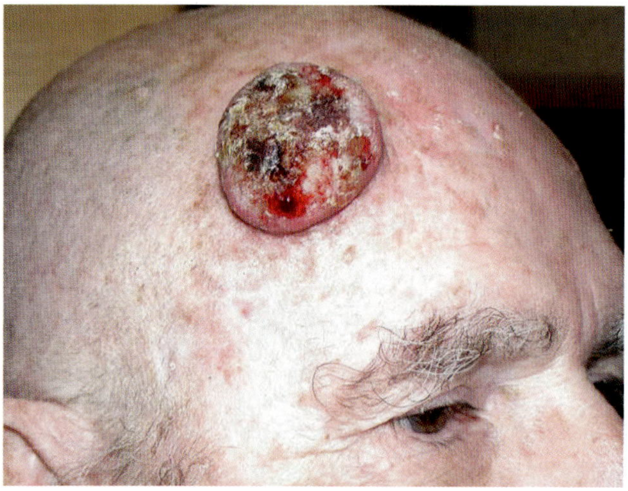

Fig. 43.7 Keratoacanthoma presenting as a crateriform keratotic tumor on the scalp in a Hispanic male

43.3 Natural History and Prognosis

SCC in skin of color is generally thought to have a worse prognosis [3]. In a case series of 163 and 175 patients, respective mortality rates for SCC in black patients were 18.4 and 29 % [3]. Mortality rates range from 17 to 30 % in other publications [2, 3]. Several reasons have been proposed for this worse prognosis, including barriers in access to care, delayed detection and treatment, inherently more aggressive disease, and false perceptions held by patients and physicians that dark skin confers complete protection against skin cancer [2, 6, 7]. Authors of one survey revealed that populations with worse morbidity and mortality from SCC are the same populations with uncertainty and false perceptions regarding this cancer [7].

Notably, SCC originating from a chronic scarring process is more aggressive, with a 20–40 % risk of metastasis, compared to a 1–4 % risk of metastasis in sun-induced SCC [2]. Furthermore, in patients under 50 years of age, 70 % of skin malignancy deaths are due to NMSC in persons of color compared with 10 % of deaths in Caucasians [1]. Additionally, SCC in skin of color frequently does not follow the progression seen in Caucasians from precursor lesions [4]. When metastases do occur, a strong correlation with tumor thickness is present, with lesions from 2.1 to 6 mm having a 4 % rate of metastases and those >6 mm with a 16 % metastatic rate [1]. Risk factors for metastatic disease include tumor diameter >2 cm, tumor depth >4 mm, location on the lip or ear or genital region, perineural invasion, aggressive histologic subtypes such as acantholytic or desmoplastic SCC, immunosuppression, recurrent lesions, rapidly growing lesions, and lesions arising out of chronic inflammation (Fig. 43.8) [1, 2]. The 10-year survival is 20 % with metastases to regional lymph nodes and <10 % with distant metastases [5].

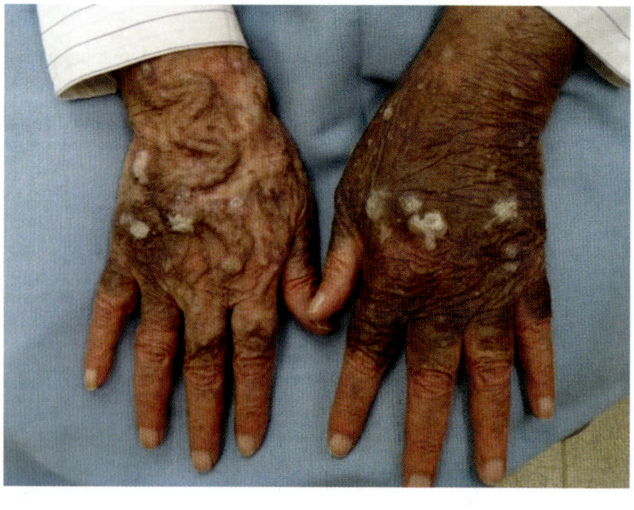

Fig. 43.8 Multiple squamous cell carcinomas on the dorsal hands in a South Asian male renal transplant patient

43.4 Histopathological Features

Histologically, the diagnosis of SCC is established when a proliferation of glassy, brightly eosinophilic keratinocytes with pleomorphic nuclei and frequent mitoses is observed [1]. The degree of nuclear atypia and keratinization varies on level of differentiation. Perineural invasion and desmoplasia may be seen in advanced SCC, and poorly differentiated SCCs may lack "overt keratinization" [1]. Actinic keratosis features the signs of chronic sun damage, including solar elastosis and squamous cell dysplasia. SCC in situ demonstrates full-thickness dysplasia that can be high grade [1].

43.5 Diagnosis and Differential Diagnosis

The diagnosis of squamous cell carcinoma is typically straightforward and is based on clinical features and histologic examination. The history and physical exam should focus on identifying clinical traits suggestive of a high-risk SCC. Presence of chronic inflammatory disease processes should alert one to perform a full skin check to evaluate for SCC in darkly pigmented individuals [3]. Lymphadenopathy should also be assessed.

Any lesion suspicious for SCC should be biopsied, including nonhealing ulcers or nodules adjacent to chronic inflammatory areas [2]. In particular, poorly healing lesions in chronic discoid lupus erythematosus metastasize at a greater rate than SCC developing from other lesions and should be biopsied immediately [5]. The type of biopsy is indicated by the characteristics of the lesion. Shave biopsies are usually adequate for superficial lesions; otherwise, deeper punch or excisional biopsies are more satisfactory for thicker lesions [3].

SCC and its associated lesions are frequently mistaken for other processes, particularly in skin of color. Specifically, SCC in situ, actinic keratosis, superficial basal cell carcinoma, psoriasis, and chronic eczema can be difficult to differentiate from one another [1]. Pigmented Bowen's disease often mimics melanoma in dark-skinned individuals [2]. Other histopathologic imitators include verruca vulgaris, warty dyskeratoma, inverted follicular keratosis, hypertrophic lichen planus, hypertrophic lupus erythematosus, atypical mycobacterial or "deep" fungal infections, granular cell tumor, and pseudocarcinomatous hyperplasia [1].

43.6 Treatment

Treatment options are similar across skin types and guidelines come from the National Comprehensive Cancer Network [1, 4]. Squamous cell carcinoma is divided into low-risk and high-risk lesions based on tumor diameter, depth, location, histologic features, and clinical traits. Low-risk lesions are treated with excision with 4–6 mm margins. Electrodessication and curettage can be used for small in situ squamous cell carcinomas in non-hair-bearing sites. High-risk lesions such as head and neck tumors, recurrent lesions, large lesions, and those with perineural involvement should be treated with Mohs micrographic surgery. Radiation may be used either adjunctively for high-risk SCC or if large perineural involvement is present, or it may be used as sole therapy if surgery is contraindicated. For metastatic disease, systemic therapy including EGFR inhibitors may be employed [1].

Keys to treatment include prevention with consistent use of sunscreen and early detection with skin exams. Unfortunately, recent surveys revealed that 65 % of African-Americans never wore sunscreen even in sunny climates and >60 % of minorities falsely believed they were not at risk for skin cancer [6]. Furthermore, patients with darker skin have been found to be significantly less likely to perform skin self-examinations or to have ever received a skin exam by a physician [8]. All patients should therefore be reminded to practice sun avoidance and sun protection.

References

1. Bolognia JL, Jorizzo JL, Schaffer JV. Dermatology, vol 1. 3rd ed. 2012. p. 1759–93. Print.
2. Gloster HM, Neal K. Skin cancer in skin of color. J Am Acad Dermatol. 2006;55(5):741–60.
3. Kelly AP, Taylor SC, editors. Dermatology for skin of color. New York: McGraw Hill; 2009. p. 291–5. Print.
4. Jackson BA. Nonmelanoma skin cancer in persons of color. Semin Cutan Med Surg. 2009;28(2):93–5.
5. Bradford PT. Skin cancer in skin of color. Dermatol Nurs. 2009;21(4):170–7, 206.
6. Battie C, Gohara M, Verschoore M, Roberts W. Skin cancer in skin of color: an update on current facts, trends, and misconceptions. J Drugs Dermatol. 2013;12(2):194–8.
7. Buster KJ, You Z, Fouad M, Elmets C. Skin cancer risk perceptions: a comparison across ethnicity, age, education, gender, and income. J Am Acad Dermatol. 2012;66(5):771–9.
8. Imahiyerobo-Ip J, Ip I, Jama S, Nadiminti U, Sanchez M. Skin cancer awareness in communities of color. J Am Acad Dermatol. 2011;64(1):198–200.

44 Dermatofibrosarcoma Protuberans

Nita Kohli and Divya Srivastava

Contents

44.1 Introduction

Dermatofibrosarcoma protuberans (DFSP) is a rare soft tissue tumor that affects 4.2 per million people in the United States each year and represents 0.1 % of all cancers [1]. Median age at diagnosis is 41 years of age, with highest age-specific annual incidence rates between ages 30 and 50 [1, 2]. It can occur in children and the elderly as well. The overall incidence of DFSP is higher in blacks than in whites and other racial groups, with black women having higher rates than black men [1].

The cause of DFSP remains unknown. Chromosomal abnormalities associated with tumor development have been discovered more recently [3]. Most DFSP tumors have a t(17; 22) translocation between collagen 1A1 (COL1A1) on chromosome 17 and platelet-derived growth factor β (PDGFβ) gene on chromosome 22. The role of trauma as a contributor to DFSP has not been definitively established; however, 10–20 % of patients report a history of prior trauma to the area [3].

N. Kohli, MD, MPH (✉)
Department of Dermatology,
University Hospitals Case Medical Center-Case
Western Reserve University, 11100 Euclid Ave, LKSD 3500,
Cleveland, OH 44106, USA
e-mail: nita.kohli@uhhospitals.org

D. Srivastava, MD
Department of Dermatology,
University of Texas Southwestern Medical Center,
5939 Harry Hines Blvd., Suite 100, Dallas, TX 75390-9191, USA
e-mail: divya.srivastava@utsouthwestern.edu

D. Jackson-Richards, A.G. Pandya (eds.), *Dermatology Atlas for Skin of Color*,
DOI 10.1007/978-3-642-54446-0_44,

44.2 Clinical Features

DFSP typically presents with an asymptomatic, slowly enlarging, flesh-colored or red-blue, firm plaque or nodule. They appear on the trunk in 50 % of cases (Fig. 44.1), followed by the proximal extremity in 20–35 % of cases, and the head and neck in only 10–15 % of cases [4]. Lesions can reach several centimeters in diameter (Fig. 44.2) with a palpable, indurated component that can extend past the visible margin of the tumor. Accelerated growth can be associated with pain, ulceration, and bleeding [3]. Often, delays in diagnosis and neglect can result in large tumors.

Bednar tumor is a rare pigmented form of DFSP. It represents less than 5 % of all cases of DFSP and is more common in blacks [1]. Clinically, it cannot be distinguished from ordinary DFSP [3].

A juvenile variant of DFSP, giant cell fibroblastoma, occurs in the first decade of life. It presents as a solitary, 2–6 cm large, slow-growing, blue-gray mass mainly on the trunk or extremities. Local recurrence is common, but metastasis has not been reported [3].

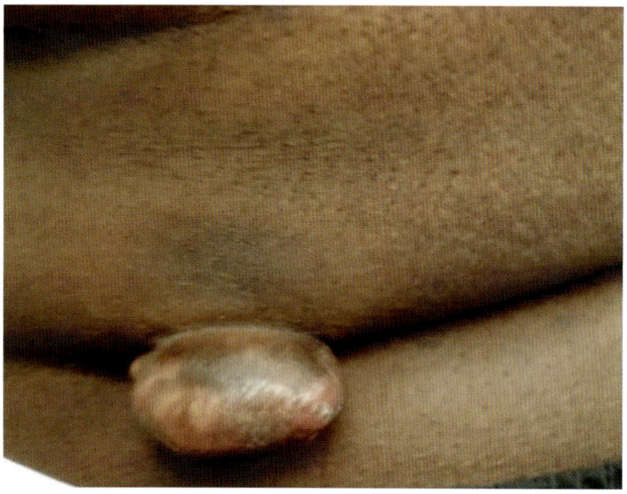

Fig. 44.1 DFSP on the lower back of an African American male

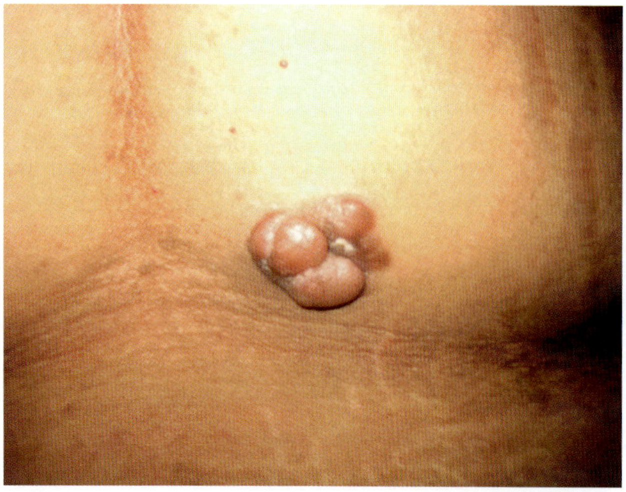

Fig. 44.2 DFSP on the mid-back of an African American female

44.3 Natural History and Prognosis

DFSP is locally aggressive and destructive, but distant metastasis is rare and has been reported in 0.5–5 % of patients [4]. If not treated, the tumor can spread locally into vital structures. Local recurrences are usually within 3 years of excision [3]. The most common site of metastasis is the lung, and nodal metastasis is rare. There is a high survival rate, with a 5- and 15-year survival of 99.2 and 97.2 %, respectively [1], and survival after distant recurrence is poor (mean 14 months, range 1–48 months) [3].

Patients with DFSP are at 25 % increased risk of developing subsequent primary malignancies compared with the general population [2]. These subsequent primary malignancies include a 21-fold increased risk of nonepithelial skin cancer (including a subsequent primary DFSP, but not including basal cell/squamous cell carcinoma) and a 5-fold increased risk of soft tissue cancer, cutaneous melanoma, and breast cancer. Overall risk of colon cancer is decreased in patients with DFSP [2]. Once a diagnosis of DFSP has been made, a complete history, review of systems, and physical examination including skin check and lymph node palpation should be performed. Patients should follow up every 3–6 months during the first 3 years and then annually thereafter [3].

44.4 Histopathology

DFSP is a low-grade sarcoma arising in the dermis, with a storiform pattern of cells with spindle-shaped nuclei. It has also been described as a fibroblastic proliferation of tumor cells arranged about a central hub, producing a cartwheel pattern [3]. This characteristic histologic pattern differentiates DFSP from other spindle cell neoplasms [3]. Tumors can penetrate into the subcutaneous fat and recurrent or older lesions may invade the fascia, muscle, nerve, or bone [3]. The tumor center is usually more cellular than the periphery. The borders are difficult to discern histologically, which accounts for inadequate excision and recurrences [3].

Bednar tumors are characterized by spindle cells in a storiform pattern mixed with melanin-containing dendritic cells, a key feature distinguishing Bednar tumor from ordinary DFSP [3]. Giant cell fibroblastoma is characterized by multinucleated giant cells adjacent to vascular-like spaces. Another histologic variant is DFSP with fibrosarcomatous change. These tumors have increased cellular atypia and mitoses. These changes are seen in approximately 7–16 % of tumors and exhibit increased local aggression, recurrence, and metastasis. However, other reports show that the prognosis is same for DFSP and DFSP with fibrosarcomatous change [4].

44.5 Diagnosis and Differential Diagnosis

Given the higher incidence of DFSP and Bednar tumor in blacks, these tumors should be included in the differential diagnosis of atypical keloids in black patients [3]. DFSP can be distinguished from dermatofibroma by its larger size, deeper penetration, and greater cellularity. Histologically, subcutaneous involvement in DFSP displays extension of spindle cells between fat cells in a honeycomb pattern, or a multilayered pattern of bundles of spindle cells oriented parallel to the epidermis [3]. In contrast, dermatofibromas have epidermal hyperplasia, small size, and occasionally hemosiderin-ringed siderophages. Immunohistochemistry is also useful in differentiation. DFSP shows CD34 positivity and Factor XIIIa negativity, whereas dermatofibromas are CD34 negative and Factor XIIIa positive.

DFSP may also appear clinically similar to lymphoma, neurofibroma, melanoma, sarcoidosis, fibrosarcoma, leiomyoma, morpheaform basal cell carcinoma, and nodular fasciitis [3]. S100 is negative in DFSP but positive in melanoma and neurofibroma. Neurofibromas have neural differentiation and mast cells and lack the storiform pattern of spindle cells seen in DFSP.

44.6 Treatment

Surgical excision is the first-line treatment for DFSP. The first resection is highly important because of local recurrent growth or metastases. DFSP exhibits tentacle-like projections (Fig. 44.3) that extend laterally between collagen bundles and deep into fascia and muscle [3]. Failure to remove these projections may account for the high local recurrence rates. Studies have shown that a 2.5 cm surgical margin to deep fascia is needed to achieve eradication with wide local excision (Fig. 44.4) [5, 6]. Mohs micrographic surgery has emerged as a treatment option for DFSP with lower recurrence rates attributed to the ability to achieve complete margin examination. However, interpretation of DFSP on frozen sections can present some challenges. Recurrence rates reported are 2 % after Mohs surgery vs. 11–50 % after wide local excision. Imatinib mesylate, a tyrosine kinase inhibitor that targets the COL1A1-PDGFβ fusion protein, has been used to shrink tumor size in some initially unresectable tumors and is indicated in recurrent and metastatic tumors [7].

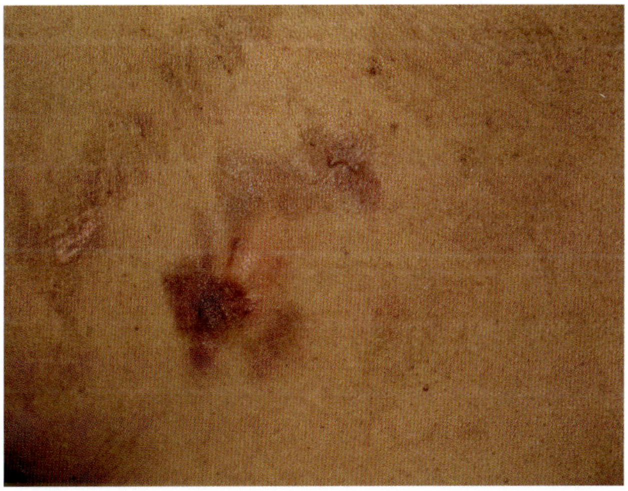

Fig. 44.3 DFSP on the chest of African American female exhibiting clinical tentacle-like projections (Photo courtesy of J.S. Bordeaux, MD, MPH)

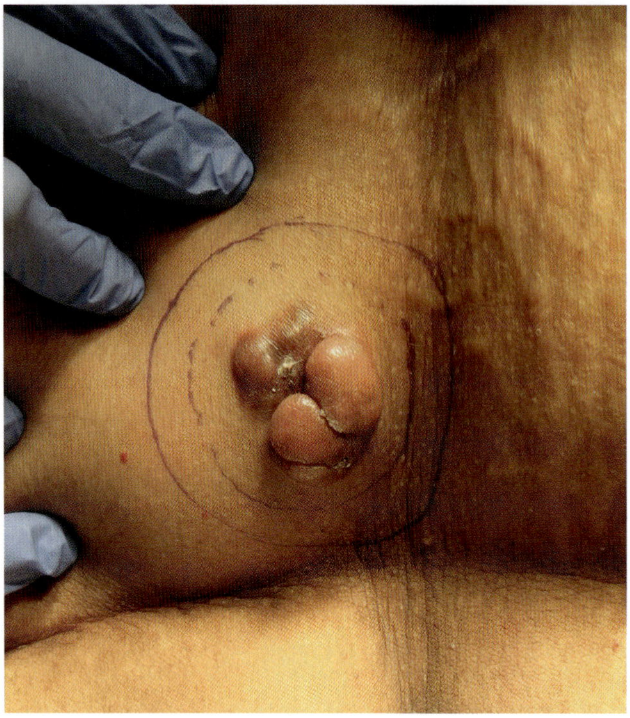

Fig. 44.4 DFSP on the mid-back of patient in Fig. 44.2 with illustrated surgical margins. The *inner circle* demonstrates palpable clinical margin. The *outer circle* delineates a 1 cm surgical margin for Mohs micrographic surgery

References

1. Criscione VD, Weinstock MA. Descriptive epidemiology of dermatofibrosarcoma protuberans in the United States, 1973 to 2002. J Am Acad Dermatol. 2007;56:968–73.
2. Kurlander DE, Martires KJ, Chen Y, et al. Risk of subsequent primary malignancies after dermatofibrosarcoma protuberans diagnosis: a national study. J Am Acad Dermatol. 2013;68(5):790–6.
3. Gloster HM. Dermatofibrosarcoma protuberans. J Am Acad Dermatol. 1996;35:355–74.
4. Bogucki B, Neuhaus I, Hurst EA. Dermatofibrosarcoma protuberans: a review of the literature. Dermatol Surg. 2012;38(4):537–51.
5. Parker TL, Zitelli JA. Surgical margins for excision of dermatofibrosarcoma protuberans. J Am Acad Dermatol. 1995;32:233–6.
6. Gloster Jr HM, Harris KR, Roenigk RK. A comparison between Mohs micrographic surgery and wide surgical excision for the treatment of dermatofibrosarcoma protuberans. J Am Acad Dermatol. 1996;35:82–7.
7. Lemm D, Muegge LO, Hoeffken K, et al. Remission with imatinib mesylate treatment in a patient with initially unresectable dermatofibrosarcoma protuberans—a case report. Oral Maxillofac Surg. 2008;12(4):209–13.

Melanoma

45

Sharif Currimbhoy and Divya Srivastava

Contents

S. Currimbhoy, BS
Department of Dermatology, University of Texas Southwestern Medical Center, 5939 Harry Hines Blvd, Dallas, TX 75235, USA
e-mail: sharif.currimbhoy@utsouthwestern.edu

D. Srivastava, MD (✉)
Department of Dermatology, University of Texas Southwestern Medical Center, 5939 Harry Hines Blvd., Suite 100, Dallas, TX 75390-9191, USA
e-mail: divya.srivastava@utsouthwestern.edu

45.1 Introduction

Melanoma affects approximately 77,000 Americans and 200,000 individuals worldwide every year and is the third most common skin cancer in patients with skin of color [1, 2]. Although patients of African American, Asian, Hispanic, and American Indian descent have a lower rate of melanoma than Caucasians, the variable presentation of lesions requires increased awareness on the part of the examining physician. The incidence of melanoma in Caucasian patients is estimated at 21.1 cases per 100,000 individuals, compared to 0.6–1.5 per 100,000 in African Americans. The rate of melanoma in Hispanics and Asians is slightly higher than in African Americans with 1.2–4.7 cases per 100,000 and 0.5–1.5 cases per 100,000, respectively [1–5]. The discrepancy in the incidence of melanoma in patients with skin of color can likely be attributed to higher melanin content in these individuals which provides a greater degree of photoprotection from carcinogenic ultraviolet radiation [3–7]. The incidence of melanoma increases with age in patients of all racial and ethnic groups, with the majority of melanomas presenting between ages 50 and 64 [4]. Patients of Hispanic, Asian, and American Indian descent are more likely to present at a younger age compared to African Americans and Caucasians [1]. With respect to gender, there is a higher rate of melanoma among females of African American, Asian, and Hispanic origin compared to Caucasians and American Indians in which a higher number of males are affected [2].

In contrast to Caucasians, risk factors such as ultraviolet radiation exposure and family history of melanoma are not thought to be significant factors for the development of melanoma in darker-skinned races [5]. Risk factors that have been implicated in the formation of melanoma in African Americans include albinism, burn scars, x-rays, history of trauma, and blistering sunburns [1, 4, 5].

D. Jackson-Richards, A.G. Pandya (eds.), *Dermatology Atlas for Skin of Color*,
DOI 10.1007/978-3-642-54446-0_45, © Springer-Verlag Berlin Heidelberg 2014

45.2 Clinical Features

The distribution of melanoma in patients with skin of color differs from that of Caucasians. While tumors in Caucasians tend to present on sun-exposed areas, such as the trunk and legs, lesions in darker-skinned patients tend to be located on non-sun-exposed regions. The "ABCDE" rule, which stands for the Asymmetry, Border irregularity, Color irregularity, larger Diameter of a melanoma lesion compared to normal nevi, and Evolution of a lesion, is often used to help distinguish benign from malignant pigmented lesions. However, this rule is less useful in patients with skin of color because of the atypical presentation of melanoma in these individuals [7]. Melanoma typically begins as a solitary, darkly pigmented, black or brown patch, papule, or nodule with irregular borders and variegated color (Fig. 45.1) [4, 5, 7]. In patients with skin of color, lesions tend to present in a more advanced stage, with a larger diameter and associated crusting, bleeding, and ulceration [5]. Lesions located on the mucosal, acral, and subungual regions account for 60–75 % of melanomas found in African American, Hispanic, and Asian populations (Figs. 45.2, 45.3, 45.4, and 45.5) [3–7]. Acral melanoma refers specifically to lesions that occur on palmar, plantar, and subungual regions [5]. Among acral melanoma, there is a strong predilection for plantar involvement, such as the sole of the foot and heel region [5, 7]. Subungual melanoma involves the nail matrix and nail bed with a predilection for the thumb and great toe nail. On examination, a longitudinal, black or brown band of pigment can usually be seen extending the length of the nail bed with dystrophy and fracture of the nail plate sometimes found in advanced disease [5, 6]. A positive Hutchinson's sign refers to pigment that spans the length of the nail and extends into the nail fold laterally or proximally and, if present, increases the likelihood of melanoma [6] (Figs. 45.6 and 45.7).

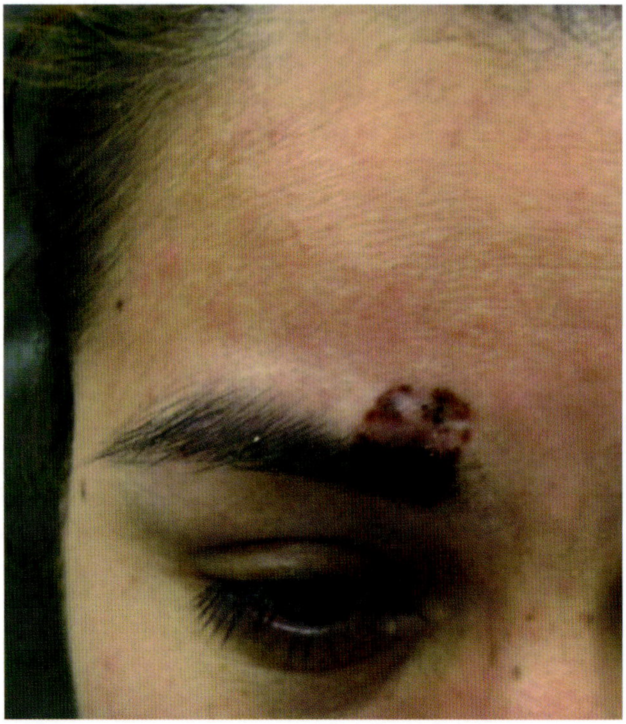

Fig. 45.1 Melanoma on the right eyebrow of Hispanic female

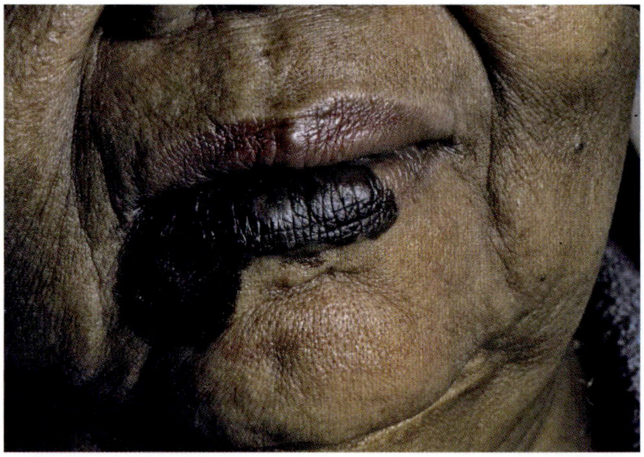

Fig. 45.2 Melanoma of the lower lip in an African American female

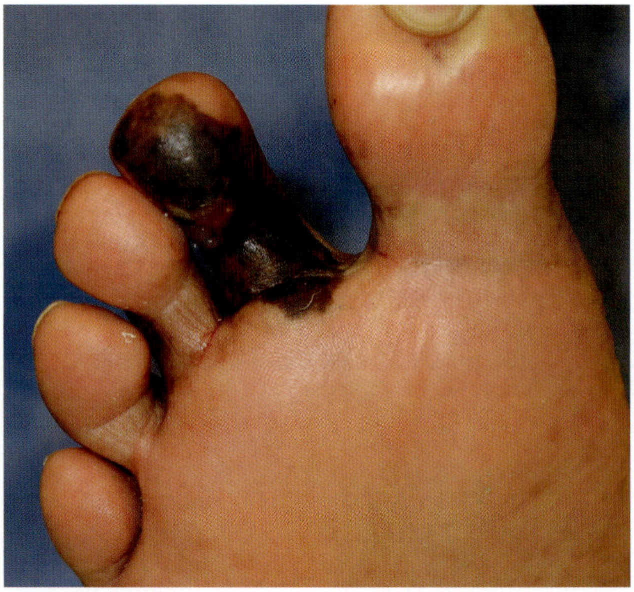

Fig. 45.3 Acral melanoma on the toe of a Hispanic male (Courtesy of Dr. Rohit Sharma)

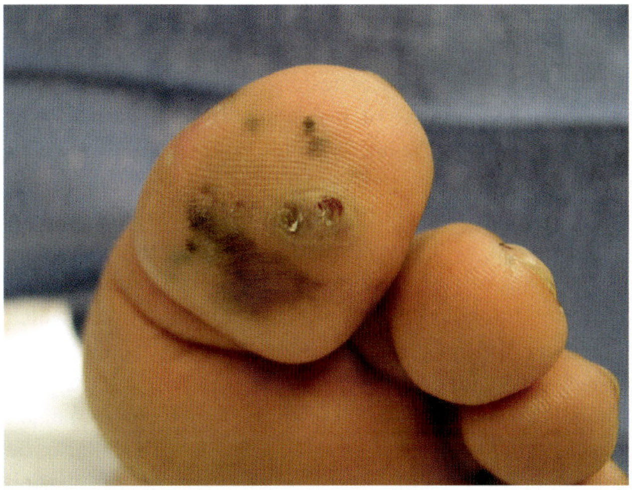

Fig. 45.4 Acral melanoma on ventral skin of great toe of a Hispanic male (Courtesy of Dr. Rohit Sharma)

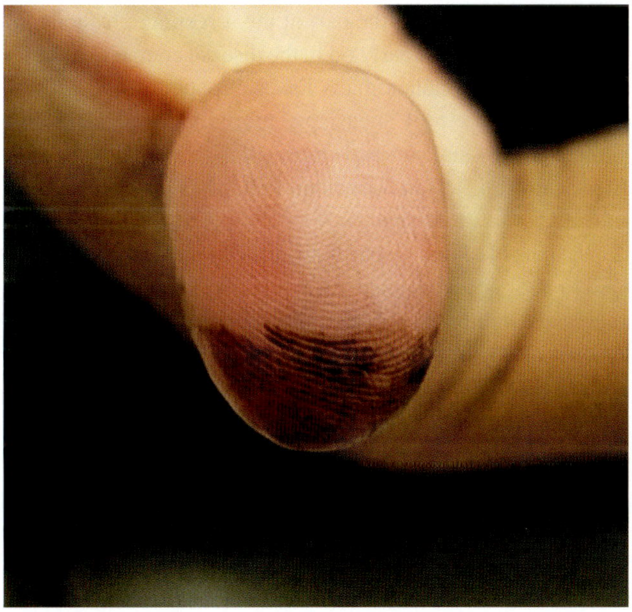

Fig. 45.5 Acral melanoma on the left thumb of a Hispanic male

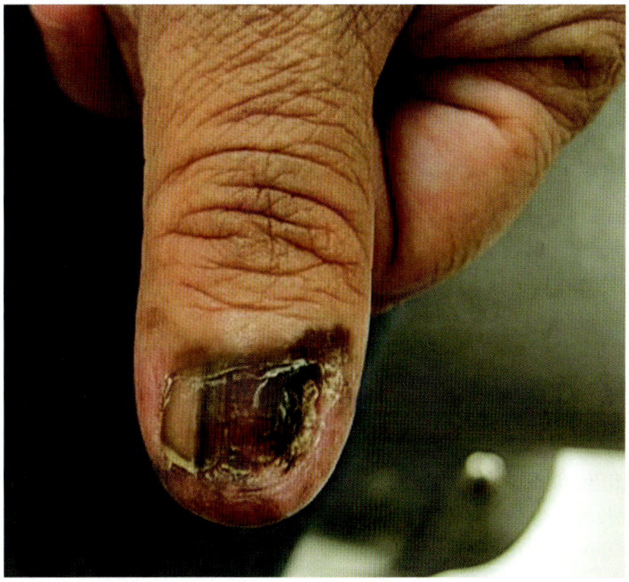

Fig. 45.6 Subungual melanoma of the thumb in a Hispanic male with a positive Hutchinson's sign on the proximal nail fold

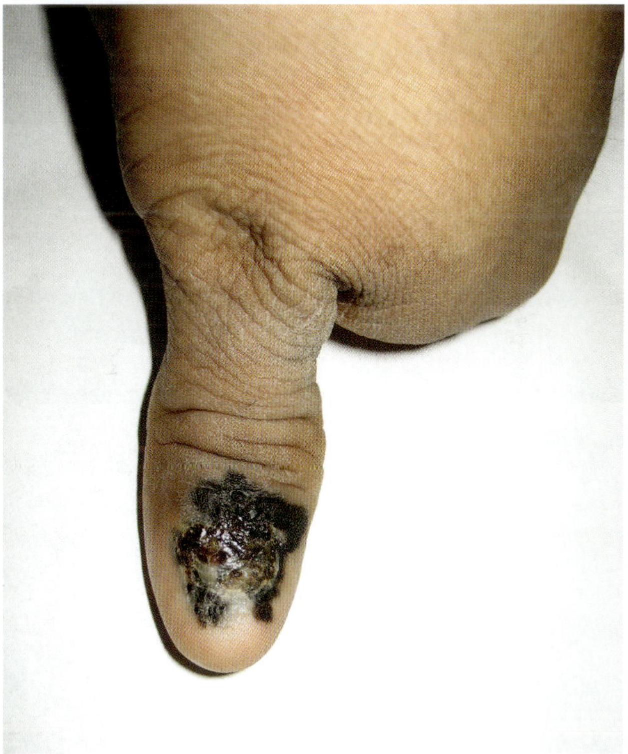

Fig. 45.7 Advanced subungual melanoma of the thumb in a Hispanic patient with a positive Hutchinson's sign on the proximal nail fold (Courtesy of Dr. Christine Liang)

45.3 Diagnosis and Differential Diagnosis

Other lesions that should be considered in the differential diagnosis for an acral melanoma include a melanocytic nevus, lentigo, seborrheic keratosis, Spitz nevus, traumatized pigmented lesion, or pigmented basal cell carcinoma. Lentigo maligna is a precursor to lentigo maligna melanoma and usually occurs on sun-damaged skin of elderly patients (Fig. 45.8). These lesions should be completely excised when possible. The differential diagnosis for a subungual melanoma includes benign longitudinal melanonychia and a subungual hematoma. Factors that suggest malignancy over a benign process include a solitary lesion, rapid progression in size, a darkly pigmented lesion with color variation, and a diameter greater than 6 mm with overlying ulceration or bleeding. In addition to these findings, a lesion width greater than 3 mm and presence of a Hutchinson's sign should increase suspicion for melanoma in subungual skin [6].

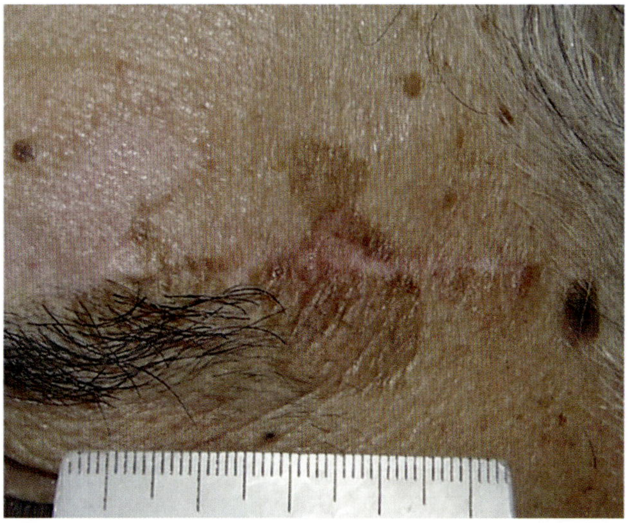

Fig. 45.8 Lentigo maligna on the left temple of a Hispanic male

45.4 Histopathological Features

Pathological evaluation of lesions should be performed to establish the presence of melanoma as well as the tumor depth for staging. The lesion should be excised entirely with clinical margins down to the level of subcutaneous fat for depth evaluation. The histological features of melanoma are characterized by an asymmetric proliferation of atypical melanocytes arising at the dermal-epidermal junction that can initially extend laterally in the epidermis after which they grow downward to penetrate the papillary dermis as single cells or nests of atypical cells [7]. Pagetoid spread, cytologic atypia, pleomorphism, hyperchromatism, increased mitosis, and prominent nucleoli may also be observed. The Breslow level refers to the depth of invasion of melanoma seen histologically and is the most important indicator of prognosis and establishment of a 5-year survival rate.

45.5 Natural History and Prognosis

An increased awareness of the variable presentation of lesions is necessary on the part of the screening physician to identify involvement early on in the disease course. Although the incidence of melanoma is lower in patients with skin of color compared to Caucasians, mortality is significantly higher. Five-year survival rates of 78.2 % in African Americans, 84.9 % in American Indians, 80.7 % in Asians, and 86.5 % in Hispanics are compared to 90.2 % in Caucasians [4]. This disparity in survival rates may be attributed to poor access to medical care, delay in diagnosis, more aggressive nature of melanoma, and difficulty in diagnosing lesions, which are typically located in less visible body sites, such as the feet [3, 4].

45.6 Treatment

Initial treatment for melanoma includes surgical excision with margins ranging from 5 to 2 cm depending on the Breslow depth of the tumor [8]. Tumors greater than 2 mm in depth are associated with a high risk of recurrence and mortality, and thus, adjuvant therapies should be considered. Interferon-α2b has been shown to inhibit the growth of tumor cells and subsequently increase survival in patients with high-risk or advanced-stage melanomas [8]. Novel adjuvant therapies for treatment of locally advanced or metastatic disease includes BRAF inhibitors such as sorafenib and vemurafenib. These compounds work by targeting the mutated oncogene, BRAF, which is identified in 60–70 % of melanomas [8]. In phase II trials, vemurafenib was found to increase overall median survival time of patients to 16 months compared to 6–10 months with other therapies [9]. Chemotherapeutic agents such as dacarbazine can be used as palliative therapy for advanced-stage or metastatic lesions; however, response is only temporary and the vast majority of patients do not achieve a long-term remission [8].

References

1. Howlader N, Noone AM, Krapcho M, Garshell J, Neyman N, Altekruse SF, Kosary CL, Yu M, Ruhl J, Tatalovich Z, Cho H, Mariotto A, Lewis DR, Chen HS, Feuer EJ, Cronin KA, editors. SEER Cancer Statistics Review. 1975–2010. http://seer.cancer.gov/csr/1975_2010/.
2. Ferlay J, Shin HR, Bray F, Forman D, Mathers C, Parkin DM. GLOBOCAN 2008 v2.0, Cancer incidence and mortality worldwide: IARC CancerBase No. 10 [Internet]. Lyon: International Agency for Research on Cancer; 2010. Available from: http://globocan.iarc.fr. Accessed on 24 Sept 2013.
3. Gloster HM, Neal K. Skin cancer in skin of color. J Am Acad Dermatol. 2006;55(5):741–60.
4. Wu XC, Eide MJ, King J, et al. Racial and ethnic variations in incidence and survival of cutaneous melanoma in the United States, 1999–2006. J Am Acad Dermatol. 2011;65(5 Suppl 1):S26–37.
5. Kelly AP, Taylor SC. Dermatology for skin of color. New York: McGraw-Hill Professional; 2009.
6. Rahman Z, Taylor SC. Malignant melanoma in African Americans. Cutis. 2001;67(5):403–6.
7. Kabigting FD, Nelson FP, Kauffman CL, Popoveniuc G, Dasanu CA, Alexandrescu DT. Malignant melanoma in African-Americans. Dermatol Online J. 2009;15(2):3.
8. Garbe C, Eigentler TK, Keilholz U, Hauschild A, Kirkwood JM. Systematic review of medical treatment in melanoma: current status and future prospects. Oncologist. 2011;16(1):5–24.
9. Boyd KP, Vincent B, Andea A, Conry RM, Hughey LC. Nonmalignant cutaneous findings associated with vemurafenib use in patients with metastatic melanoma. J Am Acad Dermatol. 2012;67(6):1375–9.

Cutaneous T-Cell Lymphoma

46

Sharif Currimbhoy and Amit G. Pandya

Contents

46.1 Introduction

Cutaneous T-cell lymphoma (CTCL) consists of several lymphoproliferative disorders of the skin that can present clinically with persistent erythematous patches, scaly plaques, and nodules that may spread to involve the peripheral blood, lymph nodes, and distal organs in advanced disease [1]. The most common forms of CTCL are mycosis fungoides (MF), with patches, plaques, or tumors of the skin, and *Sézary syndrome*, which is a leukemic form of CTCL that typically presents de novo or rarely progresses from patch/plaque stage MF [1, 2]. Other less common presentations include hypopigmented MF which is more prevalent in younger patients with skin of color [3]. CTCL is a relatively uncommon disease with an incidence estimated between 4.1 and 6.4 cases per million per year with men affected twice as commonly as women [1, 4, 5]. The median age of onset of mycosis fungoides is between 60 and 69 years of age [5]. African Americans are affected at nearly 1.7 times the rate of Caucasians and also suffer a higher rate of mortality [6, 7]. Hispanic and Asian patients, however, are affected at only half the rate of Caucasians [7]. The etiology of CTCL is unknown, although immunologic and viral causes have been proposed.

S. Currimbhoy, BS
Department of Dermatology, University of Texas Southwestern Medical Center, 5939 Harry Hines Blvd, Dallas, TX 75235, USA
e-mail: sharif.currimbhoy@utsouthwestern.edu

A.G. Pandya, MD (✉)
Department of Dermatology,
University of Texas Southwestern Medical Center,
5323 Harry Hines Boulevard,
Dallas, TX 75390, USA
e-mail: amit.pandya@utsouthwestern.edu

D. Jackson-Richards, A.G. Pandya (eds.), *Dermatology Atlas for Skin of Color*,
DOI 10.1007/978-3-642-54446-0_46, © Springer-Verlag Berlin Heidelberg 2014

46.2 Clinical Features

The clinical findings associated with MF may be fairly nonspecific early in the disease course. *Patch stage* MF typically presents with localized, erythematous, patches which may be mistaken for eczema or psoriasis [1, 2]. Lesions of *plaque stage* MF are thicker, more darkly pigmented, and dusky with the presence of scale (Figs. 46.1, 46.2, 46.3, and 46.4). Plaques may vary in shape from oval to arciform or serpiginous [1, 2, 8]. In general, MF affects sun-protected skin. The flexural surfaces, buttocks, hips, and upper thighs are typical sites of involvement in early disease with many patients complaining of severe pruritus associated with lesions [1, 2, 8]. *Tumor stage* MF is characterized by dome-shaped, red-brown nodules and tumors that may ulcerate and which can develop de novo on normal-appearing skin or from patches and plaques of MF (Figs. 46.5 and 46.6).

Sézary syndrome presents with generalized erythroderma and palpable lymphadenopathy with severe pruritus and lichenification of the skin (Figs. 46.7 and 46.8) [1, 2, 8]. Peripheral blood involvement is a hallmark of *Sézary syndrome* with the presence of abnormal circulating lymphoid cells (Sézary cells).

Hypopigmented MF is a less common variant but one that is seen mostly in patients with skin of color [3]. It presents clinically with multiple hypopigmented macules and patches distributed across the body with no associated scale or epidermal atrophy (Figs. 46.9 and 46.10).

Folliculotropic MF is a variant in which the lymphoma cells infiltrate follicles, leading to scaly follicular papules and alopecia (Figs. 46.11 and 46.12).

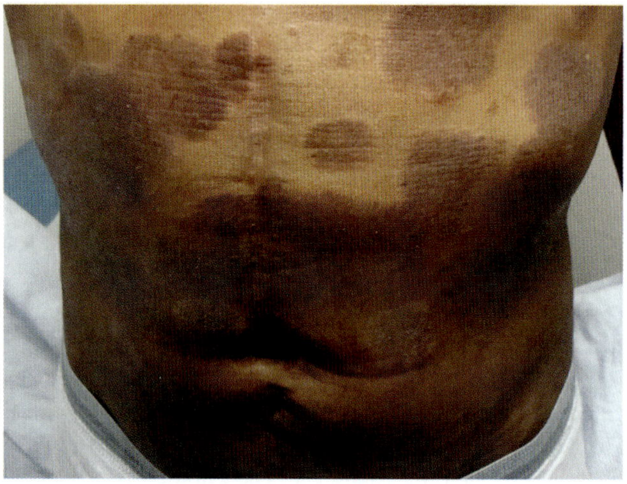

Fig. 46.1 Hyperpigmented plaques on the abdomen due to MF in an African American male

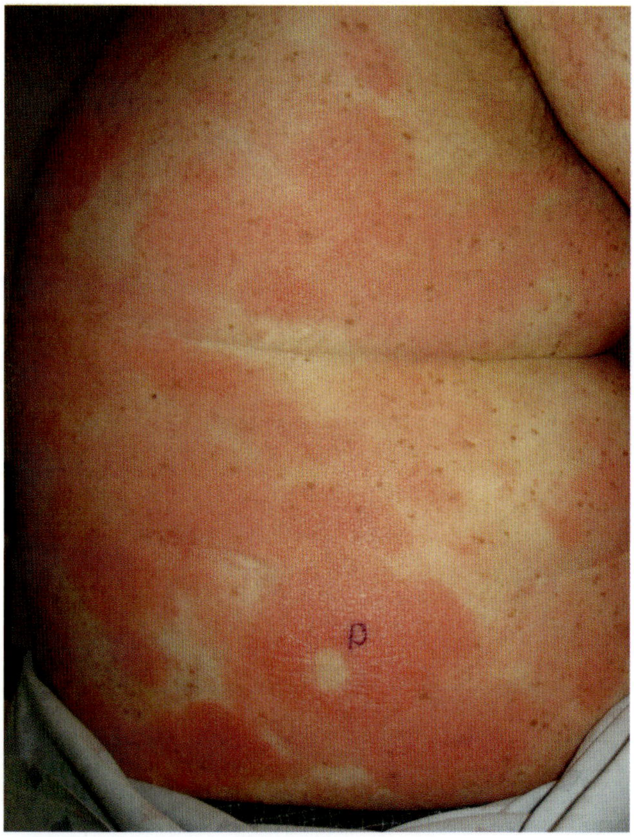

Fig. 46.2 Erythematous plaques on trunk due to MF in a Hispanic male

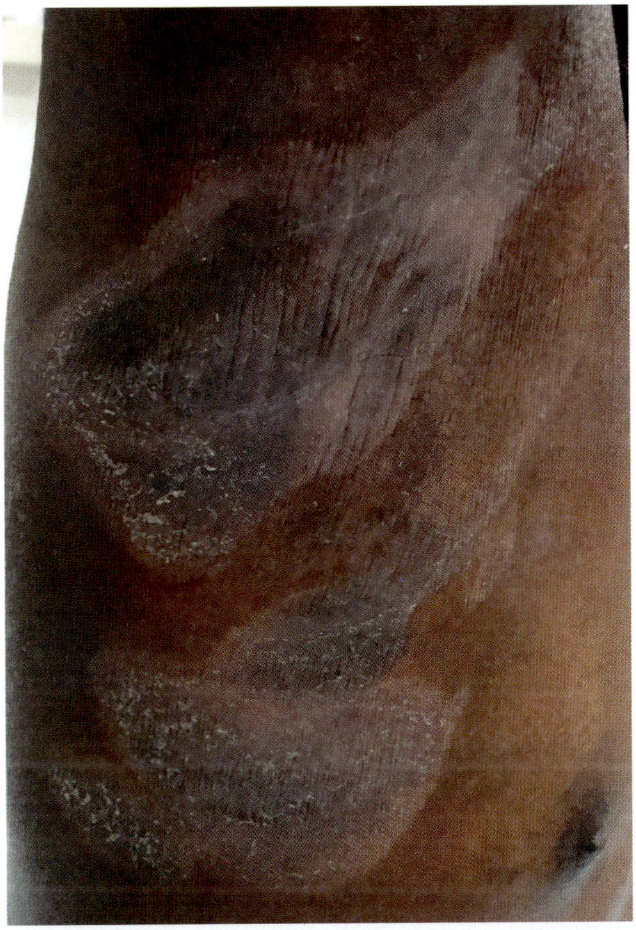

Fig. 46.3 Erythematous plaques in axilla due to MF in an African American male

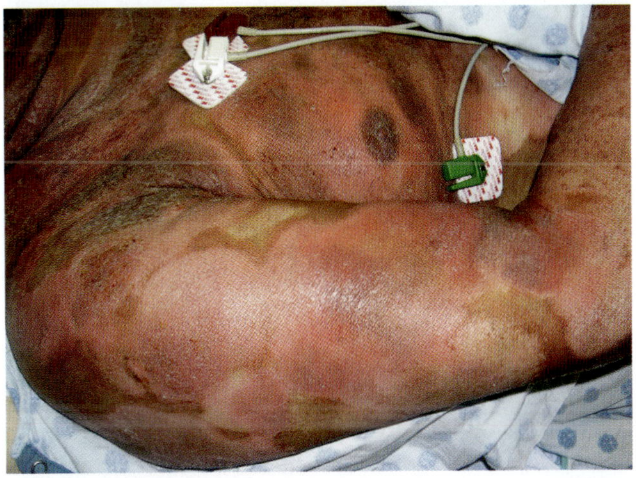

Fig. 46.4 Erythematous plaques diffusely over body due to MF in a Hispanic male

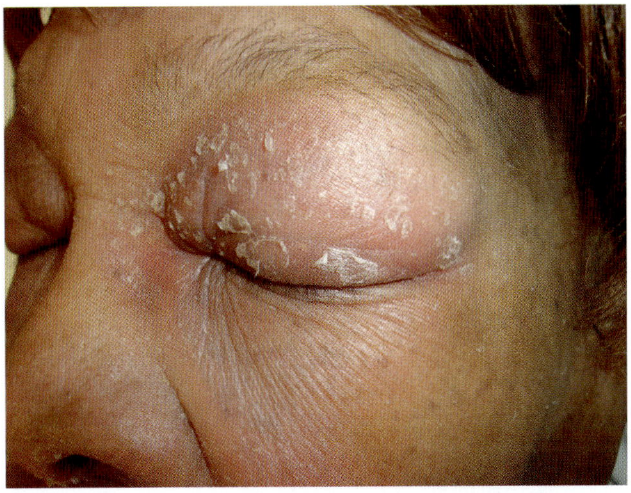

Fig. 46.5 Tumor on the eyelid due to MF in an African American female

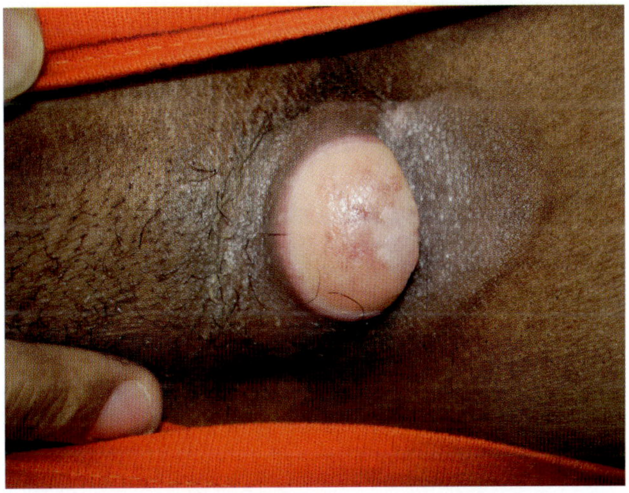

Fig. 46.6 Tumor in the axilla due to MF in an African American female

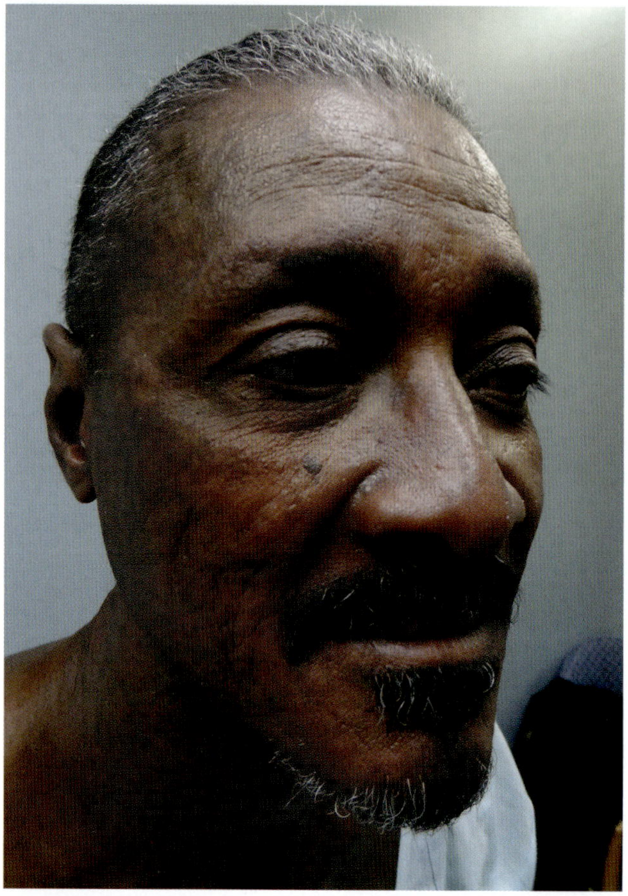

Fig. 46.7 Sézary syndrome with erythroderma on the face of an African American male

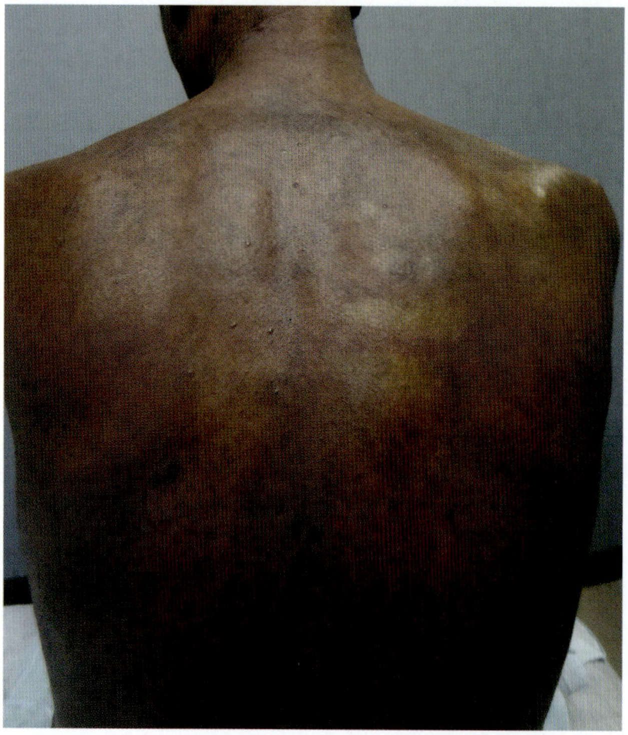

Fig. 46.8 Sézary syndrome with erythroderma on the back of an African American male

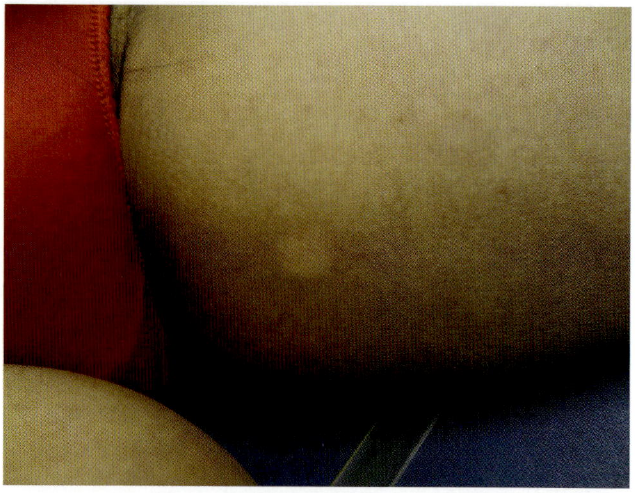

Fig. 46.9 Hypopigmented MF on the thigh of a Hispanic female

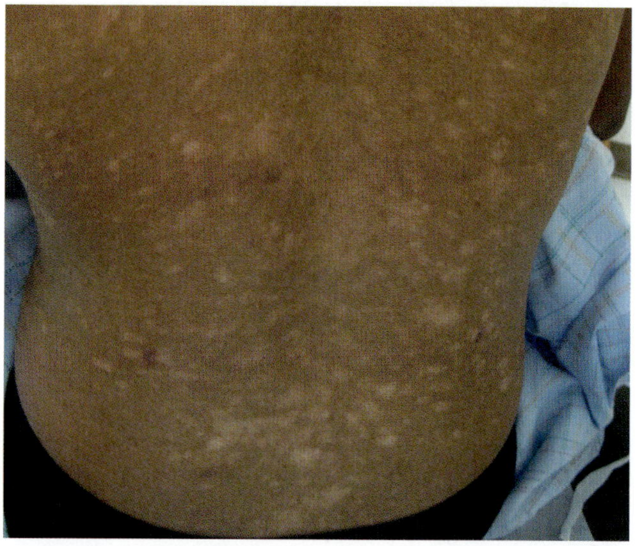

Fig. 46.10 Hypopigmented MF on the lower back of a Hispanic male

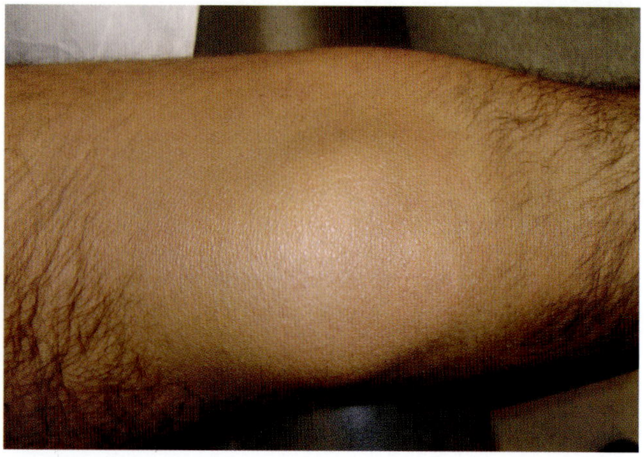

Fig. 46.11 Alopecia of the leg due to folliculotropic MF in a Hispanic male

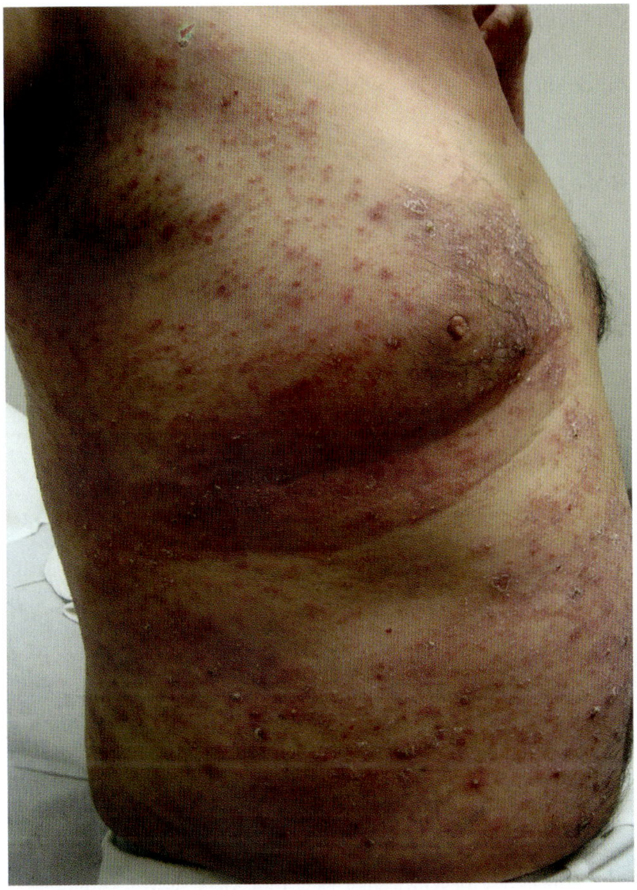

Fig. 46.12 Folliculotropic MF on the trunk of a Hispanic male

46.3 Diagnosis and Differential Diagnosis

Diagnosis of MF can be difficult during the premycotic phase and may require numerous biopsies over months to years to make the diagnosis [1, 8]. The differential diagnosis for MF includes chronic atopic dermatitis and plaque psoriasis early in disease. Palmoplantar pustulosis, sarcoidosis, ichthyosis, and drug eruption should also be considered [9]. The differential diagnosis for *Sézary syndrome* includes other causes of erythroderma, including atopic dermatitis, psoriasis, and drug eruptions.

Hypopigmented mycosis fungoides in patients with skin of color can presents similarly to other common conditions and a biopsy may be required for a definitive diagnosis. The differential for hypopigmented MF includes pityriasis versicolor, postinflammatory hypopigmentation, vitiligo, pityriasis alba, idiopathic guttate hypomelanosis, and rarely leprosy.

46.4 Histopathological Features

The histopathology of MF can be fairly nonspecific early on in the disease and numerous biopsies may be required to establish diagnosis. Microscopic examination typically reveals an epidermal infiltrate of T-cells in the epidermis without associated spongiosis and a band-like infiltrate of T-cells in the reticular dermis [1, 8, 9]. Pautrier microabscesses are aggregated collections of atypical lymphocytes in the epidermis that are often observed. Sézary cells appear as atypical lymphocytes with large, hyperchromatic, cerebriform nuclei and can be seen in the skin biopsy or a peripheral blood smear [2, 8]. The presence and number of Sézary cells in the peripheral blood should be examined as this is necessary for staging purposes. This is typically done using flow cytometry of peripheral blood. Hypopigmented MF lesions reveal a variable lymphocytic infiltrate with epidermotropism and little dermal involvement.

46.5 Natural History and Prognosis

The prognosis of CTCL depends on the stage of disease outlined by the tumor, node, metastasis, and blood stage (TNMB) system. The overall median survival for patients with MF/Sézary syndrome is 18.3 years with a better prognosis seen in Caucasians, females, younger patients, and individuals with lower clinical stage [1, 6]. Patients with early stage disease with minimal patches or plaques confined to the skin do not have a decreased overall survival compared to age-matched healthy controls [6]. Patients with patch or plaque stage MF, with no extracutaneous involvement, have a median survival between 15.8 and 21.5 [6]. The presence of cutaneous tumors, generalized erythroderma, extracutaneous organ or lymph node involvement, or transformation of MF to Sézary syndrome all carry a significantly poorer prognosis with a median survival time ranging from 4.7 to 1.4 years [1, 6]. African Americans and Hispanic females have a higher prevalence of early onset MF compared to Caucasians, with African Americans having a higher mortality and poorer prognosis compared to other races.

46.6 Treatment

Treatment for CTCL depends on the stage of disease. The treatment of choice for patients with limited cutaneous disease consists of topical corticosteroids, topical nitrogen mustard (mechlorethamine), topical retinoids, narrowband ultraviolet B (NBUVB), and psoralen plus ultraviolet A (PUVA) [10]. Systemic treatments used in more advanced-stage disease include methotrexate, interferons, and oral systemic retinoids such as bexarotene and extracorporeal photopheresis [10]. Combinations of topical and systemic agents as well as phototherapy are often employed. Novel agents for the treatment of CTCL include histone deacetylase inhibitors (HDACIs) which induce apoptosis of cells by causing DNA damage through modification of chromatin.

More potent therapies with cytotoxic chemotherapeutic agents such as gemcitabine and pegylated liposomal doxorubicin are often used for aggressive or refractory disease [10]. Drug resistance is common in advanced MF/Sézary syndrome, and although treatment with systemic chemotherapeutic agents may have a high initial response rate, remission times are often short, with disease recurrence in the span of months.

References

1. Siegel RS, Pandolfino T, Guitart J, Rosen S, Kuzel TM. Primary cutaneous T-cell lymphoma: review and current concepts. J Clin Oncol. 2000;18(15):2908–25.
2. Habif TP, et al. Skin disease, diagnosis and treatment. Edinburgh: Saunders; 2011. p. 493–7.
3. Lambroza E, Cohen S, Phelps R, Lebwohl M, Braverman IM, Dicostanzo D. Hypopigmented variant of mycosis fungoides: demography, histopathology, and treatment of seven cases. J Am Acad Dermatol. 1995;32(6):987–93.
4. Weinstock MA, Gardstein B. Twenty-year trends in the reported incidence of mycosis fungoides and associated mortality. Am J Public Health. 1999;89(8):1240–4.
5. Sun G, et al. Poor prognosis in non-Caucasian patients with early-onset mycosis fungoides. J Am Acad Dermatol. 2009;60(2):231–5.
6. Agar NS, et al. Survival outcomes and prognostic factors in mycosis fungoides/Sezary syndrome: validation of the revised International Society for Cutaneous Lymphomas/European Organisation for Research and Treatment of Cancer staging proposal. J Clin Oncol. 2010;28(31):4730–9.
7. Criscione VD, Weinstock M. Incidence of cutaneous T-cell lymphoma in the United States, 1973–2002. Arch Dermatol. 2007;143(7):854–9.
8. Kelly AP, Susan T. Chapter 44: Cutaneous T-cell lymphoma. In: Dermatology for skin of color. New York: McGraw-Hill Professional; 2009.
9. Zackheim HS, McCalmont TH. Mycosis fungoides: the great imitator. J Am Acad Dermatol. 2002;47(6):914–8.
10. Lansigan F, Foss F. Current and emerging treatment strategies for cutaneous T-cell lymphoma. Drugs. 2010;70(3):273–86.

Part VIII

Photodermatitis

Polymorphous Light Eruption

47

Prescilia Isedeh and Henry W. Lim

Contents

47.1 Introduction

Polymorphous light eruption (PMLE) is the most common of the immunologically mediated (formerly categorized as idiopathic) photodermatoses. The prevalence of PMLE ranges from 10 to 20 %, depending on the geographic location [1]. Onset is typically within the first three decades of life [2–5]. Females are two to three times more affected than males [2–5].

P. Isedeh, MD (✉)
Department of Dermatology, Henry Ford Medical Center,
Henry Ford hospital, 3031 West Grand Blvd., Suit 800,
Detroit, MI 48202, USA
e-mail: pisedeh1@hfhs.org

H.W. Lim, MD
Department of Dermatology, Henry Ford Medical Center,
Henry Ford Hospital, 3031 West Grand Blvd., Suit 800,
Detroit, MI 48202, USA
e-mail: hlim1@hfhs.org

D. Jackson-Richards, A.G. Pandya (eds.), *Dermatology Atlas for Skin of Color*,
DOI 10.1007/978-3-642-54446-0_47,

47.2 Clinical Features

PMLE lesions can present as non-scarring, erythematous, pruritic papules, vesicles, papulovesicles, plaques, or nodules [1]. Pinpoint variant of PMLE is the most common morphology seen in individuals with skin phototypes IV–VI (Figs. 47.1 and 47.2) [3]. Pinpoint PMLE is characterized by the development of pinpoint papules, 1–2 mm, on sun-exposed areas minutes or hours after ultraviolet radiation [6]. PMLE has a predilection for the arms, forearms, hands, head, and neck region.

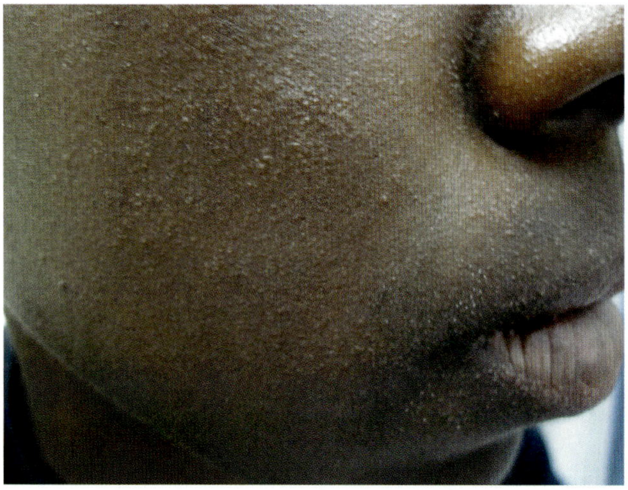

Fig. 47.1 Pinpoint papules due to PMLE located on the cheek and perioral skin in an African American male (Photograph reprinted with written permission from the *Journal of Drugs in Dermatology*)

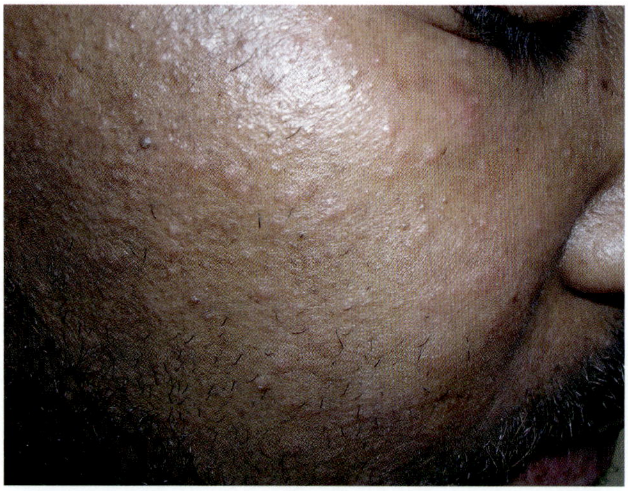

Fig. 47.2 Pinpoint papules due to PMLE on the cheek of an African American male (Photograph reprinted with written permission from the *Journal of Drugs in Dermatology*)

47.3 Natural History and Prognosis

PMLE lesions present hours to days after ultraviolet (UV) light exposure. The lesions and usually last over 1–7 days and completely resolve without scarring [3]. PMLE typically begins in the spring, improving by late summer with "hardening" due to increased tolerance of the skin [4]. These patients have decreased ability to be locally suppressed upon exposure to UV, which explains the "hardening" response seen clinically [5].

47.4 Histopathological Features

Histology of the skin lesion is considered nonspecific, revealing superficial and deep dermal inflammatory cell infiltrates [1]. Variable epidermal changes can occur that range from mild spongiosis to acanthosis [1].

47.5 Diagnosis and Differential Diagnosis

Diagnosis of PMLE is typically made through history, morphology of lesions, and clinical course; phototesting and photopatch testing are not routinely performed [6]. Selected laboratory examinations such as antinuclear antibody (ANA), anti-Ro (SSA), anti-La (SSB), plasma porphyrin levels, and in some cases biopsy of persistent lesions may assist in making the diagnosis [2]. Differential diagnoses include, but are not limited to, systemic lupus erythematosus, eczema, erythropoietic protoporphyria, solar urticaria, and actinic prurigo.

47.6 Treatment

Prevention is essential with sun avoidance, utilization of broad spectrum sunscreen, and photoprotective clothing [7]. Additionally, light tolerance or "hardening" can be accelerated using narrowband UVB phototherapy or, less commonly, psoralen plus UVA (PUVA) before the sunny period of the year [7]. Other treatment modalities include topical corticosteroids and antimalarials. Systemic corticosteroids may rarely be required in the setting of acute exacerbation of the disease or during a brief winter vacation to a sunny locale [8].

References

1. Chiam LYT, Chong W. Pinpoint popular polymorphous light eruption in Asian skin: a variant in darker-skinned individuals. Photodermatol Photoimmunol Photomed. 2009;25:71–4.
2. Tutrone W, Spann C, Scheinfeld N, Deleo V. Polymorphic light eruption. Dermatol Ther. 2003;16:28–39.
3. Kontos AP, Cuscak CA, Chaffins M, Lim HW. Polymorphous light eruption in African Americans: pinpoint papular variant. Photodermatol Photoimmunol Photomed. 2002;18:303–6.
4. Leroy D, Dompmartin A, Faguer K, Michel M, Verneuil L. Polychromatic phototest as prognostic tool for polymorphic light eruption. Photodermatol Photoimmunol Photomed. 2000;16:161–6.
5. van de Pas CB, Kelly DA, Seed PT, Young AR, Hawk JL, Walker SL. Ultraviolet-radiation-induced erythema and suppression of contact hypersensitivity responses in patients with polymorphic light eruption. J Invest Dermatol. 2004;122(2):295–9.
6. Kerr HA, Lim HW. Photodermatoses in African Americans: a retrospective analysis of 135 patients over a 7-year period. J Am Acad Dermatol. 2007;57:638–43.
7. Lehman P, Schwarz T. Photodermatoses: diagnosis and treatment. Dtsch Arztebl Int. 2011;108(9):135–41.
8. Bansal I, Kerr H, Janiga JJ, Qureshi HS, Chaffins M, Lim HW, Ormsby A. Pinpoint papular variant of polymorphous light eruption: clinical and pathological correlation. J Eur Acad Dermatol Venereol. 2006;20:406–10.

Chronic Actinic Dermatitis

48

Prescilia Isedeh and Henry W. Lim

Contents

48.1 Introduction

Chronic actinic dermatitis (CAD) is a chronic photodermatosis commonly affecting patients with skin of color. Chronic actinic dermatitis (CAD) has been reported in the North America, Europe, and Asia, but because it is under-recognized, it is likely to be prevalent worldwide [1]. Thus far, this disorder has been described in Caucasians, African Americans, Latin Americans, Japanese, Chinese, and Indians [1]. In the United States, it is more commonly seen in African Americans. Both genders can be affected, with elderly men more commonly affected with CAD [2].

P. Isedeh, MD (✉)
Department of Dermatology, Henry Ford Medical Center, Henry Ford Hospital, 3031 West Grand Blvd., Suit 800, Detroit, MI 48202, USA
e-mail: pisedeh1@hfhs.org

H.W. Lim, MD
Department of Dermatology, Henry Ford Medical Center, Henry Ford Hospital, 3031 West Grand Blvd., Suit 800, Detroit, MI 48202, USA
e-mail: hlim1@hfhs.org

D. Jackson-Richards, A.G. Pandya (eds.), *Dermatology Atlas for Skin of Color*,
DOI 10.1007/978-3-642-54446-0_48, © Springer-Verlag Berlin Heidelberg 2014

48.2 Clinical Features

CAD presents as a widespread eczematous eruption with scale and lichenification developing into infiltrated plaques occurring on sun-exposed skin of the face, scalp, posterolateral neck, upper chest, and the dorsal surfaces of the arms and hands (Figs. 48.1, 48.2, and 48.3) [1]. Affected skin can also appear erythrodermic [2]. Skin creases, finger webs, lower earlobe folds, and upper eyelids may be spared [1]. Unexposed areas of skin can also become affected, albeit less severely, after several years [1].

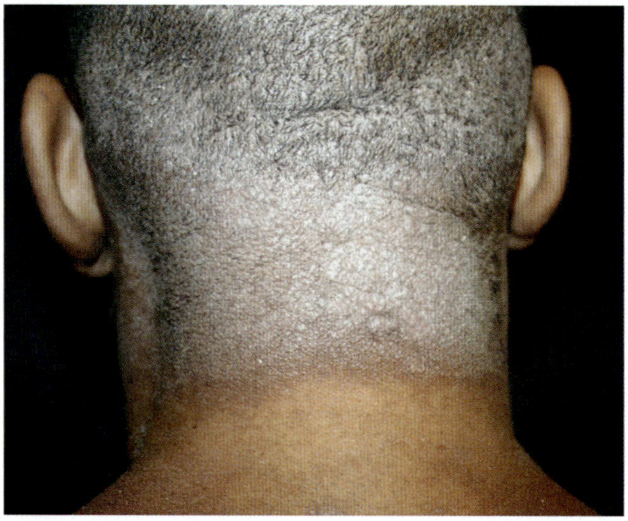

Fig. 48.1 Sharply demarcated lichenified plaques with scaling on the back of the neck of an African American male

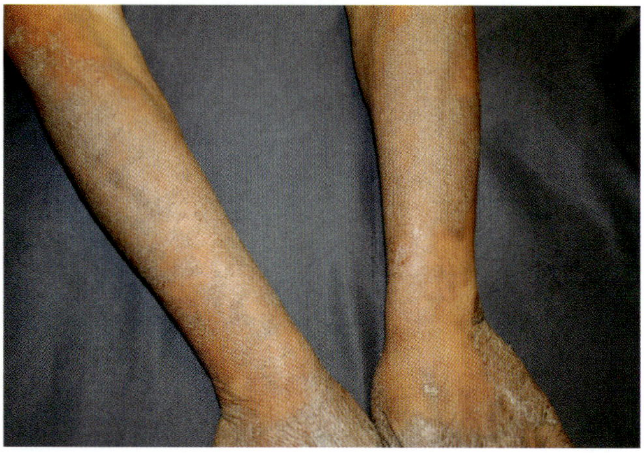

Fig. 48.3 Well-demarcated, scaly lichenified plaques with irregular borders on the dorsal surfaces of the forearms in an African American male

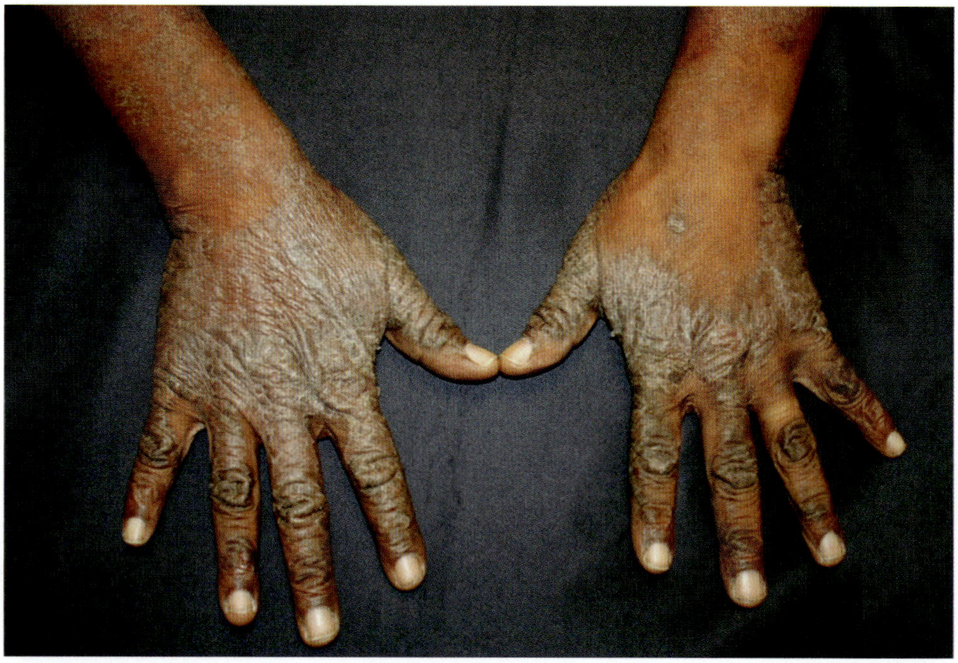

Fig. 48.2 Sharply demarcated scaly plaques with pronounced lichenification on the dorsal surfaces of the hands of an African American male

48.3 Natural History and Prognosis

Generally, when CAD is diagnosed in younger patients, there is a previous or concurrent history of atopic dermatitis [3]. This disorder is more severe during the summer months or after prolonged exposure to sunlight [3]. The etiology of CAD is unknown, but it is thought that this condition arises due to an increased susceptibility to develop delayed-type allergic responses to both endogenous photoallergens and exogenous allergens [2].

48.4 Histopathological Features

On histology, there are eczematous changes with deep dermal lymphohistiocytic inflitrates [1]. Sections obtained from infiltrated plaques show epidermotropism and Pautrier-like nests of cells, reminiscent of cutaneous T-cell lymphoma (CTCL) [1].

48.5 Diagnosis and Differential Diagnosis

The diagnosis of CAD can be made from a thorough history, morphology of lesions, and clinical course; it is confirmed by phototesting and skin biopsy [4]. The three main criteria for the diagnosis of CAD are reduction in minimal erythema dose (MED) testing to UVA, UVB, and/or less commonly, visible light; a persistent eczematous eruption primarily affecting sun-exposed skin but occasionally extending to covered areas; and histopathological changes similar to those of chronic eczema [1]. Additionally, patch testing may be helpful in the diagnosis of CAD because of the close relationship of the condition with allergic contact dermatitis, reported most commonly in patients seen in the United Kingdom [1]. Because histologic changes in CAD may be similar to those of CTCL, phototesting and Sézary count determination are helpful in differentiating these two conditions. In CAD, MEDs are abnormal, while peripheral Sézary cells are absent [5].T-cell phenotype marker studies have shown that there is a predominance of CD8+ T cells in CAD, whereas CD4+ T cells are the most commonly observed cells in infiltrates caused by CTCL [5].

48.6 Treatment

The first step in management is rigorous photoprotection [1, 5]. In addition to sunlight avoidance, known allergens should also be avoided [1, 2]. Topical corticosteroids are required during exacerbations of the disease [2]. Topical tacrolimus has been used successfully for milder conditions of the disease [2]. In severe exacerbation, systemic immunosuppressant with a short course of prednisone may be necessary. If a longer course of systemic immunosuppression is needed, mycophenolate mofetil or azathioprine can be effective in reducing symptoms and lesions [2]. Psoralen plus UVA (PUVA) therapy has also been used, but very low doses ($\leq$0.25 J/cm^2) of UVA, together with oral prednisone, are initially necessary to avoid exacerbating the disease [1, 5].

References

1. Forsyth E, Millard T. Diagnosis and pharmacological treatment of chronic actinic dermatitis in the elderly. Drugs Aging. 2010;27(6): 451–6.
2. Dawe R, Ferguson J. Diagnosis and treatment of chronic actinic dermatitis. Dermatol Ther. 2003;16:45–51.
3. Que S, Brauer J, Soter N, Cohen D. Chronic actinic dermatitis: an analysis at a single institution over 25 years. Dermatitis. 2011;22(3): 147–54.
4. Kerr HA, Lim HW. Photodermatoses in African Americans: a retrospective analysis of 135 patients over a 7-year period. J Am Acad Dermatol. 2007;57:638–43.
5. Hawk JLM, Lim H. Chronic actinic dermatitis. In: Lim HW, Honigsmann H, Hawk JLM, editors. Photodermatology. New York: Informa Healthcare; 2007. p. 170–83.

Actinic Prurigo

49

Prescilia Isedeh and Henry W. Lim

Contents

49.1 Introduction

Actinic prurigo (AP) is a chronic idiopathic photodermatosis affecting those living in North, Central, and South America [1–4]. It is most commonly seen in the mestizo population, which refers to people of mixed Indian and European ancestry, who live in Central and South America [1]. Individuals living in these areas at high attitudes, particularly greater than 1,000 m above sea level, are more likely to develop AP [1, 3]. AP has been found to have a strong association with human leukocyte antigen (HLA) subtypes [1, 2, 5, 6]. The most prevalent HLA subtype is HLA DRB1*0407 followed by HLA DRB1*0401, found in at least 60–70 and 20 % of affected patients, respectively [1, 2, 5].

AP is caused by electromagnetic radiation, predominately ultraviolet (UV) A light [2]. It has been postulated that AP is a form of autoimmune disease associated with an antigen, such as an epidermal protein that is transformed by UV exposure [7]. Langerhans cells are thought to present the UV-induced antigen to the cellular immune system, thus inducing or augmenting the inflammatory response [8].

P. Isedeh, MD (✉)
Department of Dermatology, Henry Ford Medical Center, Henry Ford Hospital, 3031 West Grand Blvd., Suit 800, Detroit, MI 48202, USA
e-mail: pisedeh1@hfhs.org

H.W. Lim, MD
Department of Dermatology, Henry Ford Medical Center, Henry Ford Hospital, 3031 West Grand Blvd., Suit 800, Detroit, MI 48202, USA
e-mail: hlim1@hfhs.org

D. Jackson-Richards, A.G. Pandya (eds.), *Dermatology Atlas for Skin of Color*, DOI 10.1007/978-3-642-54446-0_49, © Springer-Verlag Berlin Heidelberg 2014

49.2 Clinical Features

AP is characterized by intensely pruritic papules, plaques, and nodules with secondary eczematization, lichenification, and excoriations, which often heal with pitted scarring and dyspigmentation (Figs. 49.1 and 49.2) [1–5]. Vesicles are not present unless there is a secondary infection [2]. The eruption occurs on sun-exposed areas such as the face, neck, extensor forearms, dorsal surfaces of the hands, and upper aspect of the chest [1–6]. Lesions can also occur in covered areas, such as the back and buttocks, but these are often less severe [1, 2, 6]. Immediately after sun exposure, edema and erythema develops, which then subsides and slowly transitions to an eczematous phase and then a pruriginous phase [6]. Patients often experience pruritus throughout the year, but they experience flares of the disease during the spring and the summer months [1, 2, 5]. Patients with AP may also have involvement of the conjunctiva and lips [1–6]. Conjunctivitis, pseudopterygium, and cheilitis, affecting mainly the lower lips, may occur [1–6].

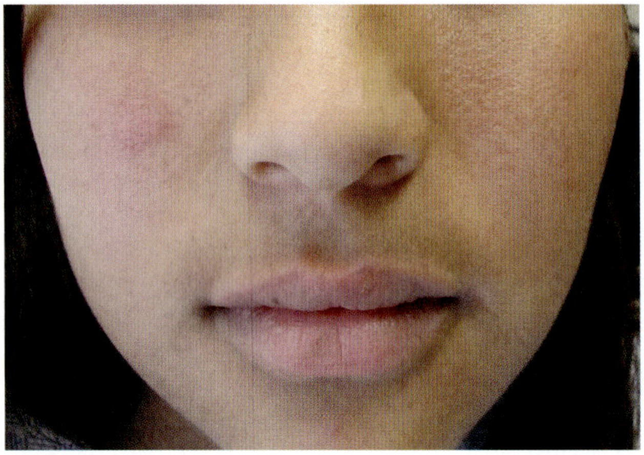

Fig. 49.1 Erythematous plaque due to actinic prurigo on the right cheek and an excoriated papule on left upper lip in a Guatemalan girl (Photograph courtesy of Tor Shwayder, M.D. and Rebecca Jansen, M.D. at Henry Ford Hospital, Detroit, MI, Department of Dermatology)

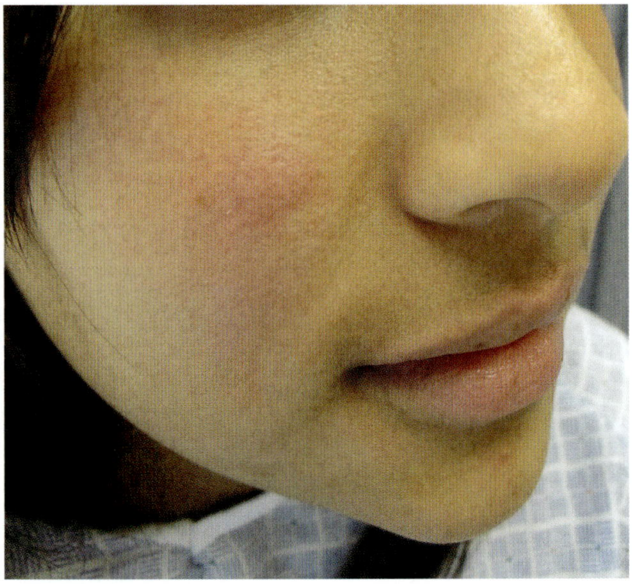

Fig. 49.2 Close-up of erythematous plaque due to actinic prurigo on the cheek of a Guatemalan girl (Photograph courtesy of Tor Shwayder, M.D. and Rebecca Jansen, M.D. at Henry Ford Hospital, Detroit, MI, Department of Dermatology)

49.3 Natural History and Prognosis

The onset of AP is during the first decade of life, predominately affecting females, with a male:female ratio of 1:2 [1–5]. AP can persist into adulthood, with only a few patients showing improvement during adolescence [2, 6]. Lesions occur predominately in the spring and summer months [2]. In temperate climates, AP may improve during the winter months, while in hotter climates, there is a tendency for the lesions to remain constant throughout the year [2].

49.4 Histopathological Features

Histology of skin lesions is usually nonspecific and nondiagnostic, showing hyperkeratosis, parakeratosis, acanthosis, and a predominantly superficial, perivascular lymphocytic infiltrate [1–4]. The presence of lymphoid follicles is commonly seen in biopsies of mucosal lesions and can be a distinguishing feature of this disorder [1–4].

49.5 Diagnosis and Differential Diagnosis

Although the biopsy of AP is nonspecific, it may be necessary to exclude other differential diagnosis such as eczema and lymphomatoid papulosis. HLA typing, antinuclear antibodies (ANA), and a porphyrin screen should be performed to exclude other photosensitive disorders such as lupus erythematosus and porphyria before phototesting [1–4].

Phototesting can confirm the diagnosis of AP as well as determine the action spectrum of the disease. The minimal erythema dose (MED) in the UVA spectrum is lowered in affected patients. [1, 2] Provocation testing is positive in approximately two-thirds of patients with AP. [1, 2] It is easier to elicit AP with provocation testing than polymorphous light eruption (PMLE). [2] In the past, AP was thought to be a variant of PMLE, but it is now considered a separate entity. [2, 5] The onset before adolescence, the persistence of lesions for more than 4 weeks, the involvement of mucosal areas, and scarring are more diagnostic of AP rather than PMLE [1, 2, 6]. Additionally, HLA typing can help distinguish these two conditions, as PMLE is not associated with HLA. [2, 4, 6]

49.6 Treatment

Photoprotection is the most important factor when treating AP. Patients are advised to wear protective clothing, sunglasses, and broad-brimmed hats [1–5].Additionally, patients are recommended to use high sun-protection factor, broad-spectrum sunscreen, and lip balm at all times. To relieve the symptom of pruritus, topical corticosteroids, emollients, and oral antihistamines may be helpful. For acute exacerbations of AP, a short course of oral corticosteroid can be effective [1–4]. Other widely used treatments include antimalarials, beta-carotene, vitamin E, and pentoxifylline, although their benefits have not been proven. Phototherapy, such as narrowband ultraviolet B (NB-UVB) and psoralen plus ultraviolet A (PUVA), has been effective in clearing and preventing new lesions in some patients [1, 2]. The NB-UVB regimen consists of treatment three times a week for approximately 5 weeks to induce hardening (resistance to photosensitivity) of the skin, but patients may have to undergo repeated courses since its effect is temporary [2]. PUVA is contraindicated in children.

The most effective treatment for the majority of patients with AP is thalidomide. It is thought that patient with AP have an overproduction of tumor necrosis factor (TNF) alpha by keratinocytes when exposed to UV, which can explain the good response to thalidomide, an anti-TNF alpha agent [2, 4]. The response to thalidomide may also serve as a marker in the diagnosis of AP [3, 4]. Thalidomide has been shown to cause rapid clearing of active lesions and reduce the number as well as severity of new lesions. The dosing of thalidomide in children is 50–100 mg/day and 100–200 mg/day in adults, with maintenance achievable with doses as low as 50 mg/week. [1, 2] Cessation of treatment without the need for ongoing therapy has been seen in some patients [1, 2]. Side effects of thalidomide include peripheral neuropathy, which is mainly a painful neuropathy, seen in 20–50 % of patients [1–6]. This side effect is thought to be largely due to the overall cumulative dose; therefore, it is imperative to taper thalidomide to the lowest required dose possible after initial control of the disease. The most feared complication of thalidomide is its teratogenic effects [1–6]. Adequate contraception is advised along with the use of barrier contraception by males [2, 3].

References

1. Chantorn R, Lim HW, Shwayder TA. Photosensitivity disorders in children: part I. J Am Acad Dermatol. 2012;67:1093.e1–18.
2. Ross G, Foley P, Baker C. Actinic prurigo. Photodermatol Photoimmunol Photomed. 2008;24(5):272–5.
3. Hojyo-Tomoka MT, Vega-Memije ME, Cortes-Franco R, Dominguez-Soto L. Diagnosis and treatment of actinic prurigo. Dermatol Ther. 2003;16:40–4.
4. Honigsmann H, Hojyo-Tomoka MT. Polymorphous light eruption, hydroa vacciniforme, and actinic prurigo. In: Lim HW, Honigsmann H, Hawk JLM, editors. Photodermatology. New York: Informa Healthcare; 2007. p. 149–65.
5. Ferguson J. Diagnosis and treatment of the common idiopathic photodermatoses. Australas J Dermatol. 2003;44:90–6.
6. Lehmann P, Schwarz T. Photodermatoses: diagnosis and treatment. Dtsch Arztebl Int. 2011;108(9):135–41.
7. Gomez A, Umana A, Trescalacios A. Immune response to isolated human skin antigens in actinic prurigo. Med Sci Monit. 2006; 12(3):BR106–13.
8. Torres-Alvarez B, Baranda L, Fuentes C, Delgado C, Santos-Martinez L, Portales-Perez D, et al. An immunohistochemical study of UV-induced skin lesions in actinic prurigo. Resistance of Langerhans cells to UV light. Eur J Dermatol. 1998;8:24–8.

Part IX

Miscellaneous

Drug Eruptions

50

Thomas Lee and Arturo R. Dominguez

Contents

T. Lee
Department of Dermatology, University of Texas Southwestern Medical Center, Dallas, TX, USA

A.R. Dominguez, MD (✉)
Department of Dermatology, University of Texas Southwestern Medical Center, Dallas, TX, USA

D. Jackson-Richards, A.G. Pandya (eds.), *Dermatology Atlas for Skin of Color*,
DOI 10.1007/978-3-642-54446-0_50, © Springer-Verlag Berlin Heidelberg 2014

50.1 Introduction

Drug eruption is a general term for a group of dermatologic disorders presenting with adverse cutaneous drug reactions. Certain drugs such as NSAIDs, antibiotics, and anticonvulsants can cause cutaneous drug eruptions with rates ranging from 1 to 5 % [1, 2]. It is thought that drug eruptions are due to hypersensitivity reactions to the drug molecules and/or their metabolites.

Recent research has revealed racial differences in HLA allele frequencies that are strongly associated with specific drug eruption disorders. For example, the HLA-B*1502 allele, present in Han Chinese, Indian, and Thai but not in Caucasian or Japanese populations, was strongly associated with carbamazepine-induced Stevens-Johnson syndrome/toxic epidermal necrolysis (SJS/TEN) [3].

50.2 Clinical Features

50.2.1 Morbilliform Rash

Because of its similarity to viral exanthems, this disorder is also known as exanthematous drug eruption. They are the most common type of cutaneous drug eruption and are characterized by a "maculopapular" appearance although the presentation can vary [1, 2]. They initially appear on the head, neck, trunk, and dependent areas [1]. The lesions then spread to the distal limbs symmetrically [1]. The rash begins as pruritic, erythematous macules that evolve into papules and finally aggregate into plaques (Fig. 50.1) [1]. Pruritus is a common complaint [1]. The mucous membranes are typically not involved.

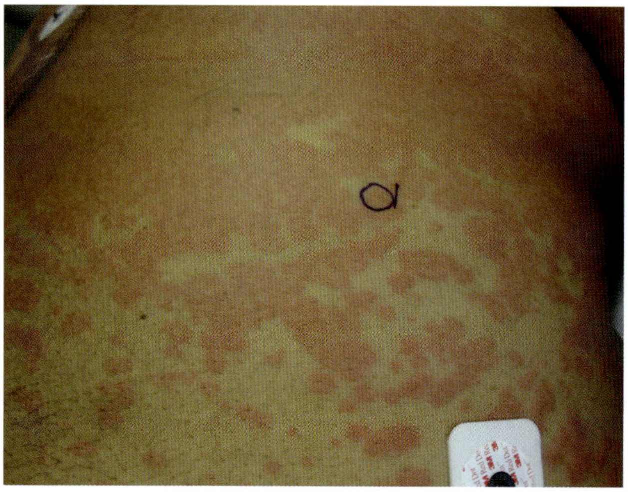

Fig. 50.1 Morbilliform drug eruption on the trunk of a Hispanic male

50.2.2 Drug Reaction with Eosinophilia and Systemic Symptoms/Drug-Induced Hypersensitivity Syndrome (DRESS/DIHS)

This syndrome is characterized by the triad of fever, skin eruption, and internal organ involvement [1, 4]. The morphology of the actual rash is variable and the presentation can include morbilliform rash, erythroderma, or pustules. Also notable is an infiltrative, indurated edema that starts in the face, upper extremities, and trunk and descends to the lower extremities [4]. The prodrome mimics a viral upper respiratory infection with associated symptoms of fever, malaise, and pharyngitis before onset of the rash [1, 4]. The lymph nodes, liver, heart, lungs, kidneys, and bone marrow can be affected [1, 4]. Patients develop atypical lymphocytosis with neutrophilia early in the disease with eosinophilia occurring later [1, 4]. Other hematologic abnormalities include agranulocytosis, thrombocytopenia, and hemolytic or aplastic anemia [1, 4] (Figs. 50.2, 50.3, 50.4, 50.5, and 50.6).

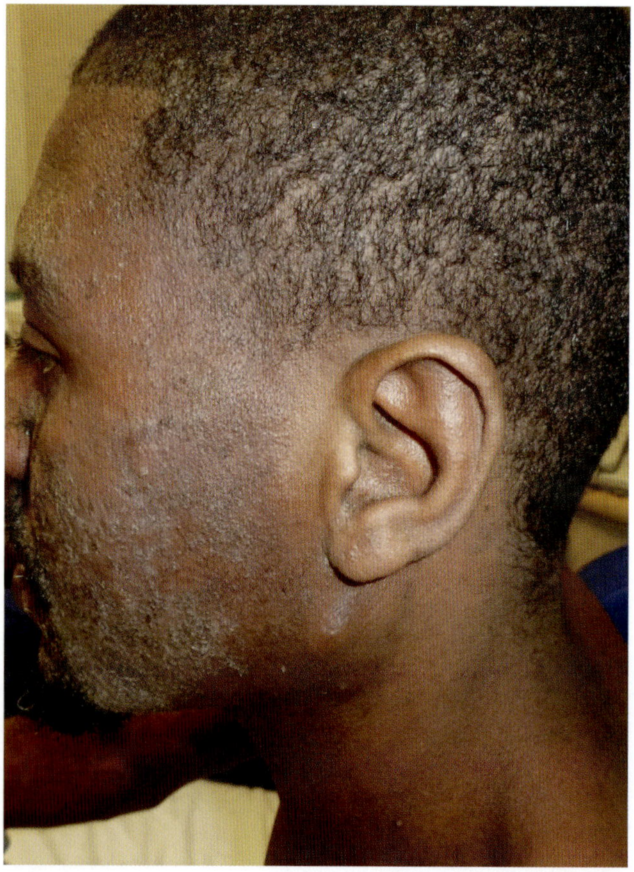

Fig. 50.2 Erythema, scale, edema, and lymphadenopathy due to DRESS in an AA male

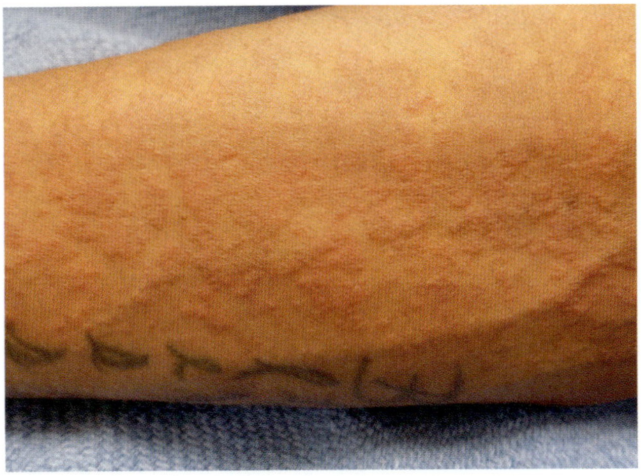

Fig. 50.3 Erythematous plaques on the arm due to DRESS in an AA male

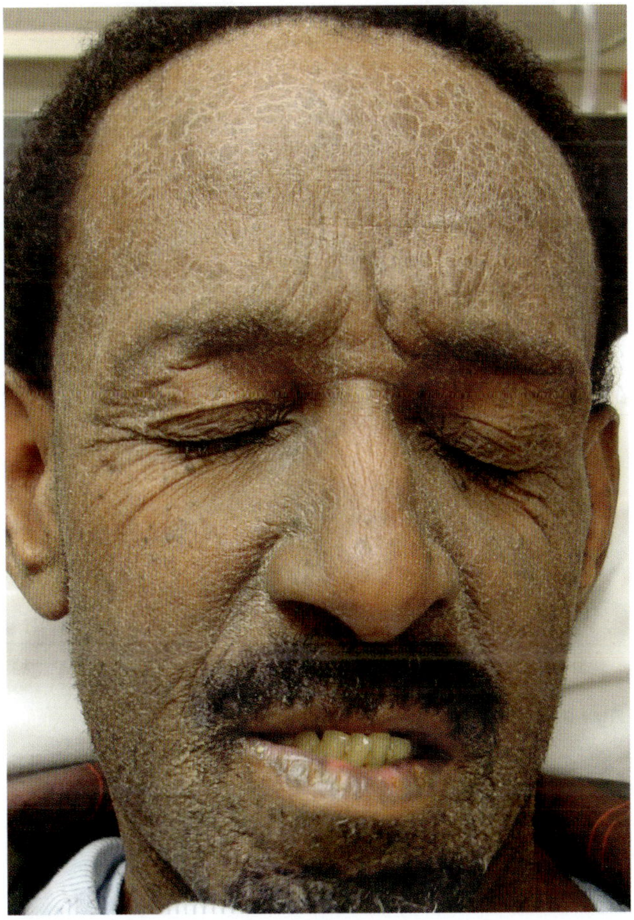

Fig. 50.4 Scale and erythema of the face in an AA patient with erythroderma due to DRESS

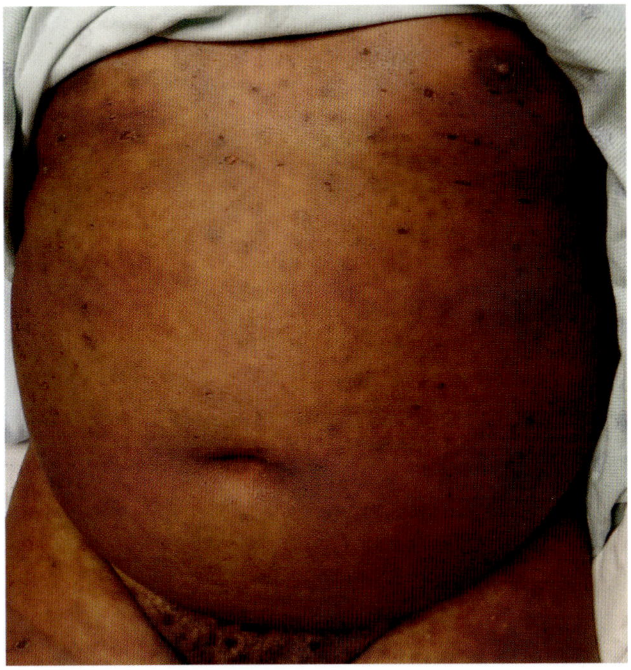

Fig. 50.5 Erythema, edema, and erosions on the trunk of an AA male with DRESS

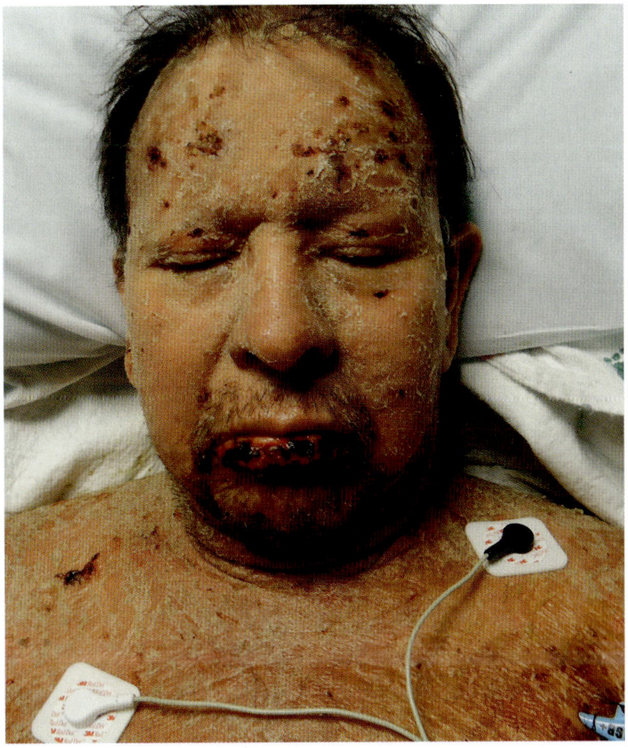

Fig. 50.6 Exfoliative form of DRESS in a Hispanic male

50.2.3 Acute Generalized Exanthematous Pustulosis (AGEP)

This drug eruption is characterized by fever and generalized, burning, or pruritic erythema followed by widespread pustules often described as "lakes of pus." [1] Edema of the face, purpura of the legs, vesicles, target lesions, and mucosal erosions may also be seen [1]. Patients have elevated neutrophil counts above 7.0×10^9/L and, in a third of cases, eosinophilia may be present [1].

50.2.4 Fixed Drug Eruptions

These are the second most common type of drug eruption, characterized by a solitary or multiple well-demarcated lesions that can occur anywhere on the body including the oral and genital mucosa [1]. The color can vary from red to red-brown, gray, blue, or violaceous [1]. Hyperpigmentation follows resolution of the skin lesions, particularly in patients with skin of color [1]. A nonpigmenting type can also occur at resolution which is associated with pseudoephedrine use [5]. There is a generalized bullous fixed eruption that can present with bullae, erosions, and dusky red patches and can mimic SJS/TEN [6] (Figs. 50.7, 50.8, and 50.9).

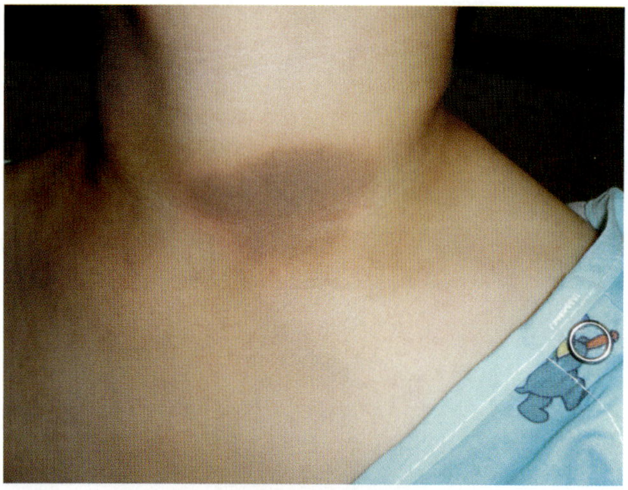

Fig. 50.7 Fixed drug eruption on the neck of a Hispanic boy

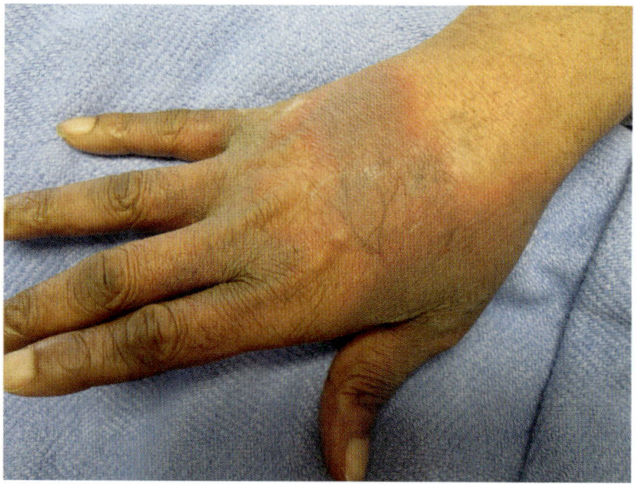

Fig. 50.8 Fixed drug eruption on the hand of an AA female

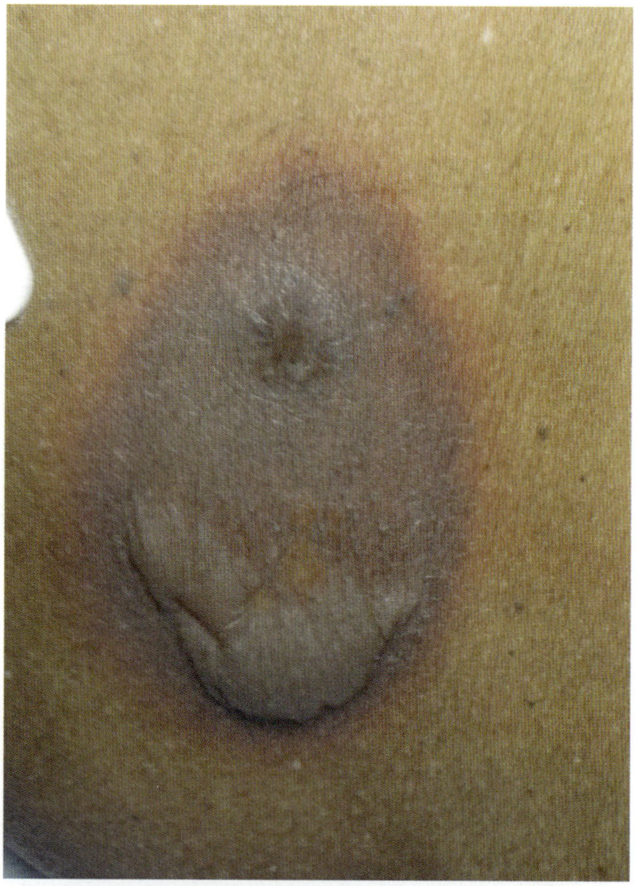

Fig. 50.9 Bullous fixed drug eruption on the abdomen of an AA male

50.2.5 Stevens-Johnson Syndrome/Toxic Epidermal Necrolysis (SJS/TEN)

A dermatologic emergency, this eruption is characterized by widespread erythematous, dusky macules and flat atypical target-like lesions. Flaccid bullae with a positive Nikolsky sign, skin erosions revealing pink and erythematous dermis, and painful inflammation and ulceration of the oral cavity occur over a period of 1 day to 2 weeks [7]. The percentage of body surface area (BSA) affected determines classification as SJS (<10 %), SJS/TEN overlap (10–30 %), or TEN (>30 %) [1, 7]. TEN with spots is classified as epidermal detachment (erosions, bullae, or Nikolsky-positive skin) of >30 % BSA with the presence of dusky macules or atypical target lesions. TEN without spots may present with generalized erythema, tender skin, and detachment of >10 % BSA but no purpuric or atypical targetoid macules and subsequently progression to sloughing of large epidermal sheets over >30 % BSA [7]. Eighty percent of cases of TEN also involve mucosal surfaces including oral, conjunctival, oropharyngeal, or genitourinary epithelia [1, 7]. Involvement of the entire gastrointestinal tract has also been reported [7]. Pulmonary dysfunction may occur in 25 % of cases and include hypoxemia, dyspnea, and bronchial mucosa sloughing [7]. Patients may also have renal and liver function test abnormalities including microalbuminuria, enzymuria, and elevated liver enzymes [7]. Anemia, leukopenia, and hepatitis are commonly seen [7]. Hypoalbuminuria, hyponatremia, encephalopathy, and myocarditis may be present [7] (Figs. 50.10, 50.11, 50.12, 50.13, 50.14, and 50.15).

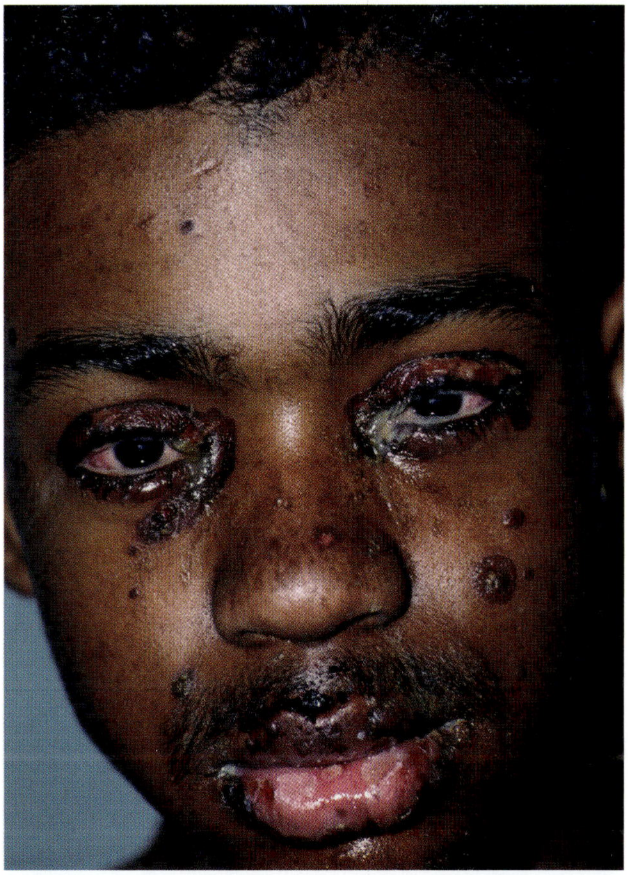

Fig. 50.11 Erosions of the lips, eyelids, and conjunctivae in an AA male with SJS (Courtesy Dr. Chauncey McHargue)

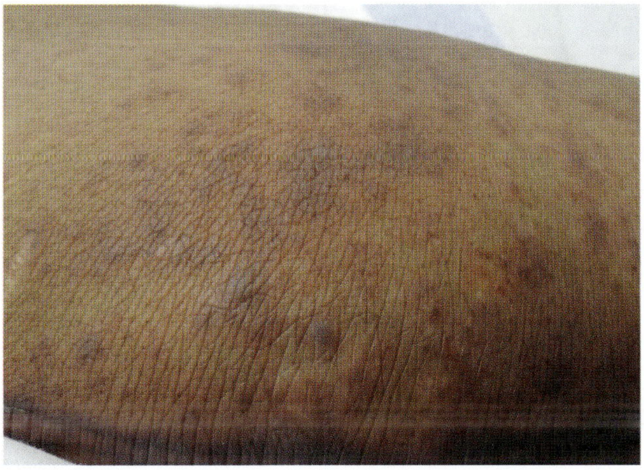

Fig. 50.10 Target lesions with dusky centers on the thigh of an AA female with SJS

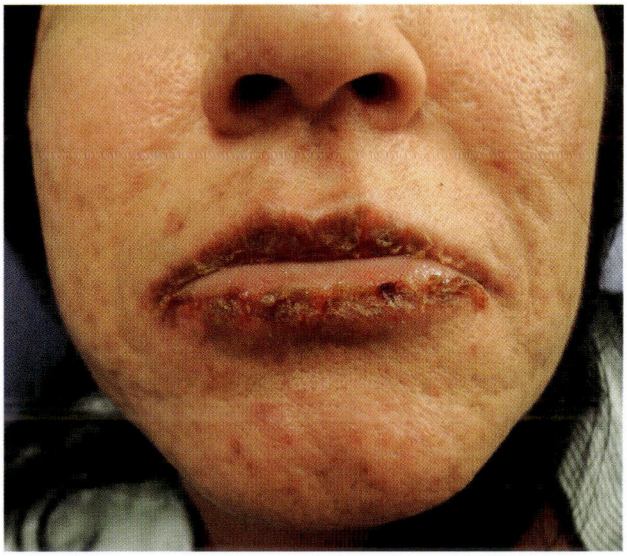

Fig. 50.12 Erosions of the lips and papules on the face in a Hispanic female with Stevens-Johnson syndrome

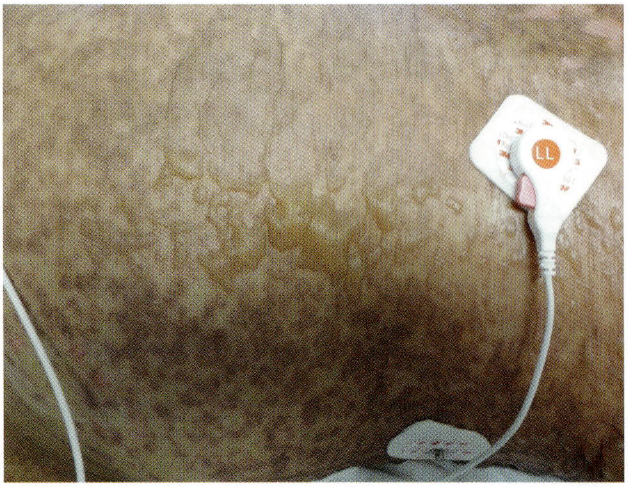

Fig. 50.13 Flaccid bullae on the trunk due to TEN in a Hispanic male

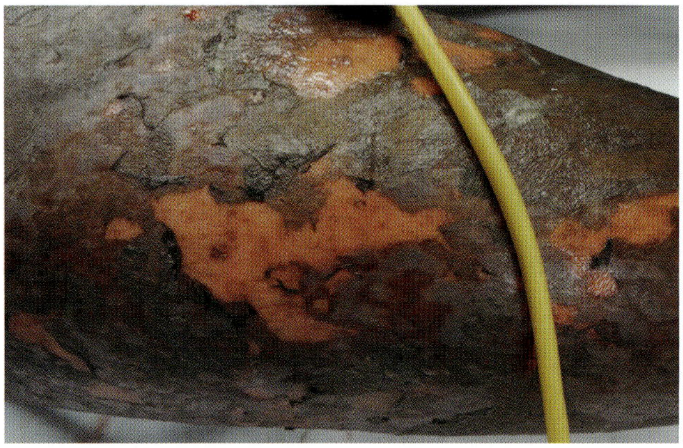

Fig. 50.14 Erosions of the thigh due to TEN in an AA male

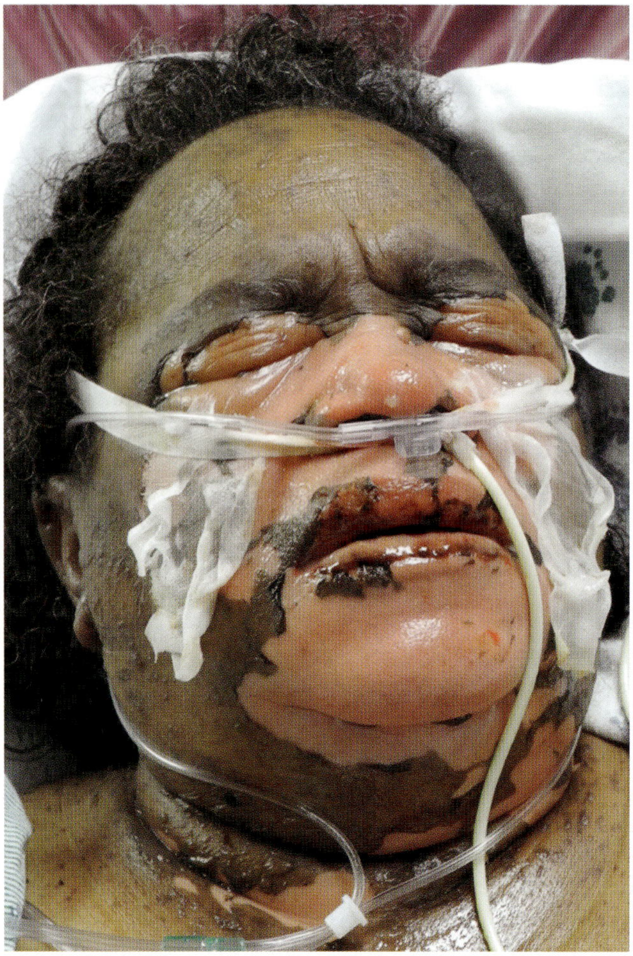

Fig. 50.15 Erosions of the face and neck due to TEN in an AA female

50.3 Natural History and Prognosis

50.3.1 Morbilliform Drug Eruption

The eruption begins 5–14 days after starting the offending drug with complete resolution of symptoms in 1–2 weeks [1]. The classic history is the patient with mononucleosis who develops a measles-like rash after using penicillin. This disorder is most commonly due to penicillin, with aminopenicillins causing eruption rates that approach 100 % in mononucleosis patients [1]. Cephalosporins, sulfonamide antibiotics, antiepileptic agents, and allopurinol are also common causes of morbilliform eruptions and not usually related to a viral infection like mononucleosis [8].

50.3.2 DRESS/DIHS

The cutaneous eruption and internal organ involvement in patients with DRESS/DIHS occur shortly after the URI-like prodrome. This disorder is notable for its long latency period ranging from 2 to 6 weeks after drug initiation [1]. Drugs associated with this disorder include the aromatic anticonvulsants (e.g., carbamazepine, phenobarbital, phenytoin), sulfonamide antibiotics, dapsone, trimethoprim, minocycline, abacavir, and allopurinol [4, 9]. This eruption is a life-threatening disorder with a mortality rate of 10 % [4, 9]. It may take weeks or even months to recover with intermittent recurrence of symptoms before full recovery [4, 9, 10]. Long-term sequelae include autoimmune phenomenon such as autoimmune thyroiditis, type I diabetes, and hemolytic anemia [4, 11].

50.3.3 AGEP

The interval time between drug use and onset of skin lesions in patients with AGEP is 2–3 days [1]. Antibiotics, especially penicillins and macrolides, are the most common offending agents. The rash begins in skin creases and sometimes the face and progresses into generalized painful or pruritic erythema within 24 h. Subsequently nonfollicular-based superficial pustules appear within these areas of erythema [1]. Pustules may coalesce and form "lakes of pus." The rash typically resolves in 10–15 days and may leave collarettes of scale. The mortality rate is 1–2 % [1].

50.3.4 Fixed Drug Eruptions

With the initial fixed drug eruption, a delay of 1–2 weeks may occur from the first exposure to the drug to the development of skin lesions [1]. Commonly associated drugs include sulfonamides, tetracyclines, NSAIDs, barbiturates, and carbamazepine [1, 8]. Lesions may persist from days to weeks and then fade slowly to residual oval, hyperpigmented patches that fade over weeks to months [1]. Subsequent reexposure to the medication results in a recurrence of previous lesions, with new inflammation occurring within 30 min to hours [1]. The reactivation of old lesions also may be associated with the development of new lesions at other sites. The generalized fixed bullous variant can be quite severe and mimic TEN with epidermal losses over 30 % BSA. A recent study reported a mortality rate of 22 % in generalized bullous fixed drug eruptions, especially in older patients [6, 12].

50.3.5 SJS/TEN

A prodrome of nausea, vomiting, diarrhea, headache, cough, sore throat, myalgias, and arthralgias can precede the rash by up to 2 weeks [1]. Mean time of rash onset after drug initiation ranges from 6 days to 2 weeks [7]. The vast majority of SJS/TEN cases are related to drug hypersensitivity followed by infections, including measles-mumps-rubella vaccination, dengue virus, *Mycoplasma pneumoniae*, and cytomegalovirus [7]. Drugs with a high risk of causing SJS/TEN include nevirapine, lamotrigine, carbamazepine, phenytoin, phenobarbital, sulfonamides, allopurinol, NSAIDs, aminopenicillins, cephalosporins, and quinolones [7]. The acute phase of TEN lasts from 8 to 12 days and is characterized by fevers, skin eruption, and mucosal lesions [1]. Reepithelialization can take up to one month with pressure sites and mucosal lesions requiring more time to heal [1]. Hyperpigmentation and hypopigmentation may take years to resolve and nail or hair loss may be permanent [7]. Dry eye syndrome, vision loss, phimosis, vaginal synechiae, dry mouth, gingival and periodontal disease, esophageal strictures, and chronic obstructive lung disease can be a long-term sequelae [1, 7]. The SCORTEN index can measure risk of death based on presence of age >40 years, concurrent malignancy, tachycardia, percent epidermal detachment, elevated BUN, elevated glucose, and low bicarbonate [13]. Calculated on the first hospital day, one risk factor in SCORTEN scoring has a mortality rate of 3.2 %, while 5 or more risk factors increases the risk of death to over 90 % [13] (Table 50.1).

Table 50.1 Clinical features, timing, and causative drugs for various drug eruptions

Drug eruption	Clinical features	Timing of rash onset after drug initiation	Drugs
Morbilliform drug eruption	Generalized macules and papules that may aggregate into plaques Appears initially on the head, neck, and trunk and then spreads to the distal limbs symmetrically No mucous membrane involvement	5–14 days	Aminopenicillins, cephalosporins, sulfonamide antibiotics, antiepileptic agents, allopurinol
DRESS	Variable rash presentation Triad of fever, rash, internal organ involvement Starts with edema of the face and upper extremities with cephalocaudal descent Early neutrophilia that evolves to eosinophilia	2–6 weeks	Carbamazepine, phenobarbital, phenytoin, sulfonamide antibiotics, dapsone, trimethoprim, minocycline, abacavir, allopurinol
AGEP	Fever and generalized, pruritic erythema leading to widespread pustules described as lakes of pus	2–3 days	Penicillins and macrolide antibiotics
Fixed drug eruptions	Solitary or multiple well-demarcated lesions Rare presentation with generalized bullae, erosions, and dusky patches	1–2 weeks	Carbamazepine, sulfonamides, tetracyclines, NSAIDs, barbiturates
SJS/TEN	Widespread erythematous, dusky macules and flat, atypical targetoid lesions Sloughing of the epidermis leaving exposed, pink dermis Bullae are Nikolsky positive. Painful mucosal erosions	6 days–4 weeks	Nevirapine, lamotrigine, carbamazepine, phenytoin, phenobarbital, sulfonamides, allopurinol, NSAIDs, aminopenicillins, cephalosporins, quinolones

50.4 Histopathologic Features

Drug reactions may show eosinophilic infiltration on histology though this is not specific for drug eruptions [1, 14].

50.4.1 Morbilliform Drug Eruption

There is focal vacuolar interface dermatitis with scattered necrotic keratinocytes at the dermoepidermal junction, dermal edema, and superficial perivascular lymphocytic infiltrate with admixed eosinophils [14].

50.4.2 DRESS/DIHS

Histologic findings are nonspecific in biopsies taken from patients with DRESS. Though the pattern can vary, the most common finding is a perivascular lymphocytic infiltrate in the papillary dermis with the possible presence of eosinophils and atypical lymphocytes [4].

50.4.3 AGEP

Histology may show spongiform subcorneal and/or intraepidermal pustules, papillary dermal edema, perivascular neutrophils and eosinophils, as well as leukocytoclastic vasculitis [14]. Unlike acute pustular psoriasis, psoriasiform epidermal changes are typically absent [14].

50.4.4 Fixed Drug Eruptions

There is basal hydropic degeneration, pigmentary incontinence, upper epidermal keratinocyte necrosis, dermal edema, vasodilation, and superficial and deep perivascular inflammation [14].

50.4.5 SJS/TEN

This is characterized by full-thickness epidermal necrosis, especially in later lesions [14]. Other late findings include subepidermal detachment, intraepidermal clefts, and intense inflammation [14]. Early lesions may show mild superficial perivascular inflammation and edema, erythrocyte extravasation in the papillary dermis, and basal keratinocyte necrosis [14].

50.5 Diagnosis and Differential Diagnosis

Drug rechallenge is helpful in demonstrating the association between the offending drug and cutaneous eruption. However, rechallenging is contraindicated in life-threatening eruptions such as DRESS and SJS/TEN [1].

50.5.1 Morbilliform Drug Eruption

Because of the similarity in appearance to viral exanthems, viral infections should be the main differential diagnosis [1]. A high fever with eosinophilia on the complete blood cell count, and the presence of facial edema, suggests DRESS/DIHS as the diagnosis [1].

50.5.2 DRESS/DIHS

As noted previously, the actual cutaneous eruption varies significantly. Internal organ involvement will distinguish this from other disorders on the differential. The RegiSCAR scoring system may be helpful in determining the probability of a diagnosis of DRESS and is dependent on factors such as degree of fever, enlarged lymph nodes, eosinophilia, atypical lymphocytes, skin involvement, organ involvement, time of resolution, and the exclusion of other potential causes [4, 9]. Erythrodermic presentations may mimic SJS/TEN, staphylococcal scalded skin syndrome, or streptococcal toxic shock syndrome.

50.5.3 AGEP

As mentioned previously, the pustules of AGEP and pustular psoriasis are morphologically similar, but the histology will show the absence of psoriasiform changes in the former [14, 15]. Patch testing with the offending drug is often strongly positive [1].

50.5.4 Fixed Drug Eruption

The differential diagnosis includes insect bites due to the solitary and specific location of the lesions [1]. Blisters can sometimes form in the center of lesions, mimicking SJS/TEN or erythema multiforme [6]. Drug withdrawal and rechallenge may be considered to help in diagnosis [1]. However, if the skin lesions were severe or generalized on presentation such as in the generalized bullous type, rechallenge is not recommended.

50.5.5 SJS/TEN

Atypical presentations with targetoid lesions as described previously can be mistaken for SJS/TEN. Erythema multiforme presents with typical three-zoned, raised target, and targetoid lesions that tend to be acral in distribution [1]. SJS/TEN lesions tend to be flat atypical targetoid lesions. Other diagnoses that can mimic TEN include staphylococcal scalded skin syndrome (SSSS), drug-induced linear IgA dermatosis, acute graft-versus-host disease (GVHD), morbilliform drug eruption, AGEP, and DRESS [16]. SSSS does not involve the mucous membranes, and erosions are limited to the granular epidermis which can be seen clinically and on biopsy [16]. Linear IgA dermatosis, usually following vancomycin use, presents as tense bullae on urticarial plaques arranged in a circular or herpetiform arrangement. Biopsy for direct immunofluorescence will reveal IgA deposits in the basement membrane region [16]. Acute GVHD with a bullous presentation can involve the mucous membranes and present histologically with full-thickness epidermal necrosis which may make it difficult to distinguish from SJS/TEN [16]. Clinical features such as acral to proximal spread, early folliculocentric distribution, diarrhea, and bilirubin elevations can be helpful [SCHWARTZ2]. Morbilliform eruptions do not involve the mucous membranes or full-thickness epidermal necrosis on histology [16]. AGEP can present with nonerosive mucous membrane changes and blisters, while DRESS can have a bullous presentation with lip erosions, but these latter lesions do not present with sloughing of epidermal sheets and histology will show absence of full-thickness epidermal necrosis [16].

50.6 Treatment

In general, treatment of drug eruptions begins with stopping the offending agent. If there are no alternative treatments and the eruption is not life-threatening, such as in morbilliform drug eruption, treating through with the offending drug with control of symptoms may be an option.

50.6.1 Morbilliform Drug Eruption

Symptomatic treatment is the mainstay therapy in this disorder. The itching and rash can be treated with oral antihistamines and topical steroids [1]. While steroid therapy may treat the pruritus, it does not shorten the duration of the skin lesions.

50.6.2 DRESS/Drug Hypersensitivity Syndrome

Systemic steroids may be started for severe internal organ involvement as well as for the rash and constitutional symptoms. [1] A 4–6-week course of oral prednisone can be given with a slow taper to prevent flares. If no improvement is noted, intravenous methylprednisolone pulse therapy, cyclosporine, or adjunctive IVIG therapy can be considered [17]. EuroSCAR has developed guidelines for the management of severe DRESS syndrome specifying appropriate diagnostic tests, treatments, and consultations [17].

50.6.3 AGEP

For patients with high fever or excessive pruritus, antipyretics, topical steroids, or oral antihistamines may be used [1]. A 7-day course of systemic corticosteroids is also an option.

50.6.4 Fixed Drug Eruptions

Withdrawing the offending agent is the treatment of choice [1]. For oral lesions, a mouthwash containing anesthetic and soothing agents may provide symptom relief. Similarly, viscous lidocaine can be used for genital lesions.

50.6.5 SJS/TEN

Patients should be admitted to the intensive care unit, especially if >10 % BSA is affected, and treated with fluid replacement, nutritional supplements, and wound care [1, 16]. Erythromycin and steroid eyedrops are helpful, but avoid silver sulfadiazine topical antibiotics or eyedrops as these can worsen SJS/TEN [1, 16]. Consult ophthalmology to monitor for vision loss and urology or gynecology for urogenital complications [1]. Long-term dental follow-up will also be needed [16]. Steroid therapy for SJS/TEN is a controversial topic as different studies have shown conflicting results [1, 16]. It is possible that once desquamation occurs, steroid use can increase infection risk which may explain the increased mortality in some studies. Studies evaluating the role of IVIG have also demonstrated mixed results with no consensus [16]. A meta-analysis initially found lower mortality in high-dose IVIG-treated TEN patients but was then found not to be statistically significant after correcting for age, BSA, and delay of treatment [16]. Small studies on plasmapheresis have shown some benefit possibly due to removal of proinflammatory cytokines [16]. Successful cases utilizing the TNF-α inhibitors infliximab and etanercept have been reported [16]. Cyclosporine, a calcineurin inhibitor which inhibits granulysin release from activated CD8+ cells, shows promise, as studies have shown decreased skin lesion progression with no increase in mortality or infection [16].

References

1. McKenna JK, Lieferman KM. Dermatologic drug reactions. Immunol Allergy Clin North Am. 2004;24:399–423.
2. Bigby M. Rates of cutaneous reactions to drugs. Arch Dermatol. 2001;137(6):765–70.
3. Aihara M. Pharmacogenetics of cutaneous adverse drug reactions. J Dermatol. 2011;38(3):246–54.
4. Husain Z, Reddy BY, Schwartz RA. DRESS syndrome: part I. Clinical perspectives. J Am Acad Dermatol. 2013;68(5):693.
5. Vidal C, Prieto A, Perez-Carral C, et al. Nonpigmented fixed drug due to pseudoephedrine. Ann Allergy Asthma Immunol. 1998;80: 309–10.
6. Lin TK, Hsu MM, Lee JY. Clinical resemblance of widespread bullous fixed drug eruption to Stevens-Johnson syndrome or toxic epidermal necrolysis: report of two cases. J Formos Med Assoc. 2002;101(8):572–6.
7. Schwartz RA, McDonough PH, Lee BW. Toxic epidermal necrolysis: part I. Introduction, history, classification, clinical features, systemic manifestations, etiology, and immunopathogenesis. J Am Acad Dermatol. 2013;69(2):173–86.
8. Kahn DA. Cutaneous drug reactions. J Allergy Clin Immunol. 2012;130(5):1225.
9. Cacoub P, Musette P, Descamps V, et al. The DRESS syndrome: a literature review. Am J Med. 2011;124:588–97.
10. Kaur S, Sarkar R, Thami GP, et al. Anticonvulsant hypersensitivity syndrome. Pediatr Dermatol. 2002;19(2):142–5.
11. Gupta A, Eggo MC, Uetrecht JP, et al. Drug-induced hypothyroidism: the thyroid as a target organ in hypersensitivity reactions to anticonvulsants and sulfonamides. Clin Pharmacol Ther. 1992;51(1):56–67.
12. Lipowicz S, Sekula P, Ingen-Housz-Oro S, et al. Prognosis of generalized bullous fixed drug eruption: comparison with Stevens-Johnson syndrome and toxic epidermal necrolysis. Br J Dermatol. 2013;168(4):726–32.
13. Bastuji-Garin S, Fouchard N, Bertocchi M, et al. SCORTEN: a severity-of-illness score for toxic epidermal necrolysis. J Invest Dermatol. 2000;115(2):149–53.
14. Ramdial PK, Naidoo DK. Drug-induced cutaneous pathology. J Clin Pathol. 2009;62:493–504.
15. Lee S, Artemi P, Holt D. Acute generalized exanthematous pustulosis. Australas J Dermatol. 1995;36(1):25–7.
16. Schwartz RA, McDonough PH, Lee BW. Toxic epidermal necrolysis: part II. Prognosis, sequelae, diagnosis, differential diagnosis, prevention, and treatment. J Am Acad Dermatol. 2013;69(2):187–204.
17. Husain Z, Reddy BY, Schwartz RA. DRESS syndrome: part II. Management and therapeutics. J Am Acad Dermatol. 2013; 68(5):709.

Index

D. Jackson-Richards, A.G. Pandya (eds.), *Dermatology Atlas for Skin of Color*,
DOI 10.1007/978-3-642-54446-0, © Springer-Verlag Berlin Heidelberg 2014

E

F

G

T